Liver Fibrosis: Mechanisms, Targets, Assessment and Treatment

Liver Fibrosis: Mechanisms, Targets, Assessment and Treatment

Guest Editors

Ralf Weiskirchen
Tilman Sauerbruch

MDPI

Basel • Beijing • Wuhan • Barcelona • Belgrade • Novi Sad • Cluj • Manchester

Guest Editors
Ralf Weiskirchen
Institute of Molecular Pathobiochemistry, Experimental Gene Therapy and Clinical Chemistry (IFMPEGKC)
RWTH University Hospital Aachen
Aachen
Germany

Tilman Sauerbruch
Department of Internal Medicine I
University Hospital of Bonn
Bonn
Germany

Editorial Office
MDPI AG
Grosspeteranlage 5
4052 Basel, Switzerland

This is a reprint of the Special Issue, published open access by the journal *Livers* (ISSN 2673-4389), freely accessible at: https://www.mdpi.com/journal/livers/special_issues/742Y9BF54R.

For citation purposes, cite each article independently as indicated on the article page online and as indicated below:

Lastname, A.A.; Lastname, B.B. Article Title. *Journal Name* **Year**, *Volume Number*, Page Range.

ISBN 978-3-7258-5441-7 (Hbk)
ISBN 978-3-7258-5442-4 (PDF)
https://doi.org/10.3390/books978-3-7258-5442-4

Contents

livers

MDPI

Editorial

Special Issue "Liver Fibrosis: Mechanisms, Targets, Assessment and Treatment"

Ralf Weiskirchen [1,*] and Tilman Sauerbruch [2,*]

[1] Institute of Molecular Pathobiochemistry, Experimental Gene Therapy and Clinical Chemistry (IFMPEGKC), RWTH University Hospital Aachen, D-52074 Aachen, Germany
[2] Department of Internal Medicine I, University Hospital of Bonn, D-53127 Bonn, Germany
* Correspondence: rweiskirchen@ukaachen.de (R.W.); tilman.sauerbruch@ukbonn.de (T.S.)

Keywords: fibrosis; hepatocytes; hepatic stellate cell; NASH/NAFLD; portal hypertension; cytokine; chemokine; therapy; extracellular matrix; cirrhosis

Fibrosis is a double-edged sword. On the one hand, it can be the final state of healed inflammation as scar tissue; on the other hand, it is frequently associated with a reduction in or loss of organ function [1,2]. Moreover, it is a surrogate parameter that indicates the progression of the disease to liver cirrhosis or even hepatocellular carcinoma. This is especially true for non-alcoholic fatty liver disease, a pandemic disorder associated with Western lifestyles and diets. To influence organ fibrosis, it is important to better understand its induction, perpetuation and termination at the molecular level. The induction of liver fibrosis may be metabolic (e.g., alcohol, diet and drugs), infectious (e.g., viruses), autoimmune (e.g., primary biliary cholangitis) or due to monogenetic defects (e.g., increased iron storage) [1,2]. The molecular mechanisms leading to final-stage fibrosis are very different depending on its pathogenesis [3,4]. This Special Issue aims to provide more insight into these processes.

We, Ralf Weiskirchen and Tilman Sauerbruch (Figure 1), cordially invite you to submit original research articles, reviews, or shorter perspective articles on all aspects related to the "Liver Fibrosis: Mechanisms, Targets, Assessment and Treatment". Expert articles describing mechanistic, functional, cellular, biochemical or general aspects of hepatic fibrogenesis are highly welcome.

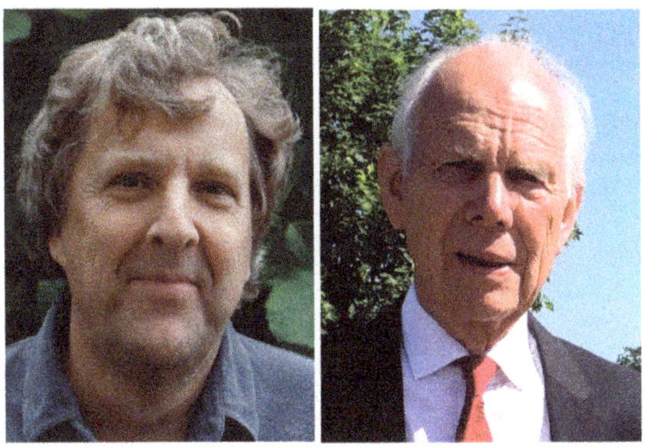

Figure 1. Editors of the Special Issue, "Liver Fibrosis: Mechanisms, Targets, Assessment and Treatment". Ralf Weiskirchen (**left**); Tilman Sauerbruch (**right**).

Relevant topics include: fibrosis, cirrhosis, hepatocellular carcinoma, NASH, NAFLD, cytokines, chemokines, extracellular matrix, fibrotic signaling, animal models, biomarkers, hepatic stellate cells, animal models of hepatic fibrosis, the translation of basic findings in hepatology to the human situation, portal hypertension, bile acids, beta-blockers, imaging of hepatic fibrosis, management and therapy of hepatic lesions. Based on our expertise, we will be happy to consider studies on all aspects of basic and clinical aspects of hepatic fibrosis.

Livers is an international, peer-reviewed, open access journal on liver science published online. Information about the submission process to this Special Issue, the types of desired publications, and guidelines for manuscript preparation are given at: https://www.mdpi.com/journal/livers/special_issues/742Y9BF54R.

Author Contributions: Conceptualization, R.W. and T.S.; writing, original draft preparation, R.W. and T.S.; writing, review and editing, R.W. and T.S.; visualization, R.W. and T.S. All authors have read and agreed to the published version of the manuscript.

Funding: R.W. is supported by the German Research Foundation (grants WE2554/13-1, WE2554/15-1, WE2554/17-1) and the Interdisciplinary Centre for Clinical Research within the Faculty of Medicine at the RWTH Aachen University (grant PTD 1-5). None of the funders had any role in the design of the study and the decision to publish this contribution.

Institutional Review Board Statement: Not applicable.

Informed Consent Statement: Not applicable.

Data Availability Statement: No new data were created or analyzed in this study. Data sharing is not applicable to this article.

Conflicts of Interest: The authors declare no conflict of interest.

References

1. Friedman, S.L.; Pinzani, M. Hepatic fibrosis 2022: Unmet needs and a blueprint for the future. *Hepatology* **2022**, *75*, 473–488. [CrossRef]
2. Acharya, P.; Chouhan, K.; Weiskirchen, S.; Weiskirchen, R. Cellular mechanisms of liver fibrosis. *Front. Pharmacol.* **2021**, *12*, 671640. [CrossRef]
3. Lurje, I.; Gaisa, N.T.; Weiskirchen, R.; Tacke, F. Mechanisms of organ fibrosis: Emerging concepts and implications for novel treatment strategies. *Mol. Asp. Med.* **2023**, *92*, 101191. [CrossRef]
4. Liedtke, C.; Nevzorova, Y.A.; Luedde, T.; Zimmermann, H.; Kroy, D.; Strnad, P.; Berres, M.L.; Bernhagen, J.; Tacke, F.; Nattermann, J.; et al. Liver fibrosis-From mechanisms of injury to modulation of disease. *Front. Med.* **2022**, *8*, 814496. [CrossRef]

Short Biography of Author

Ralf Weiskirchen, Ph.D., was born on 2 February 1964 in Bergisch Gladbach (North Rhine-Westphalia, Germany). After his school education, he studied biology and obtained his PhD with distinction at the University of Cologne in Germany. Thereafter, he worked for several years as a Research Associate at the Institute of Biochemistry, University of Innsbruck, Austria. Back in Germany, he habilitated at the Technical University of Aachen and became a full Professor in 2007 at the Aachen University Hospital. Currently, he is head of the Institute of Molecular Pathobiochemistry, Experimental Gene Therapy and Clinical Chemistry (IFMPEGKC) at the RWTH University Hospital Aachen. His major research interest is the analysis of TGF-β/BMP and PDGF signaling pathways in the pathogenesis of liver disease. In particular, he has an interest in understanding the contribution of different hepatic cell subpopulations to the formation and resolution of hepatic disease. Professor Weiskirchen maintains a variety of national and international cooperations that are focused on molecular aspects of hepatic disease pathogenesis and therapy. Moreover, his work is concentrated on the identification and evaluation of novel biomarkers that are relevant to estimating the severity or outcome of hepatic diseases.

Tilman Sauerbruch, Professor Emeritus, was born on 9 July 1946 in Lauingen on the Danube. After studying Medicine at the universities of Würzburg, Montpellier, Hamburg and Heidelberg, he trained as an internist and gastroenterologist at the University of Heidelberg and at the academic teaching hospitals of Pforzheim and Munich Schwabing. Gustav Paumgartner enabled him to enter the field of hepatology at the University of Munich, where he taught and worked as an assistant and associate professor from 1984 to 1992. Between 1992 and 2012, he was a full professor of Medicine at the University of Bonn and Head of the Medical Department I, a time during which Peter Malfertheiner, Frank Lammert, Ulrich Spengler, Jürgen Rockstroh and Jonel Trebicka were essential members of the clinic's staff. From 2012 to 2014, he was a full professor and temporary head of the Department of Gastroenterology and Endocrinology at the University of Göttingen. He is a fellow of the American Gastroenterological Association. In 2018, he was Honorary President of the International Liver Congress (ILC) of the European Association for the Study of the Liver (EASL). He is an honorary member of the German Society for Internal Medicine. In 1985 he received the Körber European Science Prize; in 2014, he received the Recognition Award of the European Association for the Study of the Liver (EASL); and in 2020, he received the Leopold Lichtwitz Medal. He tries to remain intellectually close to academic Medicine, especially hepatology.

livers

MDPI

Editorial

Special Issue "Liver Fibrosis: Mechanisms, Targets, Assessment and Treatment"

Ralf Weiskirchen [1,*] and Tilman Sauerbruch [2,*]

[1] Institute of Molecular Pathobiochemistry, Experimental Gene Therapy and Clinical Chemistry (IFMPEGKC), RWTH University Hospital Aachen, D-52074 Aachen, Germany
[2] Department of Internal Medicine I, University Hospital of Bonn, D-53127 Bonn, Germany
* Correspondence: rweiskirchen@ukaachen.de (R.W.); tilman.sauerbruch@ukbonn.de (T.S.)

Liver fibrosis is a significant challenge in hepatology, as it represents the common pathway of chronic liver injury due to various causes such as viral hepatitis, metabolic dysfunction-associated steatotic liver disease (MASLD), intoxication, alcohol-related liver disease, autoimmune conditions, and genetic disorders [1,2]. The progression of fibrosis not only indicates worsening organ dysfunction but also warns of serious complications, such as cirrhosis and hepatocellular carcinoma. The latter is the fourth-leading cause of cancer death worldwide [3]. Despite advancements in our understanding, effective antifibrotic treatments are limited, and many aspects of fibrogenesis remain unclear. This highlights the pressing need for ongoing research on the molecular mechanisms behind hepatic fibrosis, as well as improved methods for early detection and targeted intervention [4]. Given the clinical importance and biological complexity of liver fibrosis, research on the mechanisms driving fibrogenesis, new diagnostic biomarkers, and emerging therapeutic approaches is more crucial than ever [5,6].

The Special Issue "Liver Fibrosis: Mechanisms, Targets, Assessment and Treatment" was conceived to provide a comprehensive platform for cutting-edge research in this rapidly evolving field. This issue includes 10 original articles, reviews and case reports contributed by over 60 authors from a variety of countries, including Denmark, Germany, Greece, Japan, Lebanon, Poland, Sweden, Turkey, the United Kingdom, and the United States. This diversity emphasizes both the global impact of liver fibrosis and the international dedication to addressing the disease through collaborative science.

The collection begins with an Editorial by Ralf Weiskirchen and Tilman Sauerbruch, who discuss the dual nature of fibrosis as both reparative scar tissue after inflammation and a driver of progressive organ failure. They invite researchers worldwide to tackle mechanistic questions and translational challenges. Their introduction underscores how multifactorial triggers, from metabolic syndrome to infections or monogenic diseases, require equally multifaceted scientific approaches (Contribution 1).

One notable original contribution comes from Vorona et al., who present a compelling case report on MASLD arising from familial partial lipodystrophy, a rare genetic disorder. This paper not only outlines diagnostic challenges, but also showcases significant improvement following leptin replacement therapy. By summarizing current diabetes treatment options in MASLD contexts alongside their case experience, they offer valuable insights into personalized medicine for rare forms of fatty liver disease (Contribution 2).

On the immunological frontlines of fibrogenesis research is the paper of Tsomidis et al., whose extensive review dissects immune checkpoint pathways, such as programmed cell death protein 1 (PD-1)/programmed death-ligand 1 (PD-L1) and cytotoxic T lymphocyte-associated antigen 4 (CTLA-4), in both innate and adaptive immunity during hepatic fibrosis progression. They highlight how advancements in immunotherapy may soon lead to antifibrotic treatments targeting these regulatory axes (Contribution 3).

Advances in non-invasive diagnostics are exemplified by Villanueva Raisman et al., who leverage targeted mass-spectrometry-based proteomics to identify plasma protein panels capable of stratifying patients across different stages of liver fibrosis. Their approach holds promise for early detection, potentially reducing invasive biopsy, and supporting precision medicine through robust biomarker discovery (Contribution 4).

Innovations in technology are further addressed by Pyka et al., who describe their development of elastography measuring caps optimized for ex vivo assessment using porcine models. Their numerical simulations, validated with preclinical data, demonstrate improved accuracy in mechanical wave propagation analysis while minimizing tissue damage during assessment procedures relevant to transplantation medicine (Contribution 5).

Pedersen et al. compare proteomic profiles between visceral adipose tissue (VAT) and liver samples from obese individuals at various MASLD stages. While no direct MASH-specific signature emerged in VAT, several immunomodulatory proteins correlated between both tissues, suggesting shared inflammatory circuits that may influence disease trajectory (Contribution 6).

From Japan comes an important clinical study by Nagaoki et al., which addresses outcomes after hepatitis C virus eradication using direct-acting antivirals (DAAs). Through long-term follow-up they identify key risk factors—including platelet count $< 11 \times 10^4/\mu L$, high liver stiffness measurement, elevated bile acids, and an enlarged left gastric vein diameter—for the aggravation of esophagogastric varices despite virological cures. These findings offer practical guidance for surveillance protocols tailored to individual risk profiles (Contribution 7).

Kamoua et al., based in North America, deliver an up-to-date review on cutaneous manifestations associated with advanced liver dysfunction, including spider angiomas, palmar erythema, jaundice, and pruritus. They stress the value of these visible markers in aiding diagnosis and prognosis at the bedside. This article highlights the urgent need for increased clinical awareness in managing patients with liver diseases (Contribution 8).

The review by El Khoury et al. bridges basic science with cardiovascular epidemiology by examining the role of carcinoembryonic antigen-related cell adhesion molecule 1 (CEACAM1) deficiency in linking insulin resistance-driven steatohepatitis/fibrosis with endothelial dysfunction that underlies atherosclerosis. Drawing on animal models they propose CEACAM1 not only as a mechanistic bridge but also as a promising therapeutic target at the intersection of hepatic and vascular disease (Contribution 9).

Finally, Chandrasekaran and Weiskirchen provide an authoritative synthesis on MBOAT7, a lipid remodeling enzyme whose genetic variants have recently been implicated in MASLD susceptibility and progression through human association studies and mouse models. They discuss how targeting enzymes like MBOAT7 could open new avenues for future fatty liver disease therapies beyond classical targets such as PNPLA3 or TM6SF2 (Contribution 10).

Taken together, these ten contributions reflect not only scientific excellence but also remarkable international collaboration, from leading European academic centers to institutions across Asia, North America, and the Middle East. Each article offers new perspectives on fundamental biology or translational approaches toward assessment and treatment.

We express our sincere gratitude to all contributing authors whose expertise has made this Special Issue possible. We particularly recognize early-career scientists whose innovative ideas are pushing boundaries forward. Our hope is that readers will find inspiration within these pages to continue exploring one of the most pressing challenges in hepatology: understanding and ultimately reversing the complex process of liver fibrogenesis.

With ongoing advances in molecular biology, immunology, diagnostics, technology, and clinical management now converging more closely than ever before, we look forward with optimism to future breakthroughs that will transform healthcare for millions living with chronic liver disease worldwide.

Author Contributions: Conceptualization, R.W. and T.S.; writing, original draft preparation, R.W. and T.S.; writing, review and editing, R.W. and T.S. All authors have read and agreed to the published version of the manuscript.

Funding: R.W. is supported by the German Research Foundation (grant WE2554/17-1), the German Cancer Aid (project 70115581), and the Interdisciplinary Centre for Clinical Research within the Faculty of Medicine at RWTH Aachen University (grant PTD 1-5). None of the funders had any role in the design of the study or the decision to publish this contribution.

Data Availability Statement: No new data were created or analyzed in this study. Data sharing is not applicable to this article.

Acknowledgments: The authors would like to express their gratitude to all the contributors to this topic. We also want to thank the supportive team at the Editorial Office of Livers for facilitating a thorough review process and ensuring effective communication with the authors. Additionally, we are grateful for the commendable and efficient efforts of the expert reviewers who evaluated submissions promptly, fairly, and constructively. Finally, our thanks go to Byoung Kuk Jang (Keimyung University School of Medicine, Daegu, Republic of Korea) and Francesco Tovoli (Department of Medical and Surgical Sciences, University of Bologna, Italy) for helping to edit articles in cases where conflicts of interest arose.

Conflicts of Interest: The authors declare no conflicts of interest.

List of Contributions:

1. Weiskirchen, R.; Sauerbruch, T. Special Issue "Liver Fibrosis: Mechanisms, Targets, Assessment and Treatment". *Livers* **2023**, *3*, 322–324. https://doi.org/10.3390/livers3030023.
2. Vorona, E.; Sorkina, E.; Trebicka, J. Progressive Metabolic Dysfunction-Associated Steatotic Liver Disease (MASLD) from a Young Age Due to a Rare Genetic Disorder, Familial Partial Lipodystrophy: A Case Report and Review of the Literature. *Livers* **2024**, *4*, 688–695. https://doi.org/10.3390/livers4040047.
3. Tsomidis, I.; Voumvouraki, A.; Kouroumalis, E. Immune Checkpoints and the Immunology of Liver Fibrosis. *Livers* **2025**, *5*, 5. https://doi.org/10.3390/livers5010005.
4. Villanueva Raisman, A.; Kotol, D.; Altay, O.; Mardinoglu, A.; Atak, D.; Yurdaydin, C.; Akyildiz, M.; Dayangac, M.; Kirimlioglu, H.; Zeybel, M.; et al. Advancing Chronic Liver Disease Diagnoses: Targeted Proteomics for the Non-Invasive Detection of Fibrosis. *Livers* **2025**, *5*, 2. https://doi.org/10.3390/livers5010002.
5. Pyka, D.; Noszczyk-Nowak, A.; Krawiec, K.; Swietlik, T.; Opielinski, K.J. Innovative Elastography Measuring Cap for Ex Vivo Liver Condition Assessment: Numerical and Preclinical Studies in a Porcine Model. *Livers* **2025**, *5*, 3. https://doi.org/10.3390/livers5010003.
6. Pedersen, J.S.; Niu, L.; Wewer Albrechtsen, N.J.; Kristiansen, V.B.; Poulsen, I.M.; Serizawa, R.R.; Hansen, T.; Gluud, L.L.; Madsbad, S.; Bendtsen, F. Comparative Analysis of the Human Proteome Profile in Visceral Adipose and Liver Tissue in Individuals with Obesity with and Without MASLD and MASH. *Livers* **2025**, *5*, 16. https://doi.org/10.3390/livers5020016.
7. Nagaoki, Y.; Yamaoka, K.; Fujii, Y.; Uchikawa, S.; Fujino, H.; Ono, A.; Murakami, E.; Kawaoka, T.; Miki, D.; Aikata, H.; et al. Useful Predictor for Exacerbation of Esophagogastric Varices After Hepatitis C Virus Eradication by Direct-Acting Antivirals. *Livers* **2024**, *4*, 352–363. https://doi.org/10.3390/livers4030025.

8. Kamoua, R.; Reese, R.; Annamraju, R.; Chen, T.; Doyle, C.; Parella, A.; Liu, A.; Abboud, Y.; Rohan, C.; Travers, J.B. Cutaneous Manifestations of Liver Cirrhosis: Clinical Significance and Diagnostic Implications. *Livers* **2025**, *5*, 37. https://doi.org/10.3390/livers5030037.
9. El Khoury, S.; Al Harake, S.N.; Youssef, T.; Risk, C.E.; Helou, N.G.; Doumet, N.M.; Aramouni, K.; Azar, S.; Najjar, S.M.; Ghadieh, H.E. Low Hepatic CEACAM1 Tethers Metabolic Dysfunction Steatohepatitis to Atherosclerosis. *Livers* **2025**, *5*, 34. https://doi.org/10.3390/livers5030034.
10. Chandrasekaran, P.; Weiskirchen, R. The Pivotal Role of the Membrane-Bound O-Acyltransferase Domain Containing 7 in Non-Alcoholic Fatty Liver Disease. *Livers* **2024**, *4*, 1–14. https://doi.org/10.3390/livers4010001.

References

1. Acharya, P.; Chouhan, K.; Weiskirchen, S.; Weiskirchen, R. Cellular Mechanisms of Liver Fibrosis. *Front. Pharmacol.* **2021**, *12*, 671640. [CrossRef] [PubMed]
2. Dua, A.; Kumari, R.; Singh, M.; Kumar, R.; Pradeep, S.; Ojesina, A.I.; Kumar, R. Metabolic Dysfunction-Associated Steatotic Liver Disease (MASLD): The interplay of gut microbiome, insulin resistance, and diabetes. *Front. Med.* **2025**, *12*, 1618275. [CrossRef] [PubMed]
3. Robert, A.; Hunold, T.M.; Parikh, N.D. Management of hepatocellular carcinoma prior to liver transplantation: Latest developments. *Hepat. Oncol.* **2025**, *12*, 2549676. [CrossRef] [PubMed]
4. Bech, K.T.; Lindvig, K.P.; Thiele, M.; Castera, L. Algorithms for Early Detection of Silent Liver Fibrosis in the Primary Care Setting. *Semin. Liver Dis.* **2024**, *44*, 23–34. [CrossRef] [PubMed]
5. Maroto-García, J.; Moreno Álvarez, A.; Sanz de Pedro, M.P.; Buño-Soto, A.; González, Á. Serum biomarkers for liver fibrosis assessment. *Adv. Lab. Med.* **2023**, *5*, 115–130. [CrossRef] [PubMed]
6. Zhao, L.; Tang, H.; Cheng, Z. Pharmacotherapy of Liver Fibrosis and Hepatitis: Recent Advances. *Pharmaceuticals* **2024**, *17*, 1724. [CrossRef] [PubMed]

livers

MDPI

Case Report

Progressive Metabolic Dysfunction-Associated Steatotic Liver Disease (MASLD) from a Young Age Due to a Rare Genetic Disorder, Familial Partial Lipodystrophy: A Case Report and Review of the Literature

Elena Vorona [1,*], Ekaterina Sorkina [2] and Jonel Trebicka [1]

1 Medical Clinic B for Gastroenterology, Hepatology, Endocrinology and Clinical Infectiology, University Hospital Muenster, 48149 Muenster, Germany; jonel.trebicka@ukmuenster.de
2 Translational and Clinical Research Institute, Newcastle University, Newcastle NE1 7RU, UK; ekaterina.sorkina@nhs.net
* Correspondence: elena.vorona@ukmuenster.de

Abstract: Steatotic liver disease is common in the general population and is associated with higher risk for cardiovascular diseases. Early diagnosis and appropriate therapy can prevent the development of irreversible end-stage liver fibrosis and reduce liver-related and cardiovascular mortality. It is important to recognise not only the common causes of metabolic dysfunction-associated steatotic liver disease, such as type 2 diabetes mellitus or morbid obesity, but also rare conditions, because their treatment is different from conventional therapy. Here, we report a female patient with familial partial lipodystrophy, in whom the diagnosis was not confirmed until several years after the initial manifestation, which delayed the start of pathogenetic therapy. After the initiation of leptin replacement therapy, a significant improvement in liver stiffness measurement was achieved within a few months. In addition, we summarise the current treatment options for diabetes and their influence on steatosis hepatis.

Keywords: metabolic dysfunction-associated steatotic liver disease (MASLD); diabetes mellitus; hypertriglyceridemia; familial partial lipodystrophy (FPL); LMNA

1. Introduction

Metabolic dysfunction-associated steatotic liver disease (MASLD) is a heterogeneous group of disorders, characterised by intrahepatic fat accumulation and liver structure and function damage in the absence of alcohol impact.

According to the multi-society Delphi consensus statement, MASLD is diagnosed, if in a patient with steatotic liver disease, identified by liver imaging or biopsy, at least one of five cardiometabolic criteria is met and alcohol intake is excluded. The cardiometabolic criteria are defined as following [1]

(1) BMI > 25 kg/m^2 or waist circumference of more than 94 cm in males and more than 80 cm in females;
(2) Fasting serum glucose $\geq$ 5.6 mmol/L (100 mg/dL) or 2 h post-load glucose levels $\geq$ 7.8 mmol/L ($\geq$140 mg/dL) or HbA1C $\geq$ 5.7% (39 mmol/L) or type 2 diabetes or treatment for type 2 diabetes;
(3) Blood pressure > 130/85 mmHg or specific antihypertensive drug treatment;
(4) Plasma triglycerides $\geq$ 1.70 mmol/L (150 mg/dL) or lipid-lowering treatment;
(5) Plasma HDL-cholesterol $\leq$ 1.0 mmol/L (40 mg/dL) in males and $\leq$1.3 mmol/L (50 mg/dL) or lipid-lowering treatment.

The current EASL-EASD-EASO multi-society clinical practice guidelines [2] provide evidence-based recommendations on diagnosis and treatment for MASLD. As advanced liver fibrosis is a predictor of liver-associated mortality, it is recommended to rule out liver fibrosis based on laboratory scores (e.g., FIB-4) and non-invasive imaging techniques.

The most available diagnostic tool for steatosis is a combination of liver sonography with vibration-controlled transient elastography (VCTE) with liver stiffness measurement (LSM) and the assessment of the controlled attenuation parameter (CAP). This diagnostic procedure is comparable with liver biopsy in terms of sensitivity and specificity [3,4] and is widely used in the last decades. Braude et al. [4] demonstrated an association between increased all-cause mortality and liver stiffness on vibration-controlled transient elastography in patients with MASLD. Comparing CAP findings with liver biopsy analyses as the reference standard, Eddowes at al. found that patients with steatosis Grade 1 had a CAP of >302 dB/m, those with Grade 2 had a CAP of >331 dB/m, and those with Grade 3 had a CAP of >337 dB/m, whereas for LSM, the cut-off values for F2, F3, and F4 were 8.2 kPa, 9.7 kPa, and 13.6 kPa, respectively [5]. There are currently no guideline-defined CAP cut-offs, which limits the use of the CAP as a diagnostic criterion for MASLD [6–8].

Lipodystrophy syndromes can be a rare cause of MASLD, where the subcutaneous tissue is unable to properly store fat, what leads to fat accumulation in visceral organs, especially in the liver. Patients with generalised or familial partial lipodystrophy usually have low adipocyte hormone leptin levels, measured in serum, and, in most cases, severe metabolic abnormalities such as severe insulin resistance with diabetes mellitus and significant dyslipidaemia (Table 1). Since absolute or relative leptin deficiency is the cause of metabolic derailment in patients with lipodystrophy, human recombinant leptin replacement therapy (Metreleptin) has been tested in several studies in recent decades, with a significant improvement in the metabolic situation achieved and maintained in most patients [9] Metreleptin is available for causal treatment of congenital lipodystrophy, and it can be recommended in addition to diet and standard drug therapy for metabolic complications of FPL, as defined in the Multi-Society Practice Guideline for Diagnosis and Management of Lipodystrophy Syndromes [10].

Table 1. Diagnostic criteria for familial partial lipodystrophy.

Medical History	Physical Examination	Body Composition	Metabolic Status	Serum Leptin Levels	Genetic Testing
-Positive family history; -History of PCO syndrome, non-alcoholic acute pancreatitis, or liver fibrosis.	-Loss of subcutaneous fat (occurring around puberty); -Muscular hypertrophy; -Prominent veins (phlebomegaly); -Acantosis nigricans; -Eruptive xanthomas; -Hirsutism; -Cushingoid appearance; -Acromegaloid appearance; -Progeroid appearance; -Heart diseases: arterial hypertension, cardiomyopathy, arrhythmias.	-Non-alcoholic steatotic liver in a non-obese individual; -Liver fibrosisto cirrhosis; dual-energy X-ray absorptiometry (DXA) and whole-body magnetic resonance imaging can confirm a pattern of fat loss.	-High triglyceride levels; -Low HDL-cholesterol levels; -Insulin resistance/diabetes mellitus; -Renal dysfunction.	Low leptin levels (however, there are no defined serum leptin levels).	To confirm the diagnosis, genetic counselling and screening of family members are required.

Functional and structural disorders of the liver are the most common organ complication, occurring in the majority of lipodystrophy patients. In LD patients with SLD, steatohepatitis improves due to metreleptin treatment, independent of diet [11]. Also, a reduction in liver volume by 33.8% for generalised lipodystrophy and by 13.4% for partial lipodystrophy after 12 months was observed [12,13]. Akinci demonstrated that 12 months after metreleptin treatment in patients with relative leptin deficiency and partial lipodystrophy liver biopsy, the results confirmed a significant decrease in steatohepatitis. This suggests that leptin deficiency may have regulatory effects in mediating fat deposition and, as consequence, damage the liver [14].

2. Case Report

Here, we report a female patient who presented to our endocrinology outpatient clinic at the age of 30 in the eighth week of pregnancy for treatment of diabetes mellitus (Figure 1).

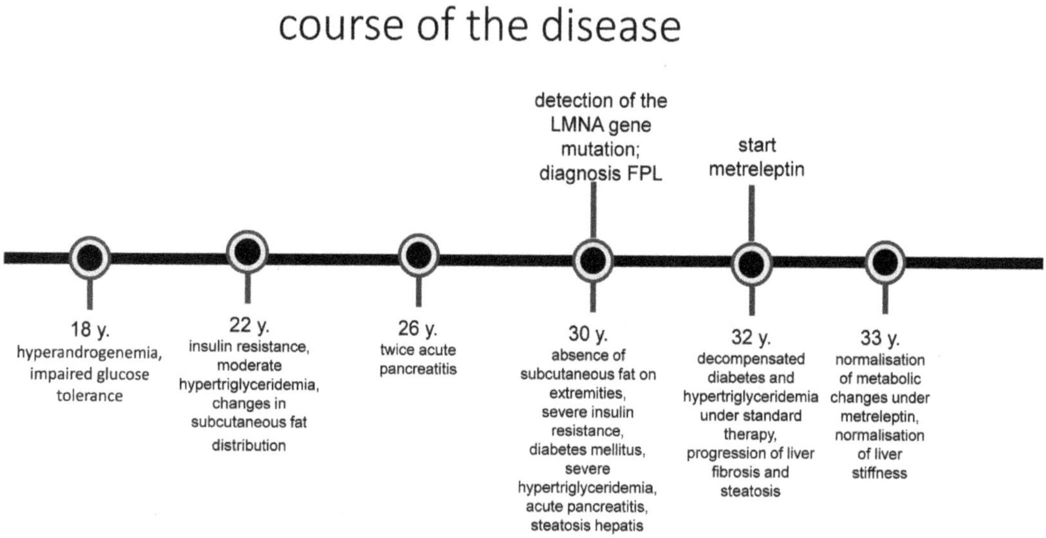

Figure 1. Course of the disease.

She had hyperandrogenaemia and impaired glucose tolerance with insulin resistance since the age of 18. At that time, her gynaecologist recommended taking oral hormonal contraception until she wanted to have children, metformin therapy (500 mg 3 times a day), and weight reduction, because of a body mass index of 27 kg/m^2, to control the hyperandrogenaemia and insulin resistance.

During her first spontaneous pregnancy at the age of 21, she was diagnosed with gestational diabetes. Postpartum, at the age of 22, she was seen in the endocrinology and diabetology department for the first time, where a fat distribution disorder with an accumulation of subcutaneous fat in the neck area with a double chin was first noticed. Furthermore, there was a slight axial and inguinal acanthosis nigricans, and her BMI was 28 kg/m^2. Hirsutism and androgenetic alopecia were not present, but the physician noted that there was prominent musculature of the lower and upper extremities, although the patient did not exercise. The laboratory tests revealed very high insulin levels (150.0 μU/mL (6–27)) with normal glucose (80 mg/dL (60–110)) as well as high lipid metabolism parameters (cholesterol: 216 mg/dL (<200); triglycerides: 700 mg/dL (<150)) and hyperandrogenaemia. Ovarian hyperandrogenaemia and hyperinsulinemia, as a sign of insulin resistance, were documented as diagnoses. A low-carbohydrate diet was recommended to reduce her insulin levels, and metformin was prescribed to improve her insulin resistance.

At the age of 26, the patient was admitted to hospital twice at intervals of 3 months due to acute pancreatitis. Very high levels of triglycerides in the serum were conspicuous. After reconvalescence, she presented to the specialised lipid clinic. The lipid disorder was classified as a "diabetogenic lipid constellation" with high LDL, low HDL, and elevated triglyceride levels because of a familial predisposition. Notably, her HbA1c of 5.9% was not significantly increased. Lifestyle modification with an increase in physical activity and a strict change in diet was recommended. Treatment with metformin 1000 mg twice daily was continued. The HbA1c value was between 6.1% and 6.7% in the years prior to presentation at our clinic.

During the first presentation in our clinic, we saw a 30-year-old pregnant patient in the eighth week of pregnancy who was overweight (BMI 30.2 kg/m^2) and had slightly elevated blood pressure (140/80 mmHg). Subcutaneous fat accumulation in the neck, throat, and facial area were very conspicuous in contrast to the muscular appearance with prominent musculature, particularly in the lower and upper extremities. There were also prominent veins on the extremities, a protruding navel, acanthosis nigricans located in the axilla and on the inner thighs, and hyperplasia of the labia pudendi. We registered absent or significantly reduced subcutaneous fat on the lower and upper extremities. The skin fold thickness was 4–6 mm on the upper arms, 10 mm on the sides of the navel, 6 mm on the thighs, and 25 mm on the scapulae. Laboratory chemistry, even if blood was taken postprandially, showed derailed lipid metabolism with dramatic hypertriglyceridemia of 8074 mg/dL (<150). The patient was admitted as an inpatient and was given a strict low-fat diet with the use of medium-chain triglyceride (MCT) diet, which led to a rapid improvement in lipid levels and was continued consistently over the course of the disease. HbA1c was only slightly elevated at 6.4%, but as the glucose levels were not within the target range for pregnancy as defined by the national diabetes guideline, insulin therapy was started.

A duplex sonography showed no evidence of relevant peripheral arterial occlusive disease of the upper and lower extremities. There was also no evidence of relevant stenosis of the extracranial arteries. Sonography of the abdomen revealed a liver with a regular contour, smooth surface, and homogeneous echo pattern but significantly enlarged and ubiquitously compacted. The liver stiffness measurement (LSM) registered a median organ density of 5.7 kPa. The assessment of the controlled attenuation parameter (CAP) revealed a high degree of steatosis hepatis (355 dB/m).

A molecular genetic analysis was initiated due to a strong clinical suspicion of familial partial lipodystrophy. A heterozygote mutation, p.(=)+(Arg482Gln), c.(=)+(1445G>A), in Exon 8 of the *LMNA* gene was detected, which confirmed the diagnosis of familial partial lipodystrophy type 2 (Dunningan type). Her fasting serum leptin levels were at the lower reference limit.

As the pregnancy progressed, the insulin dose had to be steadily increased to keep the glucose levels within the recommended target range. Due to pronounced insulin resistance, which was also aggravated by the pregnancy, the daily insulin doses reached up to almost 1000 IU. This made the patient's quality of life considerably more difficult, as subcutaneous insulin injections were very painful as she had only a thin layer of subcutaneous fatty tissue. The hypertriglyceridemia could be controlled to some extent by a strict diet with a medium-chain triglyceride (MCT) diet. Nevertheless, moderate pancreatitis occurred once during pregnancy, which was treated with analgesics and volume administration. An insulin deficiency due to pancreatitis could be excluded.

The patient delivered on time by caesarean section. Postpartum, insulin was discontinued, and therapy with metformin 1000 mg twice daily, fenofibrate 250 mg daily, and omega-3 polyunsaturated fatty acids was carried out, under which the metabolic situation remained well controlled for 1.5 years. Treatment with GLP1 receptor analogues or DPP4 inhibitors was deliberately avoided due to concerns about the recurrence of pancreatitis.

After a gastrointestinal infection, metabolic derailment occurred, and insulin therapy was restarted. In the short term, however, there was increasing deterioration in her general condition with blurred vision, a feeling of warmth, malaise, extreme muscle weakness, and hyperphagia. She was unable to exercise due to a lack of muscle strength. Laboratory chemistry revealed hyperglycemic derailment (HbA1c 8.7%) and massive hypertriglyceridemia (2437 mg/dL (<150)). The patient had to be hospitalised, insulin therapy was intensified, and SGLT2 inhibitor therapy was initiated. The transaminases were moderately elevated; sonographically, we registered hepatomegaly with a kissing phenomenon, a rounded contour, and a smooth surface, with a homogeneous but clearly condensed echo pattern. Fibroscan and CAP measurements confirmed moderate to severe liver fibrosis and stage 3 steatosis hepatis.

Thus, 1.5 years postpartum, a metabolically derailed condition of partial familial lipodystrophy was under the consistently implemented standard therapy. The guidelines for the management of lypodystrophy and the criteria for leptin replacement therapy set out in the specialist information were thus fulfilled. This therapy was absolutely necessary in view of the otherwise uncontrollable diabetes and hypertriglyceridemia. The initiation of leptin replacement therapy with metreleptin, starting according to the current recommendations of 3 mg s.c. once daily (https://myaleptainfo.eu, accessed on 10 December 2024), was discussed with the patient. It was also expected that fine-tuning of the insulin therapy in terms of dose reduction would be necessary over the course of the treatment in order to avoid hypoglycaemia. Her subcutaneous FGM3 sensor was attached for continuous glucose level monitoring.

Three months after starting treatment with Metreleptin, the patient reported a significantly improved quality of life: reduced food intake, a reduced abdominal circumference, and a reduction in insulin doses and injections. She felt much stronger, walking was now better, and she no longer had any muscle pain. The distance she could walk had increased significantly since starting the metreleptin injections. The insulin therapy could be stopped. Laboratory tests showed normalisation of the transaminases, triglyceride levels had fallen 100-fold, and her HbA1C was now within the normal range.

Six months after the initiation of leptin replacement therapy, diabetes mellitus was also well controlled (HbA1c 5.4%), and oral diabetes therapy could be de-escalated. Sonographically, we registered a normalisation of liver size, and liver stiffness had decreased significantly.

Nine months after the start of therapy, metreleptin was increased to the recommended standard dose of 5 mg s.c. due to a renewed moderate increase in triglycerides and HbA1c in an otherwise symptom-free patient. Twelve months after the start of therapy, the metabolic parameters were within the target range, and the metreleptin dosage could be maintained (Table 2).

Table 2. Changes in liver function and structure depending on metabolic parameters and therapy.

Time Point	Therapy	HbA1C 4.3–6.1%	Triglycerides <150 mg/dL	AST (10–35) ALT (10–35)	Liver Stiffness	CAP
First admission (8th week of pregnancy)	Strict MCT diet	6.4%	8074 mg/dL	N.A.	5.7 kPa	355 dB/m
1.5 years postpartum	Strict diet; insulin; metformin; empagliflozinfibrate; omega-3	8.7%	2437 mg/dL	82 U/L 84 U/L	8.7 kPa	313 dB/m
After starting metreleptin	Metreleptin; metformin; empagliflozinfibrate; omega-3	5.9% (after 3 months)	263 mg/dL (after 3 months)	12 U/L 19 U/L (after 3 months)	3.6 kPa (after 6 months)	386 dB/m (after 6 months)

AST, aspartate aminotransferase; ALT, alanine aminotransferase.

3. Conclusions

Metabolic dysfunction-associated steatotic liver disease is a common condition in the general population with the estimated prevalence up to 30% [15–17]. Several international clinical practice MASLD guidelines [2,18] emphasise the importance of early detection and evidence-based and complex treatment with regard to liver-related and cardiovascular mortality. The treatment options include lifestyle modifications, pharmacological treatment of diabetes mellitus and obesity (as we summarised in Table 3), specific therapy of fatty liver [6] and therapy of cardiovascular diseases (arterial hypertension, dyslipidaemia).

Table 3. Treatment options in type 2 diabetes mellitus and fatty liver disease.

Therapy	Modality	Advantages	Limitations
Lifestyle: -diet; -exercise	-Mediterranean diet, avoiding alcohol and smoking; -At least 150 min per week of moderate training or 75 min per week of intensive training	CVD risk improvement; weight reduction; improvement in liver injury	Multidisciplinary patient support is needed (education, behavioural therapy); low-threshold availability is needed
Metformin	500–2000 mg daily dose, 1–2 daily oral intake	Insulin resistance improvement; glycaemic control; no risk for hypoglycaemia; weight reduction; safe to use for MASLD(including compensated liver cirrhosis)	Histological improvement in steatohepatitis and fibrosis not confirmed so far; gastrointestinal side effects; hepatic function: contraindicated in hepatic decompensation; renal function: contraindicated in renal decompensation (eGFR < 30 mL/min)
GLP1-RA (glucagon-like peptide 1 receptor agonists)	Weekly subcutaneous injections	Glycaemic control; no risk for hypoglycaemia; CVD risk improvement; weight reduction; safe to use for MASH (including compensated liver cirrhosis)	Histological improvement in steatohepatitis and fibrosis not confirmed so far; gastrointestinal side effects, incl. pancreatitis; hepatic function: contraindicated in decompensated liver cirrhosis; renal function: contraindicated in end-stage renal failure (eGFR < 15 mL/min)
Dual-agonist GLP1-GIP (glucagon-like peptide 1 receptor agonists and glucose-dependent insulinotropic polypeptide)	Weekly subcutaneous injections	Glycaemic control; no risk for hypoglycaemia; weight reduction	Gastrointestinal side effects incl. pancreatitis; hepatic function: contraindicated in decompensated liver cirrhosis; renal function: contraindicated in end-stage renal failure (eGFR < 15 mL/min)
DPP4-I (dipeptidylpeptidase 4 inhibitors)	25–100 mg daily oral intake	Glycaemic control; no risk for hypoglycaemia	Histological improvement in steatohepatitis and fibrosis not confirmed so far; risk of pancreatitis; hepatic function: contraindicated in decompensated liver cirrhosis; renal function: dose reduction, if eGFR < 45 mL/min, contraindicated in end-stage renal failure (eGFR < 15 mL/min)
SGLT2-I (sodium-glucose transporter 2 inhibitors)	Daily oral intake	Glycaemic control; no risk for hypoglycaemia; CVD risk improvement; weight reduction; safe to use for MASLD; approved for heart failure and chronic kidney disease treatment	Histological improvement in steatohepatitis and fibrosis not confirmed so far; euglycemic ketoacidosis; urogenital infections; hepatic function: dose reduction in Child B cirrhosis; contraindicated in decompensated liver cirrhosis; renal function: dose reduction, if eGFR < 60 mL/min
Insulin	1–5 times daily subcutaneous injections	Glycaemic control; possible in end-stage hepatic or renal diseases	Hypoglycaemia; weight gain
Pioglitazone (peroxisome proliferator-activated receptor agonist)	daily oral intake	Glycaemic control; insulin resistance improvement; possible histological improvement in steatohepatitis	Weight gain; bone loss in postmenopausal women; fibrosis regression is not confirmed so far; not approved in all countries as indicated on label
Metreleptin (recombinant leptin) in confirmed lipodystrophy	daily subcutaneous injections; 3.0–7.5 mg	Glycaemic and lipid improvement; weight reduction; histologically confirmed improvement in steatohepatitis	Hypoglycaemia; not been studied in patients with impaired renal or hepatic function, so no dosage recommendations can be given
Resmetirom (beta-thyroid hormone receptor agonist)	daily oral intake	Histologically confirmed improvement in steatohepatitis and fibrosis	Not approved in all countries as indicated on label; contraindicated in liver cirrhosis

In the case of our patient, although the first symptoms of the disease with the phenotype typical of familial lipodystrophy manifested at a young age, the correct diagnosis could only be confirmed 12 years later, and serious and potentially fatal complications, such as acute pancreatitis, had already occurred. The multimodal therapy of the metabolic derailment was not sufficient.

The replacement of the missing hormone leptin (in combination with a diet and glucose- and triglyceride-lowering drugs) with Metreleptin is the only approved causal therapy for leptin deficiency-related consequences in patients with congenital generalised and partial familial lipodystrophy. In the case of our patient, if the situation of uncontrolled diabetes mellitus and hypertriglyceridemia, which cannot be controlled by conventional therapy, was to have persisted, further serious secondary diseases could have developed, such as progression of the existing metabolic dysfunction-associated steatotic liver disease to liver cirrhosis, with the increasing risk of hepatocellular carcinoma, progression of atherosclerosis with cardiovascular secondary diseases such as coronary heart disease to myocardial infarction, cerebrovascular disease to stroke, peripheral arterial occlusive disease, diabetic retinopathy to blindness, diabetic nephropathy to terminal kidney insufficiency requiring dialysis, and diabetes-related peripheral polyneuropathy.

In addition to the known and more common causes of metabolic dysfunction-associated steatotic liver disease, rare disorders such as familial lipodystrophy should be considered in unusual clinical presentations, as specific treatment options are available in these cases.

Author Contributions: Conceptualization E.V.; methodology E.V.; software E.V.; validation, not necessary; formal analysis not necessary; investigation, E.V.; resources, E.V.; data curation, E.V.; writing—original draft preparation, E.V.; writing—review and editing, J.T. and E.S.; visualization, E.S.; supervision, J.T.; project administration, E.V.; funding acquisition, not necessary. All authors have read and agreed to the published version of the manuscript.

Funding: This research received no external funding.

Institutional Review Board Statement: Not applicable.

Informed Consent Statement: Written informed consent has been obtained from the patient to publish this paper.

Data Availability Statement: The original contributions presented in the study are included in the article, further inquiries can be directed to the corresponding author.

Conflicts of Interest: The authors declare no conflict of interest.

References

1. Rinella, M.E.; Lazarus, J.V.; Ratziu, V.; Francque, S.M.; Sanyal, A.J.; Kanwal, F.; Romero, D.; Abdelmalek, M.F.; Anstee, Q.M.; Arab, J.P.; et al. A multisociety Delphi consensus statement on new fatty liver disease nomenclature. *Hepatology* **2023**, *78*, 1966–1986. [CrossRef] [PubMed] [PubMed Central]
2. European Association for the Study of the Liver (EASL); European Association for the Study of Diabetes (EASD); European Association for the Study of Obesity (EASO); European Association for the Study of the Liver (EASL). EASL-EASD-EASO Clinical Practice Guidelines on the management of metabolic dysfunction-associated steatotic liver disease (MASLD). *J. Hepatol.* **2024**, *81*, 492–542. [CrossRef] [PubMed]
3. Mózes, F.E.; Lee, J.A.; Selvaraj, E.A.; Jayaswal, A.N.A.; Trauner, M.; Boursier, J.; Fournier, C.; Staufer, K.; Stauber, R.E.; Bugianesi, E.; et al. Diagnostic accuracy of non-invasive tests for advanced fibrosis in patients with NAFLD: An individual patient data meta-analysis. *Gut* **2022**, *71*, 1006–1019. [CrossRef] [PubMed] [PubMed Central]
4. Braude, M.; Roberts, S.; Majeed, A.; Lubel, J.; Prompen, J.; Dev, A.; Sievert, W.; Bloom, S.; Gow, P.; Kemp, W. Liver stiffness (Fibroscan®) is a predictor of all-cause mortality in people with non-alcoholic fatty liver disease. *Liver Int.* **2023**, *43*, 90–99. [CrossRef] [PubMed] [PubMed Central]
5. Eddowes, P.J.; Sasso, M.; Allison, M.; Tsochatzis, E.; Anstee, Q.M.; Sheridan, D.; Guha, I.N.; Cobbold, J.F.; Deeks, J.J.; Paradis, V.; et al. Accuracy of FibroScan Controlled Attenuation Parameter and Liver Stiffness Measurement in Assessing Steatosis and Fibrosis in Patients with Nonalcoholic Fatty Liver Disease. *Gastroenterology* **2019**, *156*, 1717–1730. [CrossRef] [PubMed]
6. Ciardullo, S.; Vergani, M.; Perseghin, G. Nonalcoholic Fatty Liver Disease in Patients with Type 2 Diabetes: Screening, Diagnosis, and Treatment. *J. Clin. Med.* **2023**, *12*, 5597. [CrossRef] [PubMed] [PubMed Central]

7. Ciardullo, S.; Perseghin, G. Trends in prevalence of probable fibrotic non-alcoholic steatohepatitis in the United States, 1999-2016. *Liver Int.* **2023**, *43*, 340–344. [CrossRef] [PubMed]
8. Archer, A.J.; Belfield, K.J.; Orr, J.G.; Gordon, F.H.; Abeysekera, K.W. EASL clinical practice guidelines: Non-invasive liver tests for evaluation of liver disease severity and prognosis. *Frontline Gastroenterol.* **2022**, *13*, 436–439. [CrossRef] [PubMed] [PubMed Central]
9. Oral, E.A.; Simha, V.; Ruiz, E.; Andewelt, A.; Premkumar, A.; Snell, P.; Wagner, A.J.; DePaoli, A.M.; Reitman, M.L.; Taylor, S.I.; et al. Leptin-replacement therapy for lipodystrophy. *N. Engl. J. Med.* **2002**, *346*, 570–578. [CrossRef] [PubMed]
10. Brown, R.J.; Araujo-Vilar, D.; Cheung, P.T.; Dunger, D.; Garg, A.; Jack, M.; Mungai, L.; Oral, E.A.; Patni, N.; Rother, K.I.; et al. The Diagnosis and Management of Lipodystrophy Syndromes: A Multi-Society Practice Guideline. *J. Clin. Endocrinol. Metab.* **2016**, *101*, 4500–4511. [CrossRef] [PubMed] [PubMed Central]
11. Brown, R.J.; Valencia, A.; Startzell, M.; Cochran, E.; Walter, P.J.; Garraffo, H.M.; Cai, H.; Gharib, A.M.; Ouwerkerk, R.; Courville, A.B.; et al. Metreleptin-mediated improvements in insulin sensitivity are independent of food intake in humans with lipodystrophy. *J. Clin. Investig.* **2018**, *128*, 3504–3516. [CrossRef] [PubMed] [PubMed Central]
12. Brown, R.J.; Oral, E.A.; Cochran, E.; Araújo-Vilar, D.; Savage, D.B.; Long, A.; Fine, G.; Salinardi, T.; Gorden, P. Long-term effectiveness and safety of metreleptin in the treatment of patients with generalized lipodystrophy. *Endocrine* **2018**, *60*, 479–489. [CrossRef] [PubMed] [PubMed Central]
13. Oral, E.A.; Gorden, P.; Cochran, E.; Araújo-Vilar, D.; Savage, D.B.; Long, A.; Fine, G.; Salinardi, T.; Brown, R.J. Long-term effectiveness and safety of metreleptin in the treatment of patients with partial lipodystrophy. *Endocrine* **2019**, *64*, 500–511. [CrossRef] [PubMed] [PubMed Central]
14. Akinci, B.; Subauste, A.; Ajluni, N.; Esfandiari, N.H.; Meral, R.; Neidert, A.H.; Eraslan, A.; Hench, R.; Rus, D.; McKenna, B.; et al. Metreleptin therapy for nonalcoholic steatohepatitis: Open-label therapy interventions in two different clinical settings. *Med* **2021**, *2*, 814–835. [CrossRef] [PubMed] [PubMed Central]
15. Younossi, Z.M.; Golabi, P.; Paik, J.M.; Henry, A.; Van Dongen, C.; Henry, L. The global epidemiology of nonalcoholic fatty liver disease (NAFLD) and non-alcoholic steatohepatitis (NASH): A systematic review. *Hepatology* **2023**, *77*, 1335–1347. [CrossRef] [PubMed]
16. Quek, J.; Chan, K.E.; Wong, Z.Y.; Tan, C.; Tan, B.; Lim, W.H.; Tan, D.J.H.; Tang, A.S.P.; Tay, P.; Xiao, J.; et al. Global prevalence of non-alcoholic fatty liver disease and non-alcoholic steatohepatitis in the overweight and obese population: A systematic review and meta-analysis. *Lancet Gastroenterol. Hepatol.* **2023**, *8*, 20–30. [CrossRef] [PubMed]
17. Le, M.H.; Le, D.M.; Baez, T.C.; Wu, Y.; Ito, T.; Lee, E.Y.; Lee, K.; Stave, C.D.; Henry, L.; Barnett, S.D.; et al. Global incidence of non-alcoholic fatty liver disease: A systematic review and meta-analysis of 63 studies and 1,201,807 persons. *J. Hepatol.* **2023**, *79*, 287–295. [CrossRef] [PubMed]
18. Cusi, K.; Isaacs, S.; Barb, D.; Basu, R.; Caprio, S.; Garvey, W.T.; Kashyap, S.; Mechanick, J.I.; Mouzaki, M.; Nadolsky, K.; et al. American Association of Clinical Endocrinology Clinical Practice Guideline for the Diagnosis and Management of Nonalcoholic Fatty Liver Disease in Primary Care and Endocrinology Clinical Settings: Co-Sponsored by the American Association for the Study of Liver Diseases (AASLD). *Endocr. Pract.* **2022**, *28*, 528–562. [CrossRef] [PubMed]

livers

MDPI

Review

Immune Checkpoints and the Immunology of Liver Fibrosis

Ioannis Tsomidis [1], Argyro Voumvouraki [2] and Elias Kouroumalis [3,*]

1 Liver Research Laboratory, Medical School, University of Crete, 71500 Heraklion, Crete, Greece; itsomidi@gmail.com
2 1st Department of Internal Medicine, AHEPA University Hospital, 54621 Thessaloniki, Central Macedonia, Greece; iro_voum@yahoo.gr
3 Department of Gastroenterology, University Hospital, 71500 Heraklion, Crete, Greece
* Correspondence: kouroumi@uoc.gr

Abstract: Liver fibrosis is a very complicated dynamic process where several immune cells are involved. Both innate and adaptive immunity are implicated, and their interplay is always present. Multi-directional interactions between liver macrophages, hepatic stellate cells (HSCs), immune cells, and several cytokines are important for the induction and perpetuation of liver fibrosis. Detailed studies of proteomics and transcriptomics have produced new evidence for the role of individual cells in the process of liver fibrosis and cirrhosis. Most of these cells are controlled by the various immune checkpoints whose main function is to maintain the homeostasis of the implicated immune cells. Recent evidence indicates that several immune checkpoints are involved in liver fibrosis. In particular, the role of the programmed cell death protein 1 (PD-1), the programmed death-ligand 1 (PD-L1), and the role of the cytotoxic T lymphocyte-associated antigen 4 (CTLA-4) have been investigated, particularly after the availability of checkpoint inhibitors. Their activation leads to the exhaustion of CD4+ve and CD8+ve T cells and the promotion of liver fibrosis. In this review, the current pathogenesis of liver fibrosis and the immunological abnormalities are discussed. The recent data on the involvement of immune checkpoints are identified as possible targets of future interventions.

Keywords: liver fibrosis; macrophages; hepatic stellate cells; innate immunity cells; adaptive immunity cells; immune checkpoints

1. Introduction

The development of liver fibrosis (LF) is characterized by the deposition of extracellular matrix (ECM) proteins produced by myofibroblasts (MFs) of various origins including epithelial cells, mesenchymal stromal cells (MSCs), and HSCs [1]. Hepatocyte damage, irrespective of etiology, leads to the recruitment of immune cells in the liver. Quiescent HSCs (qHSCs) are activated and transformed into MFs, which are the main producers of connective tissue elements. If the insult is short term, the pro-fibrotic and anti-fibrotic mechanisms of the liver are in balance, and LF is not likely to occur. The continuous activation of the heterogenous population of hepatic MFs, mostly driven by liver macrophages, is the hallmark of chronic liver disease (CLD), but several other cells of the innate and adaptive immunity are also implicated [2,3]. The advancement of liver fibrosis leads to the final stage of cirrhosis. The pathological characteristics of cirrhosis are extensive fibrosis, the development of regenerative nodules, and the distortion of the hepatic architecture leading to overt clinical manifestations [4].

Global epidemiological data [5,6] reveal that almost 1.5 billion people suffer from CLD, leading to approximately 20,000 annual deaths, half of which are direct complica-

 https://doi.org/10.3390/livers5010005

tions of liver cirrhosis. The overall mortality from cirrhosis has increased by 47.15% in recent years [7]. The WHO's Global Burden of Diseases reports indicate that 560.4 age-standardized disability-adjusted life-years (DALYs) per 100,000 population worldwide were due to cirrhosis. In comparison, only 151.1 DALYs were due to liver cancer [8]. The most frequent causes of CLD are viral hepatitis, alcoholic liver disease, and metabolic-associated fatty liver disease (MAFLD/MASH) with heterogeneity across geographical regions [9]. Hepatitis B virus (HBV) and hepatitis C virus (HCV) are the underlying etiology of more than 60% of cirrhotic cases worldwide [10]. Less frequent etiologies that lead to fibrosis and cirrhosis include, among others, genetic diseases of iron or copper overload, cholestatic syndromes, and autoimmune diseases [4]. An important step in the clarification of the immune modulation and the therapeutic potential of the inhibition of certain immune checkpoints practically started when James Allison described the cytotoxic T lymphocyte-associated protein 4 (CTLA-4) and Tasuku Honjo described the programmed cell death protein 1 (PD-1). They were awarded the Nobel Prize for Physiology or Medicine in 2018 [11,12]. Immune checkpoint molecules are ligand–receptor pairs that exert inhibitory or stimulatory effects on immune responses. Most of the immune checkpoint molecules that have been described so far are expressed on cells of the innate and adaptive immune system, particularly on natural killer (NK) cells and T cells, respectively. They maintain the self-tolerance and modulate the immune responses of effectors in different tissues to minimize the tissue damage. Immune checkpoint proteins (ICPs) trigger the exhaustion, senescence, or apoptosis of effector immune cells [13].

It is, therefore, imperative to delineate the mechanisms implicated in the process of fibrosis. The present review will focus on the current data on the pathogenesis of liver fibrosis with emphasis on the immunological aspects and the emerging roles of the immune checkpoints.

2. A Pathogenetic Overview of Liver Fibrosis

2.1. The Fibrotic Process

For descriptive reasons, four pathological stages of fibrosis can be identified. Initially, exogenous or endogenous elements cause damage to the local liver cells and induce inflammation, followed by the large recruitment of immune cells at the site of the initial damage, thus aggravating the inflammatory response. Damaged hepatocytes or activated sinusoidal cells, by whatever cause, produce cytokines such as tumor necrosis factor-alpha (TNF-α) and IL-1, which are responsible for the recruitment of extrahepatic immune cells. In addition, they secrete pro-fibrotic factors, generating the background for the third stage. Quiescent hepatic stellate cells (HSCs) are transformed into myofibroblast-like HSCs [14,15] that lead to the fourth stage, the deposition of large amounts of ECM, and the remodeling of the liver architecture [16–18].

The ECM is composed of collagens, including type I (the most abundant protein) and type III collagens, fibronectin, elastin, and smaller amounts of several other proteins. The important components of the ECM are the basement membrane proteins such as laminin. It should be noted that myofibroblasts first secrete procollagen into the tissue, while mature collagen fibers evolve at a later extra-cellular stage through modification and cross-linking [19].

An important mechanism of fibrosis is the Epithelial-to-Mesenchymal Transition (EMT). It implies the differentiation of epithelial non-mesenchymal cells that acquire a fibroblast phenotype. Their participation in liver fibrosis has been extensively studied [20–23]. Epithelial cells undergo EMT under the influence of certain stimuli. An important one is the snail family transcriptional repressor 1 (Snail1). Hepatocytes with the deletion of the snail1 gene showed a significant decrease in EMT. Snail1 affected genes known to contribute to the progression of liver fibrosis, increasing the expression of pro-fibrotic genes such as those involved in collagen and vimentin production in the liver [24]. Moreover, the expression of Snail1 increased during the TGF-β1-induced EMT in murine hepatocytes, while the expression of the miR-30 family members was significantly down-regulated. miR-30 inhibited the EMT transformation in hepatocyte by targeting Snail1 [25]. Studies of cholestatic liver diseases have demonstrated the participation of EMT transformation in experimental and in human cholangiopathies such as biliary atresia. Cholangiocytes acquire mesenchymal markers and lose their epithelial characteristics [26–28]. The involvement of liver macrophages in EMT hepatocyte trans-differentiation has not been conclusively proved. Data from extrahepatic cancers indicate that the involvement of liver macrophages cannot be ruled out [29,30].

Recent evidence has indicated a significant role of non-coding RNAs in liver fibrosis. Myofibroblast activation is positively or negatively modulated by a number of non-coding RNAs [31]. They act on either EMT or through the ECM. ECM deposition can suppress miR-29, an important negative regulator of pro-fibrotic genes. Consequently, many such genes are recruited in the ribosomes and sustain the deposition of ECMs even in the absence of the initial stimulus. On the other hand, increased ECM stiffness activates the Hippo pathway effector Yes-associated protein 1 (YAP1), which also increases ECM deposition, thus initiating another positive feedback loop mediated by miR-21 [32]. miRNAs are implicated in liver fibrosis and stellate cell activation by targeting SMAD proteins [33]. MiR-199a promotes EMT transformation and fibrosis by increasing the expression of genes encoding procollagens and the tissue inhibitor of metalloproteinase-1 (TIMP1) [34]. MiR-32 is also pro-fibrotic in hyperglycemia in experimental conditions. Its inhibition attenuated EMT-induced liver fibrosis [35]. Several other miRNAs increase fibrosis in liver damage, affecting fibrotic pathways such as transforming growth factor-β/Smad, Wnt/β-catenin, and snail [36,37].

HSCs activation is also influenced by several anti-fibrotic miRNAs such as miR-16 and miR-19b among others that retain the quiescence of HSCs or induce either apoptosis or the de-differentiation of activated HSCs [37]. In more detail, miR-30a attenuates the EMT process by reducing TGF-β1. There is an inverse relation between mir30 and snail1, indicating that snail1 is a possible target of mir30, as mentioned before [38]. In addition, miR-30a can repress fibrosis by suppressing beclin-mediated autophagy [39].

Long non-coding RNAs (lncRNAs) are also implicated in liver fibrosis. An upregulation of lncRNA H19 in murine fibrosis activated the EMT pathway [40]. GAS5 acts as a sponge platform for miR-23a, a fact that ameliorates the progression of fibrosis [41]. The overexpression of Meg8 lncRNA was noticed during the activation of HSCs. Meg8 repressed the pro-fibrotic genes in activated HSCs and EMT, while its knockdown induced the expression of mesenchymal markers in hepatocytes [42].

In murine MASH models, the circRNA_29981 was identified as a possible regulator of HSC transformation [43]. Moreover, the mitochondrial circRNA SCAR can close the mitochondrial permeability transition pores, repressing the activation of MFs by inhibiting the mitochondrial ROS output [44].

A third important mechanism implicated in the regulation of liver fibrosis is the involvement of transcription factors such as the nuclear receptors (NRs) [45]. They mediate anti-inflammatory effects through direct interaction with other transcription factors, such as NF-κB [46,47]. They also have a fundamental role in liver regeneration and HSC activation [48,49]. The farnesoid X receptor (FXR) is better studied, and the use of FXR agonists repressed liver fibrosis in animal models by reducing HSC activation [50–52]. The details of nuclear receptors on liver fibrosis are found in recent extensive reviews [53,54].

A fourth and very important factor modulating liver fibrosis, and other forms of organ fibrosis, is the epigenetic modification of genes. They may lead to either the activation or repression of downstream proteins. Non-coding RNAs may act as epigenetic regulators. Other epigenetic modifications include DNA methylation, histone modification, and chromatin remodeling [55,56]. The DNA methylation pattern is critical in liver fibrosis [57] as it is in the activation of HSCs. The downregulation of the gene coding for the DNA methyl transferases DNMT3a and DNMT3b decreased DNA methylation followed by the suppression of HSC activation [58]. The activation of the hedgehog (Hh) pathway triggers liver EMT. The hypermethylation of the negative regulator of Hh, patched 1 (PTCH1), leads to its downregulation and an increase in liver fibrosis. Recent studies have established the anti-fibrotic efficacy of Salvianolic acid B (Sal B) that inhibits the Hh-mediated EMT [59]. In Sal B-treated cells, PTCH1 was increased due to the inhibition of DNA methyltransferase 1 (DNMT1), followed by a decrease in DNA methylation. The observed upregulation of miR-152 led to the hypomethylation of PTCH1, as DNMT1 was the direct target of miR-152 [60].

2.2. Cells Involved in Liver Fibrosis

2.2.1. Kupffer Cells and Liver Macrophages

Traditionally, Kupffer cells (KCs) included all macrophages in the liver, expressing surface markers such as F4/80 in mice or CD68 in humans. However, hepatic macrophages are a heterogeneous population, particularly after liver injury, and can be broadly divided into embryonic tissue resident KCs and monocyte-derived macrophages [61].

KCs are, therefore, liver resident macrophages initially generated in the embryo but also during adulthood [62,63]. Embryo-derived KCs (Em-KCs) persist in the liver throughout life by self-renewal [64]. In normal adulthood, bone marrow (BM)-derived monocytes can enrich the KC pool when Em-KCs are exhausted [65]. Monocyte-derived macrophages are recruited and accumulated in the liver after a damaging insult [66]. Em-KCs are CD49a+, a fact that distinguishes them from BM monocytes [67]. Em-KCs have a dual role in liver inflammation as they express both pro-inflammatory cytokines such as TNFa and anti-inflammatory cytokines such as IL-10. Em-KCs seem to be operational during normal homeostasis and promote tolerance, participating only in early liver injury, while BM-KCs act in chronic inflammation and fibrosis [68]. In the murine liver, only a few macrophages originate from BM monocytes under normal conditions [69]. Murine monocytes are divided into two phenotypes based on the presence of the lymphocyte antigen 6 complex, locus C (Ly6C). Ly6Chigh monocytes are recruited to the liver in liver injury and differentiated into BM-derived macrophages that are responsible for chronic inflammation and fibrosis. On the other hand, Ly-6Clow BM-derived macrophages promote damage resolution [70]. During early liver injury, damage-associated molecular patterns (DAMPs) and pathogen-associated molecular patterns (PAMPs), produced by the injured hepatocytes, interact with the Toll-like receptors (TLRs) on KCs. The activated KCs in turn recruit Ly-6Chigh macrophages through the release of chemokines such as CCL2 and CXCL1. Ly-6Chi macrophages sustain the activation and survival of HSCs [71], producing pro-fibrogenic mediators such as TGFβ, PDGF, and CCL2 [72]. Galectin-3 is also a lectin secreted by macrophages, which promotes HSC activation [73]. Liver macrophages also express receptors that bind the alarmin high-mobility group box 1 (HMGB1), released from injured hepatocytes. HMGB1 also activates HSC and stimulates the phenotypic responses of liver MFs [74].

The initial classification of KCs included classically activated pro-inflammatory M1 cells and alternatively activated anti-inflammatory M2 cells. LPS and IFNγ polarize KCs into M1 cells expressing inflammatory molecules such as IL-1, IL-12, TNFa, inducible nitric oxide synthase (iNOS), and a group of CXCL chemokines. On the other hand, Th2 helper T cells and IL-4 polarize KCs into M2-type expressing Arginase 1, IL-10, and PDL-1 and CCR2, CXCR1, and CXCR2 chemokines [75]. The M1/M2 balance is also dependent on production by the M2 cells of IL-10 that promotes M1 apoptosis [76,77]. M2 macrophages are additionally classified into distinct subtypes expressing different genes [78]. The M2 phenotype predominantly mediates tissue repair, but when the liver injury persists, M2 macrophages acquire a pro-fibrotic capacity [79].

In the diseased liver, macrophages frequently express both inflammation and regenerative markers with phenotypes that may change according to the local conditions and, therefore, the traditional model may not be relevant in liver damage [80,81]. A complex classification goes beyond the traditional distinction between M1 and M2 polarization [82,83]. It has been proposed that instead of the classical classification, a more detailed description should be made based on the activation stage, such as M (IL-10) or M (TGF-β) [84]. This classification is compatible with the changing roles of macrophages in liver disease that may be completely different or even opposite [19]. The fact that most macrophages do not comply with the M1/M2 model was recently verified. Two cytokines, the macrophage colony stimulating factor (M-CSF) and the granulocyte macrophage stimulating factor (GM-CSF) involved in the differentiation of KCs, indicate that the situation is more complex. In general, GM-CSF leads to M1 polarization and M-CSF to M2 polarization, but their combination with other cytokines may lead to a spectrum of macrophages expressing both M1 and M2 markers [85,86]. The murine models of liver fibrosis have shown an additional factor that participates in macrophage activation. The Notch signaling pathway is a significant regulator of macrophage differentiation. The suppression of the Notch1/Jagged1 signaling pathway may reverse M2 polarization [87]. In another model, the repression of the Notch signaling reduced the activation of HSCs and the polarization of macrophages into the M1 phenotype with the upregulation of anti-inflammatory genes and the reduction in liver fibrosis [88]. Several other macrophage-specific signaling pathways such as c-Jun N-terminal kinase (JNK), nuclear factor kappa-B (NF-kB), Janus kinase (JAK), and the signal transducer and activation of transcription (STAT) participate in liver fibrosis progression. On the opposite side, the activation of the Wnt/β-catenin signaling pathway in macrophages favors the resolution of liver fibrosis [19]. Murine studies, using single-cell RNA sequencing, identified a distinct type of hepatic bone marrow-derived macrophage with an inflammatory profile, particularly prominent in MASH [89].

The definition problem is far from being solved. Recently, in the murine livers, two types of KCs were characterized by single-cell RNA sequencing. KC1 represents the majority of KCs and is an endothelial cell-selective adhesion molecule (ESAM) negative with a low expression of CD 206. Functionally, it is tolerogenic, while KC2 (CD206hi) has pro-inflammatory potential [19]. An additional pro-fibrogenic subset of liver macrophages was characterized by the presence of the triggering receptor expressed on the myeloid cells 2 (TREM2+) CD9 + marker and was prominent in liver fibrosis, particularly in MAFLD/MASH patients [90,91]. In patients with liver fibrosis, findings analogous to the Ly6C murine macrophages were described.

The exact role of each of the described macrophage subtypes in individual liver diseases is not fully clarified. Murine alcohol-related liver disease (ALD) is exacerbated by infiltration of chemokine receptor positive macrophages, such as CCR2+ or CCR5+ [92]. Moreover, activated liver macrophages secrete vasoconstrictive agents that lead to the induction of portal hypertension and the development of liver fibrosis as they enhance HSCs transformation into MFs [64]. In addition, the activation of KCs and liver macrophages is metabolically re-programmed by endoplasmic reticulum (ER) stress present in MAFLD/MASH [93]. The additional implications of macrophage subtypes in MASH have been mentioned above.

2.2.2. Hepatic Stellate Cells

Under normal conditions, they contain retinoids and are the only site of vitamin A storage. Activated HSCs (aHSC) secrete more pro-fibrotic factors and a positive loop is operative, aggravating fibrosis [94,95]. aHSC may proliferate, produce ECM proteins, and generate inflammatory signals [31]. ECM accumulation is the outcome of the synthesis and degradation of ECM proteins. Matrix metalloproteinases (MMPs), including collagenase (MMP1) and Gelatinase B (MMP9) are zinc-dependent enzymes that degrade ECM components. The deposition of ECM in fibrosis depends on the balance between the MMPs and tissue inhibitors of metalloproteinases (TIMPs) [96]. An imbalance in the activity of MMPs and TIMPs can promote either the progression or the resolution of liver fibrosis [97]. Upon activation, HSCs lose vitamin A droplets and have different characteristics compared to quiescent HSCs such as increased expressions of alpha-smooth muscle actin and collagen type 1 alpha 1. The expression of the peroxisome proliferator-activated receptor γ (PPARγ) is reduced [1]. aHSCs are the main, but not the only, progenitors of MFs [98]. MFs may also originate from portal fibroblasts and bone marrow-derived cells [99] and by the already discussed EMT [100,101] or the complementary endothelial-to-mesenchymal (EndoTM) transition [102,103]. The activation of HSCs is mediated by either several extracellular growth factors, including the platelet-derived growth factor (PDGF), the transforming growth factor-β (TGFβ), the connective tissue growth factor (CTGF), the Wnt/β catenin pathway, chemokines, lipolysaccharide (LPS), DAMPs and PAMPs, or by nuclear mechanisms through the actions of miRNAs. Epigenetic mechanisms may also be implicated, as mentioned before, as well as a number of cellular factors such as oxidative stress and reactive oxygen species (ROS), ER stress, and the autophagic pathway [104,105].

Autophagy has attracted attention as it provides the necessary energy through a specialized form of autophagy called lipophagy that metabolizes the lipid droplets to maintain the activation of HSCs [106–108]. However, there is evidence that autophagy may also protect from liver fibrosis, acting as a double-edged sword [109–112]. Thus, PDGF inhibited autophagy, inducing the release of multivesicular body-derived exosomes and microvesicles from HSCs. Therefore, increased autophagy in HSCs represses liver fibrosis by inhibiting the release of fibrogenic extracellular vesicles [113].

HSCs are by no means a homogeneous population as believed in the past. Studies in the livers of rodents identified two transcriptomes from different populations. One was located in the portal area and the other was associated with the central vein. Interestingly, the latter was responsible for the production of collagen during centrilobular liver damage [114]. The HSC subtype of zone 1 is not transformed into MFs in liver injury but behaves as a capillary pericyte, participating in the process of sinusoidal capillarization [115]. In aging livers, HSCs with a "mixed" phenotype have been identified. They have lipid droplets indicating quiescence together with the markers of senescence and activation such as aSMA. ScRNAseq analysis indicated that even MFs are also a heterogeneous population with distinct functions [101,116].

2.2.3. The Interplay Between KCs and HSCs

As mentioned above, damaged hepatocytes release reactive oxygen species (ROS) and DAMPs. DAMPs activate Toll-like receptors (TLRs), TNFa receptors, and IL1R. The binding of DAMPs to their ligands initiates the myeloid differentiation 88 (MYD88) pathway, followed by the activation of nuclear factor kB (NF-κB) in Kupffer cells, and the transcription of the NLRP3 inflammasome. The resultant inflammatory response is due to the transcription of procaspase-1, pro-IL-18, and pro-IL-1β. ROS also initiate the transcription of NLRP3. Activated inflammasomes induce the production of IL-1β and IL-18, which in turn differentiates HSCs into myofibroblasts, promoting the development of liver fibrosis [117–119]. TNFa produced by Kupffer cells may promote fibrosis as it inhibits the apoptosis of HSCs and increases the production of TIMPs by activated HSCs [113,120].

Kupffer cells and HSCs in the murine fibrotic liver were able to recruit Ly6Chi monocytes by secreting CCL2, after the hepatocyte-specific deletion of NF-κB. Recruited monocytes further activated HSCs and aggravated fibrosis [121]. The deletion of CCL2 inhibited monocyte recruitment and attenuated liver fibrosis [121]. In addition, activated HSCs produced tissue inhibitors of metalloproteinases (TIMPs), which aggravated fibrosis by inhibiting the degradation of ECM by metalloproteinases [122].

MCP-1 secreted by macrophages increases fibrosis, interfering with macrophages and HSCs. CCR2, the receptor of MCP-1, is expressed on both Kupffer cells and HSCs. In Kupffer cells, the stimulation of CCR2 increases liver infiltration by macrophages, inducing early liver inflammation [123]. In HSCs, the stimulation of CCR2 causes an overexpression of fibrosis genes [124]. CXCL6 was found to be an initiator of TGF-β production by Kupffer cells [125]. In addition, the production of CCL2 and CCL5 by macrophages induced the fibrotic phenotype of HSC and initiated their movement toward the damaged area via their matching receptors in HSCs [126,127]. Stimulated HSCs also express CCL2 and CCL5, which participate in a positive feedback loop and aggravate liver fibrosis [128,129]. Increased levels of CXCL6 were demonstrated in the serum and liver of patients with advanced fibrosis. In vitro cell experiments indicated that HSCs were only indirectly stimulated by CXCL6, which induced TGF-β secretion by KCs [125]. Furthermore, the binding of PDGF produced by activated KCs transforms quiescent HSCs into activated HSCs [130].

Table 1 presents a synopsis of macrophage cytokines and chemokines involved in the interactions with HSCs.

Table 1. Macrophage cytokines and chemokines involved in the interaction with HSCs.

Molecules	Functions	References
TGF-β	Primarily produced by macrophages. Enhances ECM production in HSCs through Smad-dependent pathways and Smad-independent pathways.	[131,132]
PDGF	Produced by macrophages. It contributes to fibrosis progression through HSC activation.	[133]
TNF-α	Upregulates TIMP-1 production, prevents HSC apoptosis.	[134,135]
IL-1β,IL-18	Produced by pro-inflammatory macrophages through activation of the NLRP3 inflammasome. Activates HSCs, upregulates TIMP production.	[136,137]
IL-13, IL-4	Produced by M2 macrophages. Promotes the activation of HSCs.	[138]
MCP1	Activates CCR2 in Kupffer cells and HSCs.	[139,140]
CCL2 CCL5	Produced by macrophages and HSCs. Increases macrophage infiltration and fibrotic phenotype of HSCs.	[141,142]
CXCL6	Induces TGF β production by KCs and indirectly promotes fibrosis.	[143]

HSCs secrete anti-inflammatory cytokines such as IL-10 and TGF-β that initiate the polarization of macrophages toward an anti-inflammatory phenotype, leading to fibrosis resolution. However, the same anti-inflammatory macrophages can also produce cytokines such as IL-13 and IL-4, which favor the differentiation of HSCs into myofibroblasts [144]. IL-6 from either KCs or HSCs may also differentiate HSCs toward myofibroblasts [145,146]. In a murine model of ALD, the extracellular vehicles from alcohol-damaged hepatocytes increased IL1β and IL-17 expression in macrophages followed by the activation of HSCs and the exacerbation of liver fibrosis [147].

An additional mechanism of macrophage–HSC interaction was recently proposed. Cadherin-11 (CDH11) induced intercellular junctions between activated HSCs and macrophages, forming a fibrotic niche. As a result, TGF-β that is produced by macrophages activates the connected HSC, thus inducing their prolonged activation. The repression of CDH11 could derange this niche and promote fibrosis resolution [148].

2.2.4. Liver Sinusoidal Endothelial Cells (LSECs)

Liver sinusoidal endothelial cells are liver endothelial cells with the unique characteristic of the presence of fenestrae. An additional characteristic is the minimal presence of basement membrane. LSECs maintain hepatic cell-to-cell communication and are regulators of signal transduction among cells [134]. The presence of fenestrations is a distinguishing feature useful for the distinction of LSECs from other liver endothelial populations [149]. LSECs are considered to be the actual gatekeepers of the liver microenvironment [150]. Any impairment of the intercellular communications of LSECs may lead to the development of liver fibrosis [151]. Thus, vascular cell adhesion molecule 1 (VCAM1) deletion from LSECs reduces macrophage accumulation in the liver and ameliorates fibrosis, as VCAM1 is an important mediator of LSEC capillarization and hence of liver fibrosis [152].

SECs also have loose cell junctions [136]. In analogy with Kupffer cells and HSCs, LSECs are not a homogeneous population in the normal mouse liver. Their phenotype is variable in the different zones of the liver acinus. Zone 1 LSECs are CD36hi and lymphatic vessel endothelial hyaluronan receptor 1 (LYVE1) low, whereas zone 2 and zone 3 LSECs are CD36low, LYVE1hi, and CD32hi [153]. In the cirrhotic liver, seven different subpopulations of LSECs were identified by scRNA analysis [91]. The increased expression of atypical chemokine receptor 1 (ACKR1) + ve and plasmalemma vesicle-associated protein (PLVAP) + ve were described in LSECs, which are restricted to the fibrotic niche and increase the trans-migration of leucocytes [91,137]. In addition, LSECs may be transformed into endothelial–mesenchymal transition (EndMT), acquiring the phenotype of mesenchymal cells. They start producing ECM proteins that further accumulate in the sinusoids, aggravating capillarization [154,155]. The impairment of autophagy, as observed in MAFLD, increases the EndMT of LSECs and induces the inflammatory response and finally liver fibrosis [139]. The underlying molecular mechanisms involve the stimulation of Twist1 by the transcriptional regulator megakaryocytic leukemia 1 (MKL1) and the signal transducer and activator of transcription 3 (STAT3), leading to an amplification of EndMT in LSECs by TGF-β [140]. The implication of LSECs in liver fibrosis is mostly indirect through the loss of the capacity of LSECs to suppress the activation of the HSCs. This is due to the capillarization of the sinusoids that prevent secretory factors from LSECs to inhibit the activation of HSCs [31].

2.2.5. Cytokines Involved in Liver Fibrosis

Fundamental fibrogenic cytokines, such as the transforming growth factor-β (TGF-β), the platelet-derived growth factor (PDGF), the vascular endothelial growth factor (VEGF), and the connective tissue growth factor (CTGF), all act through specific receptors and participate in advanced liver fibrogenesis [16].

a. TGF-β and IL-10.

TGF-β belongs to a superfamily of 33 cytokines, including among others the isoforms of TGF-β (TGF-β1/2/3), the bone morphogenetic proteins (BMPs), the growth and differentiation factor (GDF), and activins [143].

Activated TGF-β molecules are liberated from a latent complex after liver injury. TGF-β then binds to the TGF-β type II receptor (TβRII), resulting in the recruitment of the TGF-β type I receptor (TβRI). Then, TβRII phosphorylates TβRI that in turn phosphorylates SMAD2 and SMAD3 proteins which are complexed with SMAD4, which translocate to the nucleus and regulate the transcription of target genes such as αSMA and CTGF [141,142]. TGF-β also activates non-canonical SMAD-independent pathways, such as MAPK, mTOR, PI3K/AKT, and Rho/GTPase. SMAD7 negatively regulates TGF-β, competing with SMAD3 and SMAD4 for TβRI binding [156].

There has been plenty of evidence that TGF-β is a crucial factor in liver fibrosis. The deletion or suppression of TGF-β attenuated liver fibrosis in mice, whereas the induced overexpression of TGF-β increased liver fibrosis [72,133,157]. The internalization of the type II receptor (TGFβRII) is dependent on the protein diaphanous homolog 1 (Diaph1) as the first step for the transformation of HSCs into MFs. The inactivation of Diaph1 inhibited the endocytosis and intracellular trafficking of TβRII, reducing Smad 3 phosphorylation [138]. The activation of the focal adhesion kinase (FAK) is also a vital component in TGFβ signaling. FAK protects TGFβRII from lysosomal degradation and promotes TGFβ-mediated HSC activation [158]. Almost all the secreted TGF-β1 is found in a latent form bound to the ECM, and the activation of TGF-β1 during fibrosis is site-specific [159]. The better-studied activation mechanism for TGF-β1 is the interaction of the latent complex with the αv-containing subset of integrins. Specifically, the integrins αvβ1, αvβ3, αvβ5, αvβ6, and αvβ8 bind to the latency-associated peptide (LAP) that inhibits the active molecule from binding to its receptors [160–162]. The deletion or blockade of the αvβ6 integrin protected mice from biliary fibrosis in the bile duct-ligated model [163,164]. Also, the blocking of αv-containing integrins by a small molecule ameliorated liver fibrosis, even after the establishment of fibrosis [165]. There is evidence that all TGF-β subtypes are involved in liver fibrosis. The increased levels of TGF-β1 have been found in the murine models of liver fibrosis [166], while increased mRNA levels of TGF-β1 have also been observed in fibrotic patients [143,166,167]. Both TGF-β1 and TGF-β2 induced EMT and fibrogenesis in isolated cell experiments. The upregulation of miR-200a downregulated smad-3 activity and mitigated the TGF-β-dependent EMT. TGF-β1 and TGF-β2 were shown to downregulate the expression of miR-200a. miR-200a also downregulated the expression of TGF-β2 via direct interaction with the 3′ untranslated region of TGF-β2 [168]. Interestingly, the serum levels of the TGF-β subtypes are different according to disease etiology. Serum TGF-β2 was significantly higher in viral cirrhosis but not in primary biliary cholangitis (PBC) patients compared to healthy controls. TGFβ-3 was increased in early and late PBC and decreased in viral cirrhosis. Hepatic vein subtype levels were similar to those in peripheral blood. All TGF-β subtypes were identified by immunocytochemistry in portal tract lymphocytes, sinusoidal cells, and cholangiocytes. TGF-β3 was only overexpressed in hepatocytes from PBC patients [169].

TGFβ and IL-10 regulate the induction of and prolongation of T cell exhaustion. IL-10 is often overproduced in chronic infections such as HIV, HBV, and HCV. The inhibition of IL-10 may prevent or even restore T cell exhaustion. IL-10 acts either directly on T cells through STAT-3 or indirectly by inducing APCs to increase T cell exhaustion and viral persistence. On the other hand, the inhibition of IL-10 in combination with PD-1 leads to the preservation of effector T cell responses, and the effective control of viral replication. Moreover, the use of neutralizing IL-10 antibodies along with therapeutic vaccination promoted CD8+ and CD4+ T cell responses, decreasing viral load [170].

TGF-β is also a suppressive cytokine involved in T cell exhaustion. TGF-β can ameliorate immune cell activation by activating downstream SMAD transcription factors. In acute viral infections, TGF-β is a negative regulator of effector function through the repression of T-bet (T-box expressed in T cells) leading to the upregulation of the pro-apoptotic factor Bim. In chronic viral infections, TGF-β expression and/or downstream SMAD2 activation lead to T cell exhaustion, thus promoting fibrosis [170,171]. HBV initiates the production of TGF-β and IL-10 by macrophages and inhibits TNF-α production [172]. Similarly, in chronic HBV (CHB) patients, monocytes produce more IL-10 and TGF-β and express high levels of PD-L1. Studies have demonstrated that HBsAg and HBV DNA directly promote PD-L1 expression and anti-inflammatory cytokines production from the monocytes of healthy people [173].

b. Activin A is expressed in murine hepatocytes, HSCs, and LSECs but not in KCs. Different activin receptor combinations are expressed in liver cells. HSCs do not respond to activin A due to the downregulation of type II activin receptors, while KCs respond by increasing the production of TNFα και TGFβ1. Conditioned medium from activin A-treated KCs led to HSC transformation into a pro-fibrogenic phenotype, expressing collagen and αSMA [174]. In addition, TGF-β itself stimulates the production of activin A by fibroblasts [131].

c. Other cytokines are implicated in the fibrotic process in the liver [132,175]. IL-1β has fibrogenic effects similar to TGF-β by inducing EMT, which can be blocked by a monoclonal antibody [176]. It should be noted that IL-6, TNFa, and IL-1-β synergistically act with TGF-β, because the deletion of these cytokines attenuates liver fibrosis [177–180]. Mechanistically, IL-1-β, and TNFa enhance TGF-β actions by downregulating the BMP activin membrane-bound inhibitor (BAMBI), which is a pseudo-receptor for the TGF-β type I receptor and a negative regulator of TGF-β signaling [120].

Whatever the mechanism of liver fibrosis might be, the end result is due to the balance of synthesis over the degradation of ECM, particularly collagens. This in turn is the balance between collagen-synthesizing enzymes and degradative factors such as collagenases and MMPs. The balance may be different according to the etiology of fibrosis. In alcoholic fibrosis and primary biliary cholangitis, it is the synthesis that predominates, while in viral fibrosis, it is the reduced degradation that is mainly responsible [181].

2.3. Resolution of Liver Fibrosis

The resolution of liver fibrosis requires a reduction in the number of activated HSCs and other MFs. This can be achieved through three mechanisms: the regression of activated HSCs to quiescence, the induction of senescence, and the elimination of activated HSCs and MFs through apoptosis and ferroptosis [2,31].

Activated HSCs can de-differentiate back to an inactivated phenotype by upregulating transcription factors such as peroxisome proliferator-activated receptor-γ (PPARγ), GATA-binding factors 4 and 6, and transcription factor 21 (TCF21) [182]. They may also enter senescence or may be eliminated by cell death. Both HSC apoptosis mediated by NK and CD8+ T cells [183] and ferroptosis have been reported during the resolution of liver fibrosis [116]. The induction of apoptosis is often mediated by natural killer cells (NK cells) through the production of interferon-γ (IFNγ) [184,185]. NK cells may also kill senescent MFs, in addition to activated HSCs [186]. The implication of natural killer T cells (NKT cells) in the induction of apoptosis is still controversial [187]. In that respect, it was recently reported that Artesunate (an ester from Artemisin) induced ferroptosis in HSCs and attenuated liver fibrosis in a murine model [188]. Another way to reduce liver fibrosis is the change in the phenotypes of liver macrophages [189]. This has been clearly demonstrated in murine models, as mentioned before. Pro-fibrogenic Ly-6Chi macrophages can change into Ly-6Clow anti-fibrotic macrophages, releasing anti-inflammatory cytokines such as IL- 10, restorative growth factors such as HGF, and ECM-degrading MMPs [61,72,83,190] including MMP12 and MMP13 [82,191]. Partial resolution is still feasible even if the fibrosis is advanced. The appearance of Ly-6Clow macrophages is associated with either the apoptosis of MFs induced by the macrophage production of TNF-related apoptosis-inducing ligands (TRAIL) [192] or by reversion to quiescent HSCs [193].

Many traditional Chinese medications (TCMs) have been reported to be effective in treating liver fibrosis. Single herbal extracts and TCM formulas may prevent or treat hepatic fibrosis. HSCs and oxidative stress, which are implicated in liver fibrosis, are common targets of TCMs [194,195]. However, caution should be exercised in the interpretation of the results as many papers on the clinical trials of TCMs do not comply with the acceptable design of trials [196].

Figure 1 summarizes the mechanisms of liver fibrosis.

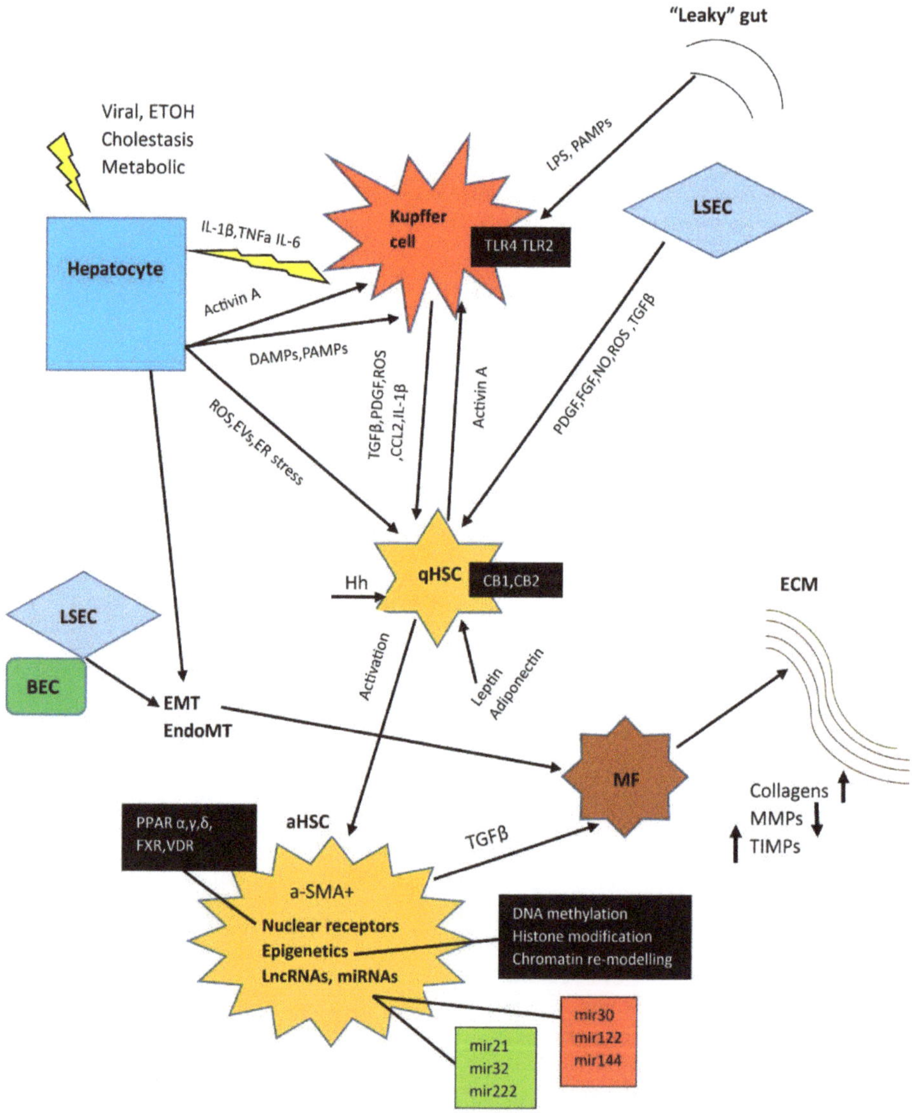

Figure 1. Cellular and molecular pathogenesis of liver fibrosis. Some elements have been omitted for clarity. For details, see text. Green box miRNAs indicate enhancement of fibrosis. Red box indicates inhibition.

BEC: Biliary epithelial cells; CB1 and 2: cannabinoid receptors 1 and 2; DAMPs: damage-associated molecular patterns; EM: epithelial-to-mesenchymal transition; EndoMT: endothelial-to-mesenchymal transition; EVs: extracellular vesicles; FGF: fibroblast growth factor; FXR: farnesoid X receptor; FGF: fibroblast growth factor; Hh: hedgehog ligand; LSECs: liver sinusoidal endothelial cells; LncRNA: long non-coding RNA; miRNA: microRNA; MMPs: matrix metalloproteinases; PAMPs: pathogen-associated molecular patterns; PDGF: platelet-derived growth factor; PPAR: peroxisome proliferator activated receptor; TIMPs: tissue inhibitors of metalloproteases; VDR: vitamin D receptor.

3. Immunology of Liver Fibrosis

3.1. The Liver as an Immune Organ

The liver, in addition to its central metabolic role, is also a significant immune organ [197,198]. It contains several components implicated in both innate and adaptive immunity. Some of them are not strictly immune cells, such as hepatocytes [199] and LSECs, but express Toll-like receptors (TLRs) and major histocompatibility complex (MHC) molecules, and participate in the maintenance of tolerance [200–203] or the biliary epithelial cells (BECs) and HSCs, which are also tolerogenic and may present antigens to T lymphocytes [135,198,204]. These cells are implicated in both innate and adaptive responses. On the contrary, liver sinusoids contain the proper cells of innate immunity such as KCs, dendritic cells, myeloid-derived suppressor cells, or lymphoid-derived cells (NKs and innate lymphoid cells). Certain cells do not comply with either the innate or adaptive immunity criteria and are defined as "innate-like", or "unconventional" lymphocytes. They include mucosal-associated invariant T (MAIT) cells, natural killer T (NKT) cells, and $\gamma\delta$-T cells. In addition, the normal liver also houses the conventional T and B lymphocytes of adaptive immunity [198].

Tolerance is a main function of the liver. An important mechanism of hepatic tolerance is the expression by several liver cells of MHC molecules not accompanied by co-stimulatory molecules. Other, equally important tolerogenic mechanisms, are the secretion of suppressor cytokines such as IL-10 and TGF-β, the inhibition of professional antigen-presenting cells (APCs), and the subjection of immune cells to programmed cell death-ligand 1 (PD-L1) [205–207]. Liver-draining lymph nodes (LNs) are also important components of the liver immune system. Portal LNs are an area of regulatory T cells (Tregs) induction, while celiac LNs are an area of T cell responses [205,208]. Moreover, cellular metabolism is associated with immune responses. A glycolytic metabolism is involved in the effector function of T lymphocytes, while fatty acid oxidation is used by non-inflammatory immune cells such as Tregs [209]. Glycolysis induced by hypoxia-inducible factor 1-alpha (HIF-1a) and oxidative metabolism induced by IL-4/STAT6 are used by either pro-inflammatory or anti-inflammatory macrophages, respectively [210–212].

3.2. Immune Factors Implicated in Liver Fibrosis

Liver fibrosis is closely linked to impaired hepatic immune responses [213]. Several experimental data indicate that the immune cells can regulate both the progression and reversal of liver fibrosis [214]. Excessive alcohol consumption, viruses, western dietary habits, or MAMPs and PAMPS originating from the microbiota of a leaky gut, may impair hepatic immune homeostasis leading to liver inflammation, fibrosis, and cirrhosis. The liver must handle antigens arriving at the sinusoids from the systemic circulation and the intestinal tract. These antigens are processed by the liver through a series of pattern recognition receptors (PRRs), such as TLRs and nucleotide-binding oligomeric domain-like receptors (NOD-like receptors), which induce either a tolerogenic response or inflammation and fibrosis [215–218].

Early in the course of chronic liver disease, damaged hepatocytes release inflammatory mediators that recruit and activate inflammatory cells, such as macrophages, lymphocytes, and NK cells [183,190,219]. Inflammation leads to a disordered crosstalk between hepatic immune cells, which drives the induction and progress of fibrosis [189,220,221]. TLRs are expressed on various hepatic cells like KCs, dendritic cells, hepatic stellate cells, endothelial cells, and hepatocytes [222]. Changes to the liver immune system leading to fibrosis include a decrease in CD8+ T cells and NK cells and an increase in CD4+ T cells infiltration accompanied by the expression of certain immune-regulatory genes [223,224].

Innate and Adaptive Immunity

Innate and adaptive immune cells are involved in hepatic inflammation, fibrosis, cirrhosis, and HCC. They have distinct roles, but at the same time, they affect each other. Adaptive immunity depends on the activation signals and cytokines secreted by the innate immune system. PAMPs from damaged hepatocytes lead to the activation of intrahepatic innate cells that initiate the recruitment of circulating immunocytes to the liver. The infiltrating cells stimulate other parenchymal and non-parenchymal cells in the liver, thus creating a perpetuating circle. The induction of pro-fibrogenic mediators such as IL-10 and TGF-β encourage liver fibrosis by activating quiescent hepatic stellate cells. The continuous supplementation of these fibrogenic stimuli promotes further disease progression toward fibrosis and cirrhosis [225].

3.3. *Innate Immunity in Liver Fibrosis*

As mentioned above, DAMPs activate innate immunity that induces fibrosis. The NLR family pyrin domain-containing 3 (NLRP3) inflammasome is a major element of the innate immunity, which functions as PRR, recognizing both PAMPs and DAMPs [226]. Kupffer cells are rich in NLRP3, and its activation leads to the secretion of several pro-inflammatory cytokines, such as IL- 1b and IL-18 [227]. Human and murine data indicate that NLRP3 activation induces caspase-1-mediated pyroptotic death and the liberation of inflammasomes that are engulfed by HSCs, leading to their activation and liver fibrosis [228].

3.3.1. Cells Involved in Innate Immunity

a. Hepatocytes. Hepatocytes may induce innate immunity as they express immune receptors that recognize PAMPs. These receptors include surface receptors such as TLR4, endosomal receptors such as TLR3, cytoplasmic receptors such as the stimulators of the IFN gene (STING) and the members of the NOD family [199,229,230]. Hepatocytes can also induce adaptive immunity. During inflammation, certain hepatocytes express MHC-II molecules and activate T lymphocytes [206,231], but as they do not express co-stimulatory molecules such as CD80 and CD86, they are not capable of generating the long-lasting activation of T cells. Importantly, hepatocytes express PD-L1 either after viral infection or under the influence of type I and type II IFN, thus mediating the apoptosis of T cells [232]. Activated hepatocytes may also induce the transformation of BM-derived monocytes into pro-inflammatory macrophages, upregulating the Yes-associated protein (YAP) and the transcriptional coactivator with a PDZ-binding motif (TAZ) [233]. YAP/TAZ is the effector in the Hippo pathway, which is a regulator of the TGF-β2-mediated fibrogenesis as indicated by data from other organs [234]. The increased expression of the transcription factor Fork head box M1 (FoxM1), and the subsequent overexpression of the CCL2 chemokine, induce hepatocyte death, leading to liver inflammation and fibrosis through macrophage recruitment [235,236].

Most of the data mentioned above come from animal experiments. However, there is evidence from liver disease patients that hepatocytes are indeed involved in inflammation and fibrosis. MHC-II molecules are expressed in the hepatocytes of alcoholic hepatitis, and activate CD4+ T cells, inducing positive lymphocytes [237]. Lipid-laden hepatocytes are more susceptible to apoptosis in patients with MASH [238]. Exosomes derived from HBV-infected hepatocyte contain miR-222 and increase fibrosis by inhibiting the transferrin receptor (TFRC) and TFRC-induced ferroptosis [239].

The autophagy pathway within the hepatocytes is also implicated in immune-mediated liver fibrosis. Autophagy protects hepatocytes from death signals [199,240] and is implicated in most chronic liver diseases [241–244]. The vitamin D receptor (VDR) promotes autophagy by regulating beclin-1, bcl-2, the mTOR elements of the autophagy pathway, and lysosomal maturation [245]. The VDR was decreased in the hepatocytes of cirrhotic patients [246]. In murine models and human cirrhosis, hepatocyte autophagy was inhibited by the miR-125a/VDR axis, leading to increased liver fibrosis [247].

Endoplasmic reticulum (ER) stress and hepatocyte senescence are two additional factors that implicate hepatocytes in the process of liver fibrosis. The accumulation of misfolded proteins in the ER activates the unfolded protein response (UPR), mediated by three ER sensors, namely PKR-like ER kinase (PERK), activating transcription factor 6 (ATF6), and inositol-requiring enzyme 1 (IRE1) to counteract the protein-folding defect [248]. Massive ER stress overcomes UPR and leads to hepatocyte steatosis and death [93,249]. ER stress can trigger C/EBP Homologous Protein (CHOP) transcription factor-dependent NLRP3 inflammasome activation and the activation of IRE1A in hepatocytes, both leading to the release of pro-inflammatory cytokines and inflammatory extracellular vesicles (EVs), therefore promoting fibrosis [199]. A strong positive correlation between senescent hepatocytes and liver fibrosis severity has been described in MASH and alcoholic liver disease patients [250,251]. In chronic viral hepatitis patients, senescence is associated with telomere shortening and the absence of telomerase in hepatocytes, favoring virus replication and liver cirrhosis [252,253]. An additional confirmation that senescent hepatocytes are directly involved in liver fibrosis was recently reported. PDGF is a potent activator of HSCs, as mentioned before. PDGF levels were significantly higher in the media from cultured senescent hepatocytes compared to control hepatocytes, and similar findings were demonstrated in serum samples from patients with cirrhosis compared to healthy controls [254].

b. Kupffer cells and liver macrophages. KCs are probably the most important cells in liver innate immunity. They are professional antigen-presenting cells (APCs) to T cells and therefore participate in the initiation of adaptive immunity [83,255]. In MASH, there is a positive correlation between the severity of inflammation and fibrosis and the number of pro-inflammatory macrophages in the periportal zone [256]. As mentioned before, early liver damage activates hepatic macrophages including the KCs. In turn, they secrete several cytokines such as TGF-β1, PDGF, TNF-α, IL-1, IL-6, and IL-10, and cytokines such as CXCL1, CCL2, and CCL5. KCs produce mediators such as ROS that induce HSC transformation and attract BM monocytes and neutrophils [183,191]. Liver macrophages, irrespective of origin, are the main sources of TGFβ and one of the leading causes of increased ECM deposition in liver fibrosis. They also maintain the survival of MFs by activating NF-kB through the secretion of IL-1β and TNFa [183,189,191,219]. In addition to these functions, Kupffer cells activated by DAMPs and PAMPs, as mentioned above, induce an increased expression of vascular adhesion molecules on LSECs [82,257].

Recruited bone marrow-derived macrophages differentiate into a Kupffer cell-like phenotype [65], approximately 60 days of repopulation after liver damage [258]. It is not clear if the newly recruited macrophages live long or whether their functional role is comparable to the original Kupffer cells [65,259].

KCs have a dual role in the immune regulation of liver inflammation and fibrosis. Depending on the microenvironment, they can acquire a pro-inflammatory phenotype (referred to as M1). M1 KCs are activated by IFNγ and lipopolysaccharide (LPS) and are characterized by the ability to present antigens and produce inflammatory cytokines such as TNFα, IL-1, IL-6, IL-12, and IL-23, promoting antiviral activity. Alternatively, KCs can acquire an anti-inflammatory phenotype (referred to as M2) characterized by their ability to balance inflammatory responses and facilitate tissue repair through the release of IL-10, IL-4, IL-13, and TGF-β and the low production of IL-12, IL-6, and TNF-α [260,261]. Furthermore, IL-17 activates Kupffer cells and lead to the upregulation of pro-fibrotic cytokines like IL-6, IL-1β, and TGF- β1 [262].

KCs differentiation into the M2 phenotype upregulates PD-L1 and galectin-9 expression in the presence of HBeAg. HBcAg upregulates TLR-2 on the surface of KCs and increases IL-10 secretion, thus upregulating CD8+ T cell exhaustion [263]. The activation of the TLR4 signaling pathway promotes M1 inflammatory differentiation that leads to the upregulation of the clearance of HBV [264]. The stimulator of interferon genes (STING) is a key adaptor in DNA-initiated innate immune activation [265]. The stimulation of KCs by STING increases the hepatic expression of interferon-inducible protein 16 (IFI 16), which binds to HBV cccDNA, inhibiting cccDNA transcription and leading to its silencing [266].

In human cirrhosis, KC numbers are similar to the normal liver [91,267], in contrast to the murine liver where extensive fibrosis and cirrhosis is accompanied by a reduction in the number of KCs [268]. The presence of KCs and the differentiation of other macrophages is influenced by stromal cells through the inhibition of monocyte maturation. This is achieved by the production of IL-6 from the stromal cells. Interestingly, the local IL-6 levels are diminished in early-stage human liver injury, implicating a protective role of IL-6 [269]. Apart from the production of TGF-β and the maintenance of the viability of MFs, KCs may be transformed into fibroblast-like cells, contributing to ECM production [270]. The KCs also promote collagen cross-linking that stabilizes collagen through the action of Lysyl-oxidase (LOX) and Lysyl oxidase-like protein-2 (LOXL2) [271]. On the opposite side, KCs produce MMP9, leading to collagen degradation [272]. KC infusion attenuated liver fibrosis in a murine model [273]. Interestingly, the T-cell immunoglobulin domain and mucin domain-4 (TIM-4) expression by KCs represses liver fibrosis [274].

Although fibrosis is the final common result in all liver diseases irrespective of etiology, the underlying participation of the involved cells may be different. Hepatitis B and hepatitis C viruses (HBVs, HCVs) activate human macrophages, but the response is different in the two viral diseases. Macrophages respond to HBV by the production of inflammatory cytokines and the stimulation of NK cells [275,276]. The response to HCV proteins is the activation of inflammasomes mediated through TLR2 activation [277,278]. HBV and HCV infection lead human macrophages to secrete immunomodulatory mediators such as IL-10, TGFβ1, PD-L1, and PD-L2 that eventually mitigate antiviral T cell response [279]. In MASH, the accumulation of fat in the macrophage [280] production of EVs from fat-containing hepatocytes, [281,282] or histidine rich glycoprotein [283,284], induces an inflammatory phenotype in liver macrophages. In ALD patients, macrophages have a fundamental role in the inflammatory response during severe alcoholic hepatitis [285,286]. In murine ALD models, increased gut permeability contributes to the recruitment of pro-inflammatory macrophages [279,287,288]. In cholestatic conditions, BM-derived macrophages are influenced by the concentration and the composition of the bile acids in the liver [289]. Chenodeoxycholic acid (CDCA) activates the NLRP3 inflammasome in the macrophages of cholestatic animals with fibrosis [290]. On the contrary, KCs have the G-protein-coupled bile acid receptor 1 (TGR5), which is a sensor for bile acids, leading to the inhibition of inflammasomes [291] and the emergence of an anti-inflammatory phenotype [292,293].

*c. **The role of HSCs***. The multiple factors implicated in the activation of HSCs are further complicated due to the interaction of HSCs with the cells of the immune microenvironment during liver fibrosis. All cells involved in both innate and adaptive immunity are communicating with HSCs either directly or indirectly [90,294]. aHSCs, apart from their fundamental contribution as ECM producers, are also pro-inflammatory cells. They produce several cytokines and chemokines such as IL-6, IL-8, and monocyte chemoattractant protein-1 (MCP-1). They also recruit monocytes and hematopoietic stem cells [15]. Inflammatory mediators produced by HSCs target the nuclear factor kappa-light-chain-enhancer of activated B-cells (NF-κB), the central regulator of the inflammatory response [295,296]. Therefore, NF-κB is a critical molecule in the inflammation and resultant fibrosis but also in the apoptosis or survival of HSCs after liver injury. Indeed, NF-κB activation is associated with an increased resistance to the apoptosis of activated HSCs [104,297].

The activation of HSCs is important in the pathogenesis of MASH. There is experimental evidence that free cholesterol accumulation in HSCs leads to their activation [298–301]. Free cholesterol in hepatocytes indirectly affects HSC activation through the stabilization of the transcriptional coactivator with the PDZ-binding motif (TAZ) with subsequent over-secretion of the pro-fibrotic factor Indian Hedgehog [302]. In chronic hepatitis B, a different mechanism is operative. aHSCs recruit large numbers of Th17 cells and promote the secretion of IL-12A and IL-22 that contribute to fibrosis [303]. On the other hand, HSCs may favor the development of tolerance in mice as they favor the expansion of FoxP3+ve Tregs or myeloid-derived suppressor cells [304,305].

HSCs also influence B-cell activity. HSCs inhibit the increased expression of activation markers on B cells and immunoglobulin production. Interestingly, blocking the interaction of PD-L1 with PD-1 mitigated the inhibition of B cells by HSCs [306].

HSCs are also implicated in inflammation and fibrosis by their involvement with the adipokines leptin and adiponectin, which act through binding to their receptors on HSCs [307–309]. Leptin is a pro-fibrotic factor that suppresses the sterol regulatory element-binding protein-1c (SREBP-1c) and activates HSCs through the β-catenin pathway [310]. Adiponectin, on the other hand, ameliorates liver fibrosis through the induction of nitric oxide (NO) and TIMP-1 production, leading to the suppression and inactivation of aHSCs [311–315]. Currently, it is not yet clear under which conditions hepatic stellate cells are pro-inflammatory and under which conditions they are tolerogenic [219].

The details of the immune regulation of fibrosis by HSCs have been extensively reviewed [2].

d. The role of liver sinusoidal endothelial cells. LSECs express TLRs and MHC molecules and are implicated in the maintenance of tolerance either through the direct inhibition of T lymphocytes by PDL1 expression or through the so-called "veto" effect, consisting of inhibiting other APCs such as dendritic cells to activate T lymphocytes by physical contact without the need for the presence of MHC [200–203,316]. The early stages of MAFLD are a clear example of the immunological role of LSECs in liver fibrosis. Lipotoxicity, adipokines, and gut-derived PAMPS lead to LSECs' de-differentiation and sinusoidal capillarization. Capillarized LSECs are transformed into a pro-inflammatory and pro-fibrotic phenotype, recruiting immune cells that cannot support the quiescence of HSCs and KCs [151,317]. Specifically, the quantity and size of LSEC fenestrae are lost, and in advanced stages they even disappear. The blood filtration in the sinusoids is impaired, and harmful components are not adequately removed, and the risk of liver injury is increased [200]. Human studies reported that the expression level of the scavenger receptor Fc gamma receptor IIb (FcγRIIb) in LSECs is negatively correlated with fibrosis and inflammation in patients with MASH. FcγRIIb is involved in the elimination of small immune complexes from sinusoids [318]. A study on patients with chronic hepatitis C showed that LSEC capillarization was observed even at the initial stages of fibrosis [319]. Moreover, there is evidence that capillarization is the result of the impaired differentiation of the bone marrow-derived LSECs [320]. An important regulator of LSECs fenestration is the bone morphogenetic protein 9 (BMP9). The role of BMP9 in liver fibrosis is controversial. The deletion of BMP9 in murine models increased liver fibrosis [321,322]. On the other hand, liver biopsies from fibrotic patients showed increased levels of BMP9 in advanced fibrosis. In murine models, BMP9 overexpression accelerated liver fibrosis, and BMP9 knockdown ameliorated fibrosis. BMP9 directly stimulated hepatic stellate cell activation via the SMAD signaling pathway to upregulate hepatic fibrosis [323]. The details of the effects of BMP9 on liver fibrosis were recently reviewed [324].

In addition to capillarization, hepatic neo-angiogenesis was also strongly related to LSECs and was associated with the development of liver fibrosis [149], possibly mediated through the vascular endothelial growth factor (VEGF) [325]. This is supported from the alterations of LSEC phenotypes made by certain drugs such as Vatalanib, a VEGFR1 and VEGFR2 inhibitor, or Lenvatinib, an inhibitor of VEGF1, VEGF2, and VEGF-A. They decreased both sinusoidal capillarization and liver fibrosis [326,327]. The beta-blocker carvedilol repressed the expression of VEGF and angiopoietin-2, leading to the attenuation of sinusoidal capillarization [328]. Moreover, HIF-1α is also implicated in LSEC capillarization and angiogenesis. MiR322/424 upregulated the expression of the HIF-1α protein in LSECs and promoted neo-angiogenesis and liver fibrosis [329]. LSECs can also directly stimulate neo-angiogenesis through the secretion of angiogenic factors. Interestingly, LSEC capillarization is a process that starts before the activation of macrophages and HSCs in liver fibrosis [134]. A detailed description of the participation of LSECs-dependent angiogenesis in liver fibrosis was recently reported [134].

LSECs are involved in the progression of liver fibrosis by two additional mechanisms. Reduced NO bioavailability has been observed in LSECs from cirrhotic rodent livers [330] due to the ROS scavenger effect of NO via the superoxide anion (O2-) and the ERK1/2-AKT axis [331]. ERK1/2 shifted the balance toward NO, favoring LSEC homeostasis, while AKT could shift the balance toward ROS, promoting liver fibrosis. A second mechanism by which NO modulates liver fibrosis is the induction of autophagy. Autophagy in LSECs increases the bioavailability of NO and eliminates the accumulation of ROS [332]. This protective action of autophagy is not sufficient at the later stages of chronic liver [333]. Autophagy acts the opposite way as well by degrading Caveolin-1 (Cav-1), leading to LECs defenestration [334]. Moreover, LSECs mediate in the transformation of macrophages into KCs. The interactions of the Notch ligand delta-like ligand 4 (DLL4) produced by LSECs binding to the Notch receptor found in macrophages is required for the induction of the KC identity. Ligands such as ICAM-1 and vascular cell adhesion protein 1 (VCAM-1) in LSECs interact with the integrins on KCs and participate in the direct interplay between KCs and LSECs [335,336].

The central role of LSECs in the regulation of liver immunology and their effects in liver fibrosis is clearly exemplified in viral diseases. In murine adenovirus infection, 90% of the virus is rapidly taken up by LSECs and only 10% is found in KCs [337]. HIV-like particles are also taken up by mouse LSECs at a rate of 100 million viral particles per minute [338]. In the duck hepatitis B virus (DHBV) model, viral particles are mostly taken up by LSECs before passing on to further infect hepatocytes [339]. In HCV, the innate sensing of the virus by LSECs leads to the release of paracrine molecules such as the pro-viral molecule bone morphogenetic protein 4 (BMP4), which promotes the viral infection of hepatocytes [340,341]. On the other hand, the direct sensing of HCV RNA in LSECs produce type I and type III interferon-containing exosomes that inhibit HCV replication [342]. The balance of the two opposite responses determines whether the HCV virus will be eliminated or will cause a sustained infection.

*e. **Mesenchymal stromal cells (MSCs)*** are fibroblast-like cells with immunomodulatory ability, as they regulate both innate and adaptive immunity and have the potential to differentiate into hepatocyte-like cells (HLCs) [343–346]. MSCs express a specific set of surface markers, such as CD73, CD90, and CD105 [347]. MSCs produce the hepatocyte growth factor (HGF) and IL-6, which inhibit monocyte differentiation into dendritic cells and the activation of KCs. They also secrete a variety of other growth factors that help the proliferation of healthy cells and protect the destruction of other cells [348–350]. They also produce IL-10 and mitigate the activation of T cells [351]. MSCs secrete prostaglandin E2 (PGE2) to transform M1 macrophages into M2 macrophages [352]. MSCs repress the proliferation of CD8+ T lymphocyte and promote Th1-to-Th2 conversion [353]. It should be noted that the anti-fibrotic potential of MSCs is dependent on autophagy and senescence. Intact autophagy maintains anti-fibrotic activity, while reduced autophagy that coincides with advanced age is associated with a reduction in MSC numbers and function, promoting liver fibrosis [354]. The scRNA analysis of cirrhotic human livers identified four subpopulations of mesenchymal cells. Mes (1) was identified as vascular smooth muscle cells, Mes (4) expressed mesothelial markers, Mes (2) resembled HSCs, but they were not present in the cirrhotic niche, and Mes (3) distinguished by PDGFRA were pro-fibrogenic. Mes (3) cells were increased in cirrhotic livers [91,137]. Extensive reviews on MSCs were recently published [355–357].

f. ***Natural killer (NK) cells.*** They bear the activating receptor NKG2D and are capable of HSC elimination, inducing apoptosis and IFNγ secretion [358–360]. IFNγ secreted by NK cells directly inhibits HSC activation and ECM synthesis [361] and amplifies the killing capacity of NK cells against HSCs by increasing the expression of the NKG2D receptor [362]. The decreased numbers and function of NKs have been demonstrated in the murine models of cirrhosis [363] and cirrhotic patients [364–366]. These findings confirmed the anti-fibrotic effects of NK cells. Four immunity-related genes in NK cells, including interferon regulatory factor 8 (IRF8) and REL, are involved in liver fibrogenesis [224].

NK cells are classified into two subpopulations. The vast majority, over 90%, express low levels of CD56 (CD56dim), while the minority express high levels of CD56 (CD56bright). The first is more cytotoxic and a better immunomodulator [367]. In acute viral hepatitis, they both exhibit an antiviral effect either by the direct killing of infected cells or by the activation of viral-specific T cells secreting IFN-γ and TNF-a [368]. NK cell function is defective in patients with chronic hepatitis B (CHB), participating in persistent HBV infection and the development of fibrosis [172]. A further mechanism of NK dysfunction in the particular group of HBeAg+ve patients with CHB is the induction by HBeAg of IL-10 secretion from Tregs, leading to an increased expression of the inhibitory receptor NKG2A on NK cells [369]. Among the many immune abnormalities found in MAFLD, a reduction in CD56bright NK cells and an elevation in CD56dim with less expression in the activating receptor NKG2D was described in patients, offering an additional explanation for the progress of liver fibrosis in MAFLD [370]. A recent observation shed more light on the role of NK cells in MAFLD. Uncoupling protein 1 (UCP1) participates in the leak of protons from the mitochondrial inner membrane. Reduced levels were found in NK cells from patients with MAFLD. Sustained high-lipid administration in mice decreased UCP1 expression and promoted NK cell necroptosis and was involved in the progression to fibrosis [371]. Patients with primary sclerosing cholangitis (PSC) showed considerably higher serum levels of IFNγ and elevated numbers of hepatic CD56bright NK cells. Murine knockout experiments confirmed that increased IFNγ turned the phenotype of hepatic NK cells into increased cytotoxicity, while its absence ameliorated liver fibrosis in PSC [372].

g. ***Neutrophils.*** There are very few resident neutrophils in the healthy liver, but there is a rapid recruitment from the circulation in the diseased liver [373]. Neutrophils participate in the liver inflammatory response through the secretion of pro-inflammatory cytokines and the production of extracellular neutrophil traps (NETs). They activate KCs and recruit other types of immune cells [374–376]. In mice, the elimination of neutrophils ameliorates the development of hepatic fibrosis [377]. The characteristic neutrophil infiltration into the liver during alcoholic hepatitis is associated with the upregulation of the glycoprotein lipocalin-2 (LCN2) in the neutrophils. A deficiency of bactericidal activity and myeloperoxidase secretion was also found in these patients [92]. The liver-infiltrating neutrophils are also implicated in the immune response in the fibrotic progression in MASH [378,379].

3.3.2. LSECs as Gatekeepers of Innate and Adaptive Immunity

LSECs have a central role in the regulation of both the innate and adaptive immunity being the gatekeepers of the overall liver immune response. Thus, in normal livers, LSECs prevent HSC activation through vascular endothelial growth factor (VEFG)-induced nitric oxide (NO) production. In addition, normal LSECs can reverse activated HSCs back to quiescence through unidentified mechanisms. Decapillarized LSECs isolated from normal rat livers can suppress HSC activation, but capillarized LSECs from cirrhotic rats lose this function. The interaction between LSECs and Kupffer cells is not clarified so far. However, in the fibrosis model, there is evidence that the crosstalk between LSECs and Kupffer cells results in a loss of fenestration and increased CD31 expression [380]. In addition, fenestrated LSECs inhibit liver inflammation by having antioxidant activity. In contrast, capillarized or defenestrated LSECs caused by factors such as ROS production or through lipotoxicity have low antioxidant activity and can induce liver inflammation and promote HSC activation.

It should be noted that the fenestrations of LSECs allow for effector CD8+ T cells to recognize viral antigens expressed in hepatocytes and produce antiviral cytokines by cellular protrusions that extend through the fenestration in a diapedesis-independent manner. This mechanism is obviously lost along with the fenestrae in liver fibrosis, and the effector function of antigen-specific T cells is decreased [381].

Furthermore, LSEC death produces PAMPS that can promote liver inflammation, fibrosis, and cirrhosis acting on KCs and macrophages [317]. LSECs are also implicated in adaptive immunity. They can restrict the entry of immune complexes and leucocytes into liver tissue. Most importantly, LSECs can act as antigen-presenting cells (APCs) and regulate lymphocyte action because they constitutively express MHC class I and II, CD54 (ICAM-1), CD4, CD11, and CD106 (VCAM-1) molecules as well as co-stimulatory molecules CD40, CD80, and CD86, which are necessary for the antigen presentation to T cells. LSECs express MHC- I receptors and present antigens to CD8+ cytotoxic T cells. At low antigen concentrations, this presentation leads to the tolerogenic deletion of CD8+ T cells, but at high antigen concentration, leads to a memory effector T cell phenotype. In HBV infection, CD8+ T cells attach to the sinusoids and then search for infected hepatocytes through LSEC fenestrae. CD8 T cells actively cross the LECS barrier once they sense an infected hepatocyte and release TNFa that in turn eliminates the infected hepatocyte. Moreover, LSECs also present antigens to CD4+ T cells through MHC class II receptors, inducing suppressor Treg cells [200,382].

3.4. Adaptive Immunity T Cells

Cells of adaptive immunity are the many subpopulations of the T lymphocyte family and the B cells. Virtually all lymphocytes originating from naive CD4+ cells participate in the regulation of liver fibrosis. T cells are classified into conventional T cells and innate-like T cells (unconventional T cells). Unconventional T cells consist of natural killer T (NKT) cells, $\gamma\delta$ T cells, and mucosal-associated invariant T (MAIT) cells [383,384]. Conventional T cells can be further subdivided into CD8+ cytotoxic T lymphocytes (CTLs), regulatory T (Treg) cells, T follicular regulatory (Tfr) cells, and CD4+ T helper cells, including Th1, Th2,

Th9, Th17, Th22, and T follicular helper (Tfh) cells [385,386]. TNF-α-producing CD4+ T cells are dominant in HBV infection, participating in the progression of liver damage. A sequential increase in IFNγ-producing CD4 T cells characterizes patients with elevated levels of viral clearance [387].

A distinct type of T cell is the tissue resident memory (TRM) T cell that is important as a first-line defense in the liver. These consist of CD8+ and CD4+ cells and they do not circulate [385]. Their storing effector ability of hepatic TRM cells makes them critical in chronic liver diseases. The proliferation of liver TRMs is modulated by cytokines such as interleukin IL-2, IL- 15, IL-10, and TGF-β. Liver TRM cells are antiviral in chronic viral hepatitis. Importantly, the number of liver TRMs positively correlates with inflammation in patients with obesity [388]. A detailed description of the role of the T cell subclasses in liver fibrosis has been published [386].

APCs are classified into professional and non-professional. All professional APCs express the MHC-II molecules and include macrophages, dendritic cells (DCs), and B-lymphocytes. The MHC family consists of MHC-I and MHC-II receptors. MHC-I presents antigens to CD8+ cytotoxic T cells, while the MHC-II molecules induce CD4+ T cell activation [213]. Hepatocytes express MHC-II molecules and co-stimulators, and they may act as an atypical APC to promote T cell activation [389,390]. This has been demonstrated in the liver samples of patients with alcoholic hepatitis (AH) and MASH, where increased levels of MHC-II were observed in close association with MHC-II-producing hepatocytes [237]. Although DCs belong to the cells of innate immunity, they connect the innate and the adaptive immunity [391]. Hepatic DCs (HDCs) are less than 1% of total liver myeloid cells and are subdivided into plasmacytoid and myeloid subpopulations. Myeloid HDCs are further classified as type 1 and type 2 [392,393]. In the healthy liver, HDCs are tolerogenic [394], but they stimulate CD4 +T cells during liver diseases [393]. The majority of HDCs are localized at the portal vein area, with a few localized at the central vein area [395], while their numbers are significantly increased in MASH patients [396]. In the murine models of liver diseases, HDCs have no effect on the survival of HSCs in contrast to macrophages [71]. Animal and human data indicate that other cell types express the MHC-II molecules and act as atypical APCs. They include mast cells, basophils, eosinophils, neutrophils, and innate lymphoid cells (ILCs) [397].

T cell response after the presentation of antigens involves the recognition of the antigen by the T cell receptors (TCRs) on the surface of either CD4+ or CD8+ cells acting in collaboration with the CD3 co-receptor [398]. Other co-stimulatory molecules such as OX40L are required for proper antigen recognition by the T cells [399–401]. TCRs comprise two different heterodimers: TCRα/TCRβ or TCRγ/TCRδ [402]. A reduction in TCR subtypes was found in the liver of fibrotic animals, while the deletion of TCRβ aggravated liver fibrosis [403].

Current evidence indicates that T cell immunity influences the fibrosis process [386]. Earlier studies reported that the transfer of CD8+ve T cells contributed to liver fibrosis. CD8+ve T cells directly activated HSCs in murine models [404]. IL-21 promotes the antiviral activity of HBV-specific CD8+ T cells by promoting the production of IFNγ, granzyme B, and CD107a and decreasing PD-1 and TIM-3 production [405]. In addition, IL-2 promotes the proliferation of CD8+ T cells by activating the mTOR pathway to restore dysfunctional CD8+ T cells [406]. IL-33 initiates the proliferation of HBV-specific CD8+ T cells and upregulates PD-1 production, promoting HBV clearance. Not unexpectedly, the plasma levels of IL-33 are low in patients with CHB [407].

The severity of liver fibrosis was positively correlated with intrahepatic CD4+ve T cell apoptosis [408]. CD4+ve T cell activity is involved in the progression of liver fibrosis, by secreting cytokines such as IL-4, IL-10, and IFN-γ, and by stimulating other immune cells such as NK cells [224,366,409]. An analysis of T cell distribution in a small number of viral cirrhosis patients found that CD4+ve T cells, but not CD8+ve cells, were decreased in cirrhotic tissue. This is in contrast to a larger and more detailed study, which reported that a reduction in CD8+ve and NK cells and an infiltration of CD4+ve memory T cells contributed to immune changes in cirrhosis [224,366,409]. The impairment of CD4+ve T cells is implicated in the evolution of liver fibrosis in MASH. An accumulation of liver CD4+ve T cells was demonstrated in human disease and murine MASH models [410–412]. CD4+ve T cells were critical in the progression of liver fibrosis after the transfer of human T cells to a specific murine model of MASH. Moreover, the depletion of human CD4+ve T cells attenuated fibrosis in the humanized MASH mice, confirming the significance of these cells in the pathogenesis of MASH [410].

As mentioned before, the group of CD4+ve T lymphocytes includes different subgroups without a uniform behavior in liver fibrosis.

T helper 1 (Th1) cells are pro-fibrotic, producing cytokines such as IFN-γ, IL-2, and TNF-a [413]. An indirect support for the role of Th1 cells in liver fibrosis came from an INFγ knockout murine model of MASH, where the attenuation of fibrosis was observed [414]. These results are in line with the clinical observations that MASH patients have increased hepatic IFNγ-producing CD4+ve T cells [415,416].

Th2 cells are anti-inflammatory, eliciting a protective immune response [417]. Th2 cells produce cytokines such as IL-4, IL-5, and IL-13 [418,419]. Increased serum levels of IL-13, accompanied by the increased hepatic expression of its receptor IL-13Ra2, were reported in MASH patients. Moreover, the IL-13-mediated killing of IL-13Ra2+ve cells suppressed liver fibrosis in a rat model of MASH, supporting the involvement of the IL-13/IL-13Ra2 pathway in MASH [420]. Paradoxically, the administration of IL-33 increased liver fibrosis in a murine model of MASH, despite the fact that IL-33 promotes a Th2 response [421].

Th1 and Th2 cells communicate with LSECs through different adhesion molecules to exert opposite effects in liver fibrosis. The interaction of Th1 cells and LSECs facilitates the reduction in LSEC fenestrae and increases LSEC angiogenesis, finally aggravating liver fibrosis, while the interaction of Th2 cells and LSECs attenuates fibrosis [422,423].

TGF-β and IL-6 are the mediators of the differentiation of T cells into Th17 cells [179,424]. The IL-17 cytokine family consists of six members, namely IL-17A-F [425]. Murine Th17 cells have strong pro-fibrogenic and pro-inflammatory potentials [183,426–428]. Th17 cells can trigger hepatic inflammation possibly due to the recruitment of macrophages by the IL-17-dependent upregulation of the chemokine CXCL10 [429,430]. However, the role of Th17 cells in liver fibrosis is not clear. There are reports supporting the pro-fibrotic potential of IL-17 [417,431–433]. Other studies support an opposite effect after blocking IL-17 [429,434]. Th17 cells play a crucial role in inflammation, hepatic fibrosis, and HCC development. Th17 cells secrete IL-17 in the presence of IL-6, IL-1β, IL-12, and IL-23, acting through binding to its receptor [435]. Almost all liver cells including hepatocytes, HSCs, BECs, KCs, and LSECs express IL-17R [436]. Moreover, Th17 cells also secrete IL-22 and granulocyte macrophage colony-stimulating factors. These cytokines increase the production and recruitment of neutrophils. Increased numbers of Th17 cells in HBV patients are associated with fibrosis and cirrhosis [437,438]. IL-17 activates MDCs and monocytes to release inflammatory cytokines and recruit neutrophils to the liver [439]. Moreover, there is a negative correlation between disease severity and the methylation level of the IL-17 promoter [440]. The Th17/Treg cell ratio increases and positively correlates with liver injury in patients with a chronic HBV infection [441].

T helper 22 cells are characterized by the production of IL-22 in the absence of IL-17 [442]. The differentiation of the Th22 cell is mediated by IL-6 and TNFa and is inhibited by TGF-β. Evidence supports an anti-fibrotic effect for IL-22 that would be beneficial in MASH [443,444]. However, there is a concern that IL-22 treatment may be a risk for hepatocellular carcinoma development through the activation of STAT3 [445].

There is an interaction of the different cytokines produced by several sources in the modulation of liver fibrosis [446]. For example, the pro-fibrotic cytokine IL-17A was also produced by neutrophils and mast cells [427,447,448]. Th17A promotes the secretion of TGF-β but also promotes the expression of TGF-βRII on fibroblasts, therefore increasing the effect of TGF-β [426,428,449], a similar effect with the Th17-associated cytokine IL-22 [447]. TGF-β in turn induces the expression of IL-17A in collaboration with the IL-1, IL-6, or TNFa [450]. The cytokines IL-4 and IL-13 are also important inducers of fibrosis in association with an eosinophil and M2 macrophage environment [451]. IL-13 induces the production of TGF-β by macrophages [452], but it may increase fibrosis independently of TGF-β [452,453] by a direct effect on myofibroblasts [454].

One should remember that the immune mechanisms of liver fibrosis vary according to the underlying etiology, and results are often contradictory. T cells are no exception. Thus, in MAFLD, activated NK cells attenuate fibrosis progression [455–457]. Single-cell transcriptome analysis showed that CD4+ve T cells, CD8+ve T cells, and γδ T cells are increased in the liver with MASH [458]. Alcohol exposure impairs the balance between different T cell subpopulations, leading to a reduction in naïve CD4+ve T cells and CD8+ve T cells [459]. CD8+ve T cell activation and infiltration are considered as the effector mediators of bile duct damage in PBC. Research has demonstrated that specific cytotoxic CD8+ T cells are indeed increased in PBC patients [460,461]. A comprehensive review on the role of Th cells in liver fibrosis has been recently published [430].

One of the most important players in the process of inflammation and fibrosis is a subset of CD4+ve cells originating from the thymus and peripheral organs that are called ***regulatory T cells (Tregs).*** They suppress the proliferation and activity of CD4+ve and CD8+ve T cells through co-inhibitory molecules such as the cytotoxic T lymphocyte antigen 4 (CTLA-4) or by secreting suppressor cytokines such as IL-10 and TGF-β [462,463]. Tregs express the transcription factor Fork head box protein 3 (FOXP3). Within the liver, both myeloid and plasmacytoid HDCs are responsible to transform naive CD4+ve T cells into Tregs by expressing the membrane checkpoint programmed cell death 1 ligand 1 (PD- L1) and by releasing IL-10 and kynurenine [462].

In hepatic steatosis, increased oxidative stress leads to the apoptosis and reduction in hepatic Treg cells, and leads to a lowered suppression of inflammatory responses [464]. Moreover, Tregs were reported to be more sensitive to apoptosis in steatohepatitis [412]. Decreased numbers of hepatic Tregs were described in the animal models of MAFLD [411,464–466]. An additional explanation is that in fatty livers, adipokines affect Treg cells. Increased leptin production from adipose tissue reduces Treg differentiation, stimulating dendritic cells to polarize CD4+ve cells into Th1 and Th17 cells instead of Tregs [467]. In disagreement with these findings, a recent study found increased numbers of Tregs in the livers of high fat- and high carbohydrate-fed mice. Moreover, the elimination of Tregs inhibited the progression of MASH [468]. In another model of MASH, increased intrahepatic Tregs were found, but when Tregs were transferred, they aggravated MASH, indicating that Tregs increase the metabolic inflammation [469]. In the bile duct ligation model, the elimination of Tregs aggravated liver fibrosis in association with the decreased production of IL-10 [470]. However, Tregs also secrete TGF-β, a well-known promoter of liver fibrosis [142]. To make things more complicated, Tregs were increased in chronic HCV and repressed liver fibrosis [471] but promoted fibrosis in another study of chronic HCV [472]. Despite these contradictory findings, most available evidence indicates that Treg cells are anti-fibrotic, secreting the immunosuppressive IL-10 [419]. An earlier study may offer some explanation. In chronic HBV, it is the significance of the balance between

Tregs and Th17 cells that is important and not the absolute number of the individual cells. Both Tregs and Th17 cells in the peripheral blood were increased, but it was the ratio of Treg/Th17 that was correlated with liver fibrosis. Moreover, experiments with isolated human HSCs indicated that Tregs from HBV patients inhibited the activation of HSCs, while recombinant IL-17 increased HSC activation [473].

Tregs are increased during persistent HBV infection [474], downregulating the effector T cells and recruiting innate immune cells to the infected liver, leading to incomplete viral clearance. IL-1β upregulates Treg activation and produces inhibitory cytokines such as IL-10, IL-35, and TGF-β, which are key mediators of Treg function. IL-10 inhibits host anti-HBV activity, leading to the increased replication of HBV. Increased IL-10 levels are correlated with HBV DNA and liver inflammation [475]. HLA-DQ promotes the suppressive function of Tregs [476], while decreased PD-1 expression mitigates the immunosuppressive ability of Tregs and promotes the antiviral activity of effector T cells [477].

HBsAg-specific Tregs intervene with Tfh-dependent HBsAb dysregulation by limiting the differentiation of HBsAg-specific Tfh cells, resulting in insufficient HBsAb production [478]. Tfh cells are implicated in B cell response. They participate in the development of germinal centers from which high-affinity memory B and long-lived plasma cells originate. B cells and plasma cells are required for a protective antibody response [479].

IL-35 is mainly secreted by regulatory T cells and regulatory B cells, which contribute to immune tolerance and viral persistence during chronic HBV infection [480]. IL-35 modulates CD4+ and CD8+ T cells, and induces immunosuppression in chronic HBV infection and non-viral hepatitis-related HCC [481,482]. IL-35 increases PD-1 expression through the JAK1/TYK2/STAT1/STAT4 pathway [483].

In summary, it is clear that Tregs are implicated in the development of liver fibrosis. Tregs activity may either be protective or promotive at different stages of fibrosis development or at different combinations with other interleukins, acting as a two-edged sword. Signaling through the mammalian target of the rapamycin (mTOR) pathway is involved in the protective function of Tregs [484].

Liver B cells are also involved in the immunological response during liver fibrosis through the production of antibodies and the presentation of antigens [485]. It seems that B cells favor the induction and progression of liver fibrosis [484], but most data are derived from pulmonary fibrosis. However, the elimination of B cells attenuated CCl4-induced fibrosis progression in mice [486], while B cell accumulation in the livers of MASH patients correlates to hepatic inflammation and fibrosis [487].

A particular subset of B cells are the ***B regulatory cells***. Bregs in patients with CHB are high, reaching a peak at the immune-active stage. There is a negative correlation with the levels of IL-17 and IFN-γ-secreting Th1 and Th17 cells and CD8+ cells, and a positive correlation with IL-4-producing Th2 cells [488,489]. Bregs can dysregulate T cell function through IL-10, TGF-β, and IL-35. IL-35 levels correlate with the deterioration of liver cirrhosis. The progression of inflammation favors the elevation of Bregs to prevent excessive immune responses, but this may prove detrimental contributing to the persistence of HBV [480,490,491].

Table 2 presents a synopsis of cytokines involved in immune responses in liver diseases.

Table 2. A synopsis of cytokines involved in immune responses in liver diseases.

Cytokines	Functions	References
TNF-α	Inhibit HBV replication, provide antiviral immunity, induce inflammation.	[432,461]
TGF-β	Impair NK cell function, promote fibrosis and HCC.	[131,132,177]
IL-10	Inhibit cytokine production, regulate T cell immunity, develop persistence of HBV infection.	[481,482,484]
IL-13	Induce inflammation, liver fibrosis. and cirrhosis.	[471,472]
IL-6	Produced by macrophages. Induce inflammation and fibrosis. Inhibit HBV replication; inhibits HBV entry.	[200,202,203]
IL-18, IL-1β	Pro-inflammatory. Activate HSCs. IL-1β induces the phosphorylation of Smad2/3 to promote the transformation of hepatocytes to EMT. IL-18 rs187238 GG genotype increases the risk of HCC in a healthy population and the risk of cirrhosis in CHB carriers.	[137,199,202]
IL-17	Exacerbate inflammation, induce liver fibrosis and cirrhosis.	[436,450,451]
IL-21	Produced by activated CD4+ T cells. Activate T and B cells. Maintenance of specific CD8+ T-cell functions and control of viremia. Increased levels may promote cirrhosis and exacerbate liver injury.	[424]
IL-22	Inhibit liver inflammation and fibrosis.	[462,463]
IL-27	Higher levels in patients with liver cirrhosis or hepatocellular carcinoma. Compensate the function of IL-21 by supporting Tfh-B cell function, required for protective antibody response.	[424]
IL-33	Induce liver damage and fibrosis, activate Tfh cells, and enhance humoral immunity; suppress HBV replication.	[426,433,440]
IL-35	Development of fibrosis, cirrhosis, and HCC. Inhibit HBV-specific CD8 T cells cytotoxicity. Inhibit cytokines and induce antiviral immunity.	[492–494]
IFN-γ	Antiviral immunity. Inhibit HBV replication; induce inflammation.	[432,434]

3.5. Unconventional T Cells

They are a heterogeneous group of lymphocytes belonging to the immune system of the liver. The better-studied subpopulations of unconventional T cells include mucosal-associated invariant T (MAIT) cells, γδ T cells, and NKT cells. In the peripheral circulation, they represent almost 10% of T cells. In the liver, however, they are the majority of T cells [379,495]. There are plenty of MAIT cells in the human liver (15–45% of the total T cells), but they are scarce in the liver of mice. On the other hand, invariant NKT (iNKT) cells are <1% of the total T cells in the human liver as opposed to 30–50% in the murine liver [68]. From a functional point of view, NKT cells can be considered as the murine equivalent of human MAIT cells [496].

NKT cells are subdivided into type I NKT (iNKT) cells and type II NKT cells [497], with the former being important in the pathogenesis of several liver diseases [367,498]. In HBV-related cirrhosis, peripheral iNKTs are over-activated and may be partly responsible for the progression of fibrosis [499]. High cholesterol uptake destroys the function of NKT cells through lipid oxidation during the evolution of MAFLD toward cirrhosis. At the early stages of MASH, a reduction in NKT cells has been reported, while in advanced MASH, NKT cells are anti-fibrotic [500,501]. Patients with PBC have increased numbers of Il-17A-producing iNKT cells. The levels of 17A correlate with fibrosis severity [492]. However, this suggestion has been recently disputed in a murine model of PBC, where it was IL-21 and not IL-17A that was associated with disease progression [502]. But again, one should remember the differences in liver NKT cells between humans and mice in every effort to explain these differences.

γδ-T cells have a TCR with two γ and δ chains instead of α and β and comprise 15–25% of all intrahepatic T cells. They are mostly located in portal tracts and areas of bile duct fibrogenesis [493,495]. The activation of γδ T cells does not require an antigen presentation by MHC molecules in contrast to αβ T cells. Therefore, they are referred to as MHC-unrestricted, which may not be absolutely true as some targets of γδ-TCR include the class I MHC molecules [494]. These cells are IL17A producers [503]. γδ-T cells were increased in the liver of the murine models of MAFLD, and their deletion or depletion ameliorated steatohepatitis and accelerated damage repair [504,505]. Interestingly, the gut microbiota may act synergistically with γδ-T IL17+ve cells in disease progression [506]. In contrast to these findings, a transfer of normal γδ T cells ameliorated liver inflammation by increasing the apoptosis of activated HSCs in the methionine–choline-deficient diet of chronic liver disease [507].

Innate lymphoid cells (ILCs). They are subdivided into three groups based on cell surface markers, the transcription factors that regulate their function, and the production of characteristic cytokines [508]. ILC1s consist of IFNγ-producing cells, and they are T-bet dependent, while ILC2s express type 2 cytokines such as IL-5 and IL-13 and are dependent on GATA-binding protein 3 (GATA3) for their function. ILC3s produce IL-17 and IL-22 and depend on the transcription factor retinoic acid receptor-related orphan receptor γt (RORγt) for their function [508–511]. Recently, a revision has been proposed to include conventional NK (cNK) cells and lymphoid tissue-inducer cells [512,513]. An intrahepatic accumulation of ILC3 cells with pro-fibrotic activity was reported in the CCl4-induced liver fibrosis model. The transfer of ILC3s after the elimination of resident ILC3s increased ECM deposition and liver fibrosis, indicating a pro-fibrogenic role of ILC3 [119,510,512,514]. In addition, a positive relation between the severity of liver fibrosis and the proportion of intrahepatic ILC2 was described. The pro-fibrotic effect of ILC2 was mediated by the overproduction of IL-13, which in turn was induced by IL-33 production from hepatocytes and Kupffer cells [515].

Mucosal-associated invariant T (MAIT) cells in circulation vary between 1 and 10% of total T cells but in the liver may increase up to 45% of intrahepatic T lymphocytes [516]. In patients with either alcohol-related or MAFLD cirrhosis, circulating MAIT cells were reduced, but they were increased in the fibrous septa. Most MAIT cells (80%) from both healthy controls and cirrhotics were CD8+ve, while 20% were double negative (CD8−CD4−). In animal models, the enrichment of mice with MAIT cells promoted liver fibrosis. MAIT cells also enhanced the fibrogenic functions of MFs and MB-derived macrophages [517]. Decreased peripheral MAIT cells with an impaired production of IFN-γ and TNF-α were also described in MAFLD patients. MAIT cells were also increased in the liver and were positively correlated with MAFLD severity. But in contrast to the previous findings, a protective role of MAITs was suggested, as activated MAIT cells in vitro induced M2 macrophage phenotype, and in MAIT-deficient animals, steatosis and inflammation was aggravated [518].

3.6. Extrahepatic Factors

The first and most important extrahepatic factor that is implicated in inflammation and fibrosis is the lymphocyte and monocyte recruitment in the liver. This is dependent on an adhesion cascade influenced by intercommunications between parenchymal and non- parenchymal cells. An example is the liberation of DAMPs by damaged hepatocytes leading to the overproduction of pro-inflammatory mediators by Kupffer cells, which increase adhesion molecule expression by LSECs. Lymphocyte recruitment across activated

LSECs involves a firm adhesion on the LSEC surface. Lymphocytes then move along the luminal endothelium until a signal makes them migrate through LSECs through either a paracellular or a transcellular route. Chemotactic factors secreted from activated HSCs direct lymphocytes into the final position within the liver tissue [200].

The dysfunctional gut–liver axis is the second extrahepatic factor that is seriously involved in liver fibrosis. It leads to a "leaky gut" through which bacterial products obtain access to the portal blood and activate liver macrophages, leading to fibrosis. The intestinal barrier is the first line of defense against human intestinal microbiota. The translocation of bacteria is further inhibited by the junctional complex of the intestinal epithelium and by immune cells infiltrating the lamina propria. In gut dysbiosis, as found in chronic liver diseases, all these elements are compromised, allowing abnormal translocations to the liver [519,520]. Different receptors expressed in liver cells can discriminate between gut commensal and pathological antigens. When dangerous signals are detected, APCs, including hepatocytes, recruit immune cells to eliminate pathogen,s maintaining immune homeostasis. On the other hand, when the massive translocation of PAMPs and DAMPs from the impaired intestinal barrier reach the liver, tolerance is replaced by an inflammatory and fibrogenic microenvironment. Innate immunity has the leading role, while adaptive immunity may sometimes be protective. Most relevant research has been based on investigations contacted in relation to MAFLD/MASH [519,521,522]. Other extrahepatic factors include the regulation of liver immunity by other organs. Thus, the spleen affects the composition of liver immune cells. Spleen lipocalin-2 represses the macrophage-induced activation of HSCs. The lung may also affect liver immune regulation, possibly via TNFa modulation of the inadequately studied lung–liver axis. The role of adipose tissue has already been presented. Activated adipose macrophages can migrate to the liver in MASH. Finally, the brain regulates liver immune responses through the liberation of catecholamine and acetylcholine from efferent sympathetic and vagus nerve fibers. They respond to hepatic inflammatory signals transmitted to the central nervous system [523].

3.7. The Interaction of Innate and Adaptive Immunity

The extensive interaction between innate and adaptive immunity was already mentioned in the subchapters of individual cells. However, there are certain discrete bridges that mediate the interplay between innate and adaptive immunity in liver fibrosis.

A first bridge is the activation of $\gamma\delta$T cells acting as a connecting point between the innate and adaptive immunity, as they express TCR$\gamma\delta$ that recognizes antigens and also produce inflammatory cytokines such as IL- 17A after stimulation [524]. The second bridge of the interplay between innate and adaptive immunity became evident in MASH investigations. Lipid toxicity and oxidative stress damage the hepatocytes, as mentioned before. Both innate immune response and adaptive immunity contribute to MASH-associated inflammation. Innate immunity may lead to fibrosis via PRRs, including TLRs and NLPR3 inflammasomes, that recognize PAMPs and DAMPs. T cell-mediated adaptive immunity also promotes fibrosis in MASH via cytotoxicity and cytokines. KCs are the bridge between the innate and the adaptive responses here. The third bridge is provided by hepatocytes, which, in addition to their functions as innate cells, also express MHC-II molecules and co-stimulators, acting as atypical APCs to induce CD4+ve T cell activation and their Th1 or Th17 cell polarization [213]. IFNγ and other Th1 cell cytokines provide the fourth bridge, as they increase the stimulation of liver macrophages to release M1 pro- inflammatory cytokines and chemokines that further increase the recruitment of monocytes and lymphocytes. Macrophages and dendritic cells release B cell-stimulating cytokines, such as the B cell-activating factor (BAFF), which are fundamental for B cell maturation into plasma cells. The fifth bridge is the secretion by both the hepatocytes and macrophages of IL-15 that improves the survival of CD8+ve T cells and in association with CXCL16, promotes liver NKT cell survival [412,484,525].

Figure 2 summarizes the immune mechanisms implicated in liver fibrosis.

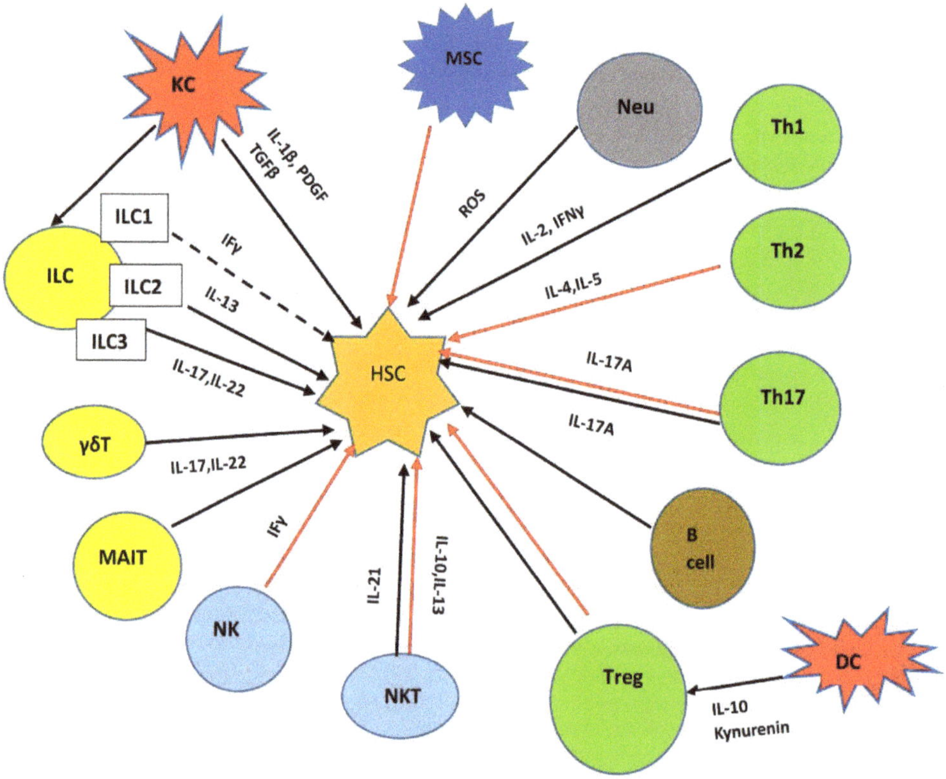

Figure 2. Immune cells and mediators involved in the pathogenesis of liver fibrosis. For details, see text. Black arrows: activation of HSCs. Red arrows: inhibition of HSCs. Dotted arrow: Not investigated. DCs: dendritic cells; ILCs: innate lymphoid cells; KCs: Kupffer cells; MAITs: Mucosal-associated invariant T cells; MSCs: Mesenchymal stromal cells; Neu: Neutrophils; ROS: reactive oxygen species.

4. Immune Checks in Liver Fibrosis

4.1. Immune Checkpoint

Immune checkpoint proteins (ICPs) have attracted extensive interest, as they are critical suppressors of the immune responses in a variety of tumors. However, they have a wider potential because they maintain immune tolerance in health by repressing T cell activation and proliferation [526–529]. ICPs which are expressed in tumor cells trigger the exhaustion, senescence, or apoptosis of effector immune cells [530,531]. The best-studied inhibitory immune checkpoints are CTLA-4, PD-1, and PD-L1. CTLA-4 is a molecule that is upregulated on the surface of activated T cells to break their over-stimulation by the TCRs. CTLA-4, also known as CD152, is a strong competitor of the TCR co-stimulatory molecule CD28 and binds to CD80 (B7-1)/CD86 (B7-2) with a stronger binding affinity compared to CD28, thus inhibiting T-cell activation [532]. CTLA-4 is mostly located in intracellular vesicles and is translocated to the cell membrane after T cell activation [533].

The upregulation of PD-1 has also been reported on activated T cells. PD-1 is mostly located at the membrane of cells [533] and binds to its ligand, PD-L1, transmitting inhibitory co-stimulatory signals that prevent T cell activation. The pro-oncogenic and immunosuppressive phenotype of the tumor microenvironment is characterized by the overexpression of PD-L1 by cancer cells and the overexpression of PD-1 and CTLA-4 by T cells [534,535]. Anti-PD-1 and anti-CTLA-4 monoclonal antibodies are two types of extensively used inhibitors of immune checkpoints (ICBs) [536].

PD-1 is expressed in several immune cells, including almost all subtypes of T cells, B cells, NK cells, macrophages, DCs, and monocytes [537–540]. High levels of PD-1 were an important characteristic of T cell exhaustion [537]. Resting effector T cells do not express PD-1, but after stimulation by antigens, there is a strong expression of PD-1 [541]. PD-1 downregulation follows the elimination of stimulation signals, otherwise the high levels are maintained [542]. Cytokines such as IL-10 and TGF-β also initiate the expression of PD-1 [543,544]. In addition, PD-L1 is induced by several inflammatory mediators such as IFN-γ, a fact that links PD-L1 expression with persistent inflammation [545,546]. The binding of PD-L1 to PD-1 inhibits the proliferation and differentiation of T cells into inflammatory populations, including Th1, Th2, and Th17 cells. This interaction also inhibits the function of CD8+ve cells. Moreover, this interaction upregulates the differentiation of T cells into Tregs [547].

CTLA-4 molecules were upregulated in CD4+ve and CD8+ve T cells in CHB according to recent studies, while the constitutive expression of CLTA-4 was reported in Tregs. CTLA-4 inhibition produced inconclusive results, as T cell proliferation and cytokine production were upregulated in some studies, while others confirmed this only after the inhibition of CTLA-4 in combination with other inhibitory receptors. CTLA-4 is also involved in T cell exhaustion in CHB, but the existing evidence is inadequate at this moment [548].

Macrophages are also modulated by ICPs. PD-1 expression in macrophages is negatively correlated with the presence of M1-polarized tumor-associated macrophages (TAMs) and their phagocytic capacity against tumor cells [549,550].

An important aspect of ICP function is the effect of post-translational modification by glycosylation. During glycosylation, glycan molecules are covalently attached to proteins or lipids by an enzymatic site-specific mechanism that affects the functions of ICPs such as biosynthesis and interactions [551]. No studies have addressed the significance of the glycosylation of ICPs in liver fibrosis and cirrhosis, but there is evidence that this may be important. Epithelial–mesenchymal transition (EMT) is a process that is involved in liver fibrosis, as mentioned before. The glycosylation of PD-1 has been studied in cancer stem cells, where the roles of EMT and N-glycosyl-transferase STT3 were explored. EMT upregulated PD-L1 expression in cancer stem cells by the EMT/β-catenin/STT3/PD-L1 signaling axis. The elimination of both STT3 isoforms suppressed EMT-mediated PD-L1 induction [552].

4.2. Association of Immune Checkpoints with Liver Fibrosis

4.2.1. The PD-1/PD-L1 Axis and CTLA-4

In recent years, the role of the PD-1/PD-L1 axis in liver fibrosis has attracted attention, but the data are still scarce and not conclusive. Most data are coming from the fibrosis progression in other organs, mainly the lung. However, they confirm that a close relationship exists between PD-1/PD-L1 signaling and liver fibrosis. The PD-1/PD-L1 interaction increases fibrosis by promoting important fibrogenic mechanisms such as macrophage polarization, T cell activation, and the trans-differentiation of epithelial cells. The upregulation of PD-L1 induces EMT, and signals that initiate EMT can also promote the expression of PD-L1, creating a positive loop [553]. Recent data indicated that an immune dysregulation of the PD1/PD-L1 immune checkpoint may be implicated in liver fibrosis [554]. There is evidence that PD-L1 inhibitors, such as pembrolizumab and nivolumab, used to treat several cancers, have a potential effect on fibrosis treatment as they reduce fibroblast activation and ECM deposition [555]. Murine studies reported that the Golgi membrane protein 1 (GOLM1) is highly upregulated in carbon tetrachloride-induced liver fibrosis. GOML1 triggered PD-L1 expression and increased fibrosis by activating the EGFR/AKT/STAT3 signaling pathway [556]. The above data indicate that the PD-1/PD-L1 signaling favors the progression of liver fibrosis. On the other hand, reports have suggested that the indirect activation of PD-L1 signaling attenuates liver fibrosis [557].

Blocking PD-L1 inhibits the production of IL-10 and differentiation into Tregs and restores in part the function of CD4+ T cells [558] and HBV-specific CD8 T cells [559]. Continuous HBsAg and HBeAg exposure led to the exhaustion of many CD8+ve T cells and a gradual upregulation of PD-L1 and CTLA-4 expression. PD-1 inhibition alone could not completely restore the exhaustion, which was achieved only after a combined PD-1/CTLA-4 inhibition [559,560]. Interestingly, lower TLR2+ve monocytes and increased PD1 + CD8 + T cell proportions may contribute to viral breakthrough (VBT) in HBV patients switched to IFNa after the failure of nucleoside/tide (NUC) analogs. The combination of TLR2 activation and the PD1/PDL1 pathway blockade may repress HBV replication and prevent VBT through increased cytokine production and the recovering of CD8 T-cell function [561]. PD-L1 antagonists may block HBV replication by initiating cytokine production and by promoting the cytotoxic effects of CD8+ T cells, mostly in patients with low HBV DNA and negative HBeAg [562].

The investigation of specific disease entities offered more evidence that ICPs are implicated in liver fibrosis. In acute viral hepatitis, PD-1 and CTLA-4 are increased during the symptomatic phase, and decreased during recovery. PD-1 and CTLA-4 have protective effects as inhibitory molecules to stop the destruction by cytotoxic T cells in self-limited viral hepatitis. In HBeAg-negative chronic asymptomatic HBV carriers, ICPs are highly expressed on Th1, Th2, Th17, and Tregs [439,563].

Moreover, in chronic HCV, hepatocytes express high levels of PD-L1, leading to the generation of Tregs and follicular regulatory T cells and the liberation of extracellular vesicles rich in TGF-β [564]. The T cell response to chronic infection is suppressed, and liver fibrosis is promoted [565]. In addition, PD-L1 expression mediates the transformation of M2 macrophages in liver fibrosis [566]. A recent clinical study demonstrated that serum PD-1 levels were higher in patients with HCV infection compared to normal controls and gradually increased along with the severity of liver fibrosis [567]. In another clinical study, peripheral blood and splenic CD4+ve and CD8+ve T-cells expressed higher levels of PD-1, mucin domain-containing protein 3 (Tim-3), and CTLA-4 in HCV patients with cirrhosis and portal hypertension compared to normal [568].

Investigations in other organs confirm the association of checkpoints with the process of fibrosis. Several findings link the PD-1/PD-L1 axis with idiopathic pulmonary fibrosis (IPF), as abnormalities of this axis were reported in many cells implicated in IPF pathogenesis [569]. Interestingly, a recent report indicated that anti-PD-L1 antibodies mitigated the ECM deposition of TGF-β1-induced lung fibroblasts by downregulating the PI3K/Akt/mTOR signaling pathway, which is critical in autophagy regulation [570]. These findings are important as the mechanism of PD-L1 in hepatic fibrosis has many similarities with pulmonary fibrosis, mainly in connection with EMT induction in the lung and the liver. PDL1 can induce the production of TGF-β in liver fibrosis. In agreement with pulmonary fibrosis, EMT pathways involving TGF-β, such as Smad and PI3K/AKT, are also active in liver fibrosis [156,571–573]. PDL1 also activates HSCs, leading to the production of several factors involved in hepatic fibrosis, as presented above [574]. Finally, PD-L1 favors the transformation into M2 macrophages, which in turn suppresses E cadherin and increases vimentin in hepatocytes, thus promoting EMT [575] in direct analogy with drug-induced pulmonary fibrosis, where the upregulation of PD-L1 promoted fibrosis through the inhibition of vimentin degradation [576]. Mechanistically, PD-L1 directly upregulated the serum and glucocorticoid kinase 2 (SGK2) and activated the SGK2/β-catenin signaling pathway to induce EMT and the transformation of liver cancer cells into a stem cell phenotype [577].

However, there are differences between liver and pulmonary fibrosis. PD-L1 on liver fibrosis is mostly immunomodulatory. Thus, in an earlier paper on chronic persistent HCV disease, it was demonstrated that HCV-specific CD8 T cells from the liver expressed high levels of PD-1 and a significant impairment of their function. CTLA-4 was also upregulated in PD-1+ve T cells from the liver but not from the blood of persistently infected HCV patients. Interestingly, the impaired function of CD8+ve cells was synergistically reversed by a combined PD-1/CTLA-4 blockade, but not by blocking PD-1 or CTLA-4 alone, indicating that both PD-1 and CTLA-4 pathways participate in the virus-specific T cell exhaustion in chronic HCV [578]. Although reported data suggests a similar role of CTLA-4 in T cell exhaustion, the documentation is weak to support the role of CTLA-4 in T cell exhaustion in chronic HBV infection, as mentioned above [548].

Another approach to clarify the role of ICPs in liver fibrosis is to delineate the association of ICPs with the functions proved to participate in the fibrotic process. ICPs are implicated in the function of critical cells in the regulation of liver fibrosis such as MCS, macrophages, and HSCs.

Thus, PD-L1 expression is involved in the immunomodulation mediated by the mesenchymal stromal/stem cells (MSCs) as well. PD-L1 on the surface of MSCs interacts with PD-1 on the surface of T cells through direct cell-to-cell communication, inhibiting the functions of T cells. PD-L1 may also be secreted, inhibiting T cell function without the close contact of cells. MSCs may transfer PD-L1 in extracellular vesicles, again affecting T cells from a distance. Signal transmissions from MSC PD-1 create a positive loop, enhancing their immunomodulatory potential. On the other hand, anti-PD-L1 antibodies can reduce immunomodulation mediated by MSCs [579].

Further immunomodulation by IPCs in liver fibrosis may be mediated via PD-1 induction in monocytes and macrophages through TLR signaling and cytokines such as TNF-α, IL-1β, and IL-6 [580,581]. Furthermore, PD-1 expression in macrophages may repress innate inflammatory responses [582,583]. PD-L1 activation sends negative signals to macrophages, inducing an immunosuppressor cell phenotype [584]. The overexpression of PD-L1 in macrophages and peripheral monocytes has been demonstrated in chronic viral infections in the liver [232,585]. A study of patients with cirrhosis showed that liver macrophages overexpressed the immune-suppressive proteins PD-L1, MARCO, and CD163. Monocytes from patients also overexpressed PD-L1, which was related to disease severity and the presence of infections. A blockade of PD-L1 with anti-PD- L1 antibodies restored liver macrophage functions [267]. These findings have been confirmed in an acetaminophen-induced acute liver injury murine model. Reduced bacterial clearance by KCs expressing PD-1 was observed during liver injury. During resolution, KCs expressed higher levels of PD-1 and lymphocytes expressed higher levels of PD-L1. The suppression of PD-1 expression by anti-PD-1 improved KC bacterial clearance. Increased PD-1 expression in monocytes and increased PD-L1 expression in lymphocytes of peripheral blood were found in patients with acute liver failure. Moreover, PD-L1 plasma levels were positively correlated with sepsis and mortality. Interestingly, PD-1 in vitro blockade restored monocyte functionality [586,587].

Activated hepatic stellate cells from human livers induce the apoptosis of activated T cells through the expression of PD-L1. Human HSCs have strong immunoregulatory activity via the B7-H1-mediated induction of apoptosis in activated T cells [588]. Murine HSCs suppressed the upregulation of activation markers on B cells together with the repression of their proliferation and their cytokine production. Interestingly, the elimination of the interaction of PD-L1 with PD-1 decreased the ability of HSCs to suppress B cell activation [306]. Several recent reports have clearly demonstrated that senescent HSCs display an increased expression of PD-1/PD-L1 proteins. An increase in the level of the PD-L1 protein in senescent cells is able to suppress their immune surveillance and inhibit their elimination by cytotoxic CD8+ve T cells and NK cells [186,589–592]. ICPs also affect TGF-β function. PD-L1, produced by HSCs, is necessary for HSC activation by protecting the two TGF-β receptors from degradation. The extracellular domain of PD-L1 protects the TβRII protein, while the 260-RLRKGR-265 motif on PD-L1 protects the TβRI mRNA [593].

4.2.2. Other ICPs Involved in Liver Fibrosis

Apart from the better-studied PD-1/PD-L1 and CTLA-4, additional ICPs have the potential to be involved in fibrosis, although the data are inadequate.

The B7 homolog 3 protein (B7-H3), also designated as CD276, is a critical ICP of the B7 immunoglobin superfamily [594]. B7-H3 is expressed on APCs and is involved in T-cell-mediated immunity. The aberrant expression of B7-H3 in several cancers is associated with a poor prognosis and increased angiogenesis [595]. B7-H4 is also a member of the same B7 superfamily. It was also found on professional APC, preventing T cell activation and was also associated with poor prognosis [596,597].

ICPs such as LAG-3, TIM-3, and CD39 on CD8+ve T cells were increased in patients with chronic HBV. The ability of CD8+ve cells to secrete TNFa, IFNγ, and perforin was downregulated [598]. TIM-3 levels positively correlated with HBV DNA levels [599]. Lymphocyte activation gene 3 (LAG-3), also designated as CD223, has been a promising target in the treatment of hepatocellular carcinoma (HCC). In patients with HCC, LAG-3 expression in Tregs and NK cells is implicated in tumor immune evasion by interacting with MHC-II molecules. Its overexpression is associated with T cell exhaustion in synergy with PD-1 and increased angiogenesis [600].

The increased expression of TIM-3 and galectin-9 also led to the inhibition and apoptotic deletion of T cells. Th cells expressing TIM-3 have a limited production of IFN-γ and TNF-α after the recognition of HBV peptides and are sensitive to galectin-9-initiated cell death. The expression of TIM-3 on peripheral T cells parallels disease progression and markers of liver damage including increases in ALT, AST, bilirubin, and international normalized ratio (INR) [600]. The inhibition of TIM-3 initiated the proliferation of HBV-specific CD8 T cells and upregulated antiviral cytokine secretion [601].

Kynurenine (Kyn) is another important IPC modulator of immune responses via its aryl hydrocarbon receptor (Ahr). For Kyn synthesis, two enzymes are implicated, the indoleamine 2,3-dioxygenase (Ido) and the tryptophan 2,3-dioxygenase (Tdo). Ido is responsible for 90% of tryptophan catabolism. Although Kyn is increased in various liver disorders, the exact involvement of Kyn in liver damage has not been clarified as Ido1, Ido2, and Tdo are activated in several cell types. However, Ido1 deficiency aggravated liver fibrosis in the CCL4-induced liver injury murine model [602]. Moreover, liver fibrosis in the same model was mitigated in Ido2−/−, indicating that the inhibition of kyn or ido 2 may ameliorate hepatic fibrosis [603].

4.3. Therapeutic Implications of Checkpoint Inhibitors in Liver Fibrosis

Despite the increasing evidence that checkpoint inhibitors are involved in the regulation of inflammation and liver fibrosis, there are very few clinical data and some experimental observations on their use in these two conditions.

A blockade of inhibitory checkpoints including PD-1, CTLA-4, 2B4, TIM-3, and galectin-9 alone or in combination has emerged as a potential therapeutic approach to restore T and B cell functions in CHB [478,558,604–607]. In studies of HBV-infected mice and blood from patients with a chronic HBV infection, a Tfh cell response to HBsAg was required for HBV clearance, and this response was blocked by Treg cells. Inhibiting Treg cell activity using neutralizing antibody against CTLA4 restored the ability of Tfh cells to clear HBV infection. This approach might be used in future clinical trials for the treatment of patients with chronic HBV infection [478].

However, there are sufficient data from the extensive use of ICPs in the treatment of HCC. It is known that the great majority of HCC cases have a background of fibrosis and cirrhosis. Therefore, data on HCC treatment may offer an overview of the use of these drugs in advanced liver disease. The results of clinical trials for HCC may be extrapolated in the future treatment of liver fibrosis, at least as far as safety is concerned.

The published results of anti-PD1/PD-L1 monotherapy for HCC with nivolumab, pembrolizumab, durvalumab, and camrelizumab indicate a non-impressive overall survival of 13.2–16.9 months. More favorable were the results of the combinations of ICPs with tyrosine kinase inhibitors. Atezolizumab, a PD-L1 inhibitor, combined with bevacizumab showed a 56% reduced risk of death compared to sorafenib. Camriezumab combined with alpatinib had an overall survival of 22.1 months compared to 15.2 months for sorafenib [608]. The Himalaya trial evaluated the STRIDE regimen consisting of a single dose of tremelimumab with a dose of durvalumab every 4 wks. A significant but again not impressive increase in overall survival of 16.4 months vs. 13.8 months for sorafenib was reported [609]. Other combination treatments of anti-PD-1 with ipilimumab and tremelimumab (CTLA-4 IPCs inhibitors) are in progress [610].

Interestingly, a systematic review of systemic therapies in HCC from 2002 to 2020 revealed that immunotherapies were more effective in viral etiologies as compared to non-viral etiologies, possibly because the immune responses are more vigorous in viral infections compared to non-viral etiologies [611].

An additional interesting approach was recently reported. Coagulation factor Xa (FXa) and its receptor proteinase-activated receptor-2 (PAR-2) promote tumor metastasis in several forms of cancer. The combination of the anti-coagulation drug rivaroxaban and an anti-PD-1 antibody induced synergistic antitumor effects in experimental models. Most importantly, rivaroxaban improved the objective response rate of HCC patients and prolonged the overall survival time [612].

Whatever the survival benefits might be, adverse events (AEs) do happen, including immune-related adverse events (irAEs) such as rash and pruritus, diarrhea and colitis, hypothyroidism and hypophysitis, pneumonitis, and psychiatric disorders [613,614]. The reactivation of HBV has also been observed [615]. ICP inhibitors combined with angiogenesis inhibitors may reduce incidence and mortality for most irAEs [616].

5. Conclusions

Liver fibrosis is the end result of almost all chronic liver diseases. However, the underlying mechanisms are different in many respects according to etiology. There has been great progress in the cellular and molecular biology of liver fibrosis, and it is now accepted that the sinusoids are a fundamental field in fibrosis induction and progress. Kupffer cells and the hepatic stellate cells are the most important cells of innate immune response implicated in fibrosis. They are the masterminds of the immune regulation of fibrosis as they interact with each other, assisted by other immune cells such as lymphocytes and liver endothelial cells. Kupffer cells are implicated in the activation of HSCs that in turn are the producers of ECM through a complex network of cytokines and chemokines. At the same time, both Kupffer cells and HSCs are responsible for the resolution of fibrosis through a network of inhibitory cytokines and the production of degrading metalloproteases. It is also well documented that adaptive immunity and its very many cells are critical components in the regulation of fibrosis as are cells of an intermediate nature such as MAIT cells and $\gamma\delta$ T cells that interact with elements of both innate and adaptive immunity. Recently, a hotspot of research is the role of the immune checkpoints (ICPs), as they are the main controllers of the excessive immune responses, and their inhibition is currently in clinical use in an effort to overcome the immune evasion masterminded by several cancers. There is increasing evidence that ICPs are involved in the regulation of liver fibrosis; therefore, a new chapter in anti-fibrotic therapy may start as many new ICPs are described and the role of the better-studied PD-1/PD-L1 and CTLA-4 is intensively researched. They are effective in non-fibrotic viral liver disease as well, but their application will be limited. The current antivirals are very effective and more cost-efficient, and it is not reasonable to replace them. There are sufficient data on the safety of ICP inhibitors, alone or in combination with other drugs, from extensive trials on the treatment of HCC, indicating that trials on the treatment of liver fibrosis are justified, and possibly a new era on immunotherapy of this difficult-to-treat liver disease is ahead.

Author Contributions: Conceptualization, E.K.; literature review, I.T. and A.V.; writing—original draft preparation, I.T., E.K. and A.V.; supervision, E.K. All authors have read and agreed to the published version of the manuscript.

Funding: This research received no external funding.

Institutional Review Board Statement: Not applicable.

Informed Consent Statement: Not applicable.

Data Availability Statement: Not applicable.

Conflicts of Interest: The authors declare no conflicts of interest.

References

1. Kisseleva, T. The origin of fibrogenic myofibroblasts in fibrotic liver. *Hepatology* **2017**, *65*, 1039–1043. [CrossRef] [PubMed]
2. Higashi, T.; Friedman, S.L.; Hoshida, Y. Hepatic stellate cells as key target in liver fibrosis. *Adv. Drug Deliv. Rev.* **2017**, *121*, 27–42. [CrossRef] [PubMed]
3. Koyama, Y.; Brenner, D.A. Liver inflammation and fibrosis. *J. Clin. Investig.* **2017**, *127*, 55–64. [CrossRef]
4. Ginès, P.; Krag, A.; Abraldes, J.G.; Solà, E.; Fabrellas, N.; Kamath, P.S. Liver cirrhosis. *Lancet* **2021**, *398*, 1359–1376. [CrossRef]
5. Devarbhavi, H.; Asrani, S.K.; Arab, J.P.; Nartey, Y.A.; Pose, E.; Kamath, P.S. Global burden of liver disease: 2023 update. *J. Hepatol.* **2023**, *79*, 516–537. [CrossRef]
6. Moon, A.M.; Singal, A.G.; Tapper, E.B. Contemporary Epidemiology of Chronic Liver Disease and Cirrhosis. *Clin. Gastroenterol. Hepatol.* **2020**, *18*, 2650–2666. [CrossRef]
7. Ye, F.; Zhai, M.; Long, J.; Gong, Y.; Ren, C.; Zhang, D.; Lin, X.; Liu, S. The burden of liver cirrhosis in mortality: Results from the global burden of disease study. *Front. Public. Health* **2022**, *10*, 909455. [CrossRef]
8. Jepsen, P.; Younossi, Z.M. The global burden of cirrhosis: A review of disability-adjusted life-years lost and unmet needs. *J. Hepatol.* **2021**, *75*, 3–13. [CrossRef]
9. Smith, A.; Baumgartner, K.; Bositis, C. Cirrhosis: Diagnosis and Management. *Am. Fam. Physician.* **2019**, *100*, 759–770.
10. Alberts, C.J.; Clifford, G.M.; Georges, D.; Negro, F.; Lesi, O.A.; Hutin, Y.J.; de Martel, C. Worldwide prevalence of hepatitis B virus and hepatitis C virus among patients with cirrhosis at country, region, and global levels: A systematic review. *Lancet Gastroenterol. Hepatol.* **2022**, *7*, 724–735. [CrossRef]
11. Dobosz, P.; Dzieciątkowski, T. The Intriguing History of Cancer Immunotherapy. *Front. Immunol.* **2019**, *10*, 2965. [CrossRef] [PubMed]
12. Kroemer, G.; Zitvogel, L. Immune checkpoint inhibitors. *J. Exp. Med.* **2021**, *218*, 20201979. [CrossRef] [PubMed]
13. Zhang, Y.; Zheng, J. Functions of Immune Checkpoint Molecules Beyond Immune Evasion. *Adv. Exp. Med. Biol.* **2020**, *1248*, 201–226.

14. Pinheiro, D.; Dias, I.; Ribeiro Silva, K.; Stumbo, A.C.; Thole, A.; Cortez, E.; de Carvalho, L.; Weiskirchen, R.; Carvalho, S. Mechanisms Underlying Cell Therapy in Liver Fibrosis: An Overview. *Cells* **2019**, *8*, 1339. [CrossRef]
15. Bourebaba, N.; Marycz, K. Hepatic stellate cells role in the course of metabolic disorders development—A molecular overview. *Pharmacol. Res.* **2021**, *170*, 105739. [CrossRef]
16. Zhang, D.; Zhang, Y.; Sun, B. The Molecular Mechanisms of Liver Fibrosis and Its Potential Therapy in Application. *Int. J. Mol. Sci.* **2022**, *23*, 12572. [CrossRef]
17. Weiskirchen, R.; Weiskirchen, S.; Tacke, F. Recent advances in understanding liver fibrosis: Bridging basic science and individualized treatment concepts. *F1000Res.* **2018**, *7*, 921. [CrossRef]
18. Rockey, D.C.; Bell, P.D.; Hill, J.A. Fibrosis--a common pathway to organ injury and failure. *N. Engl. J. Med.* **2015**, *372*, 1138–1149. [CrossRef]
19. Gao, C.C.; Bai, J.; Han, H.; Qin, H.Y. The versatility of macrophage heterogeneity in liver fibrosis. *Front. Immunol.* **2022**, *13*, 968879. [CrossRef]
20. Zhao, Y.L.; Zhu, R.T.; Sun, Y.L. Epithelial-mesenchymal transition in liver fibrosis. *Biomed. Rep.* **2016**, *4*, 269–274. [CrossRef]
21. Park, J.H.; Park, B.; Park, K.K. Suppression of Hepatic Epithelial-to-Mesenchymal Transition by Melittin via Blocking of TGFβ/Smad and MAPK-JNK Signaling Pathways. *Toxins* **2017**, *9*, 138. [CrossRef] [PubMed]
22. Li, T.Z.; Kim, S.M.; Hur, W.; Choi, J.E.; Kim, J.H.; Hong, S.W.; Lee, E.B.; Lee, J.H.; Yoon, S.K. Elk-3 Contributes to the Progression of Liver Fibrosis by Regulating the Epithelial-Mesenchymal Transition. *Gut Liver.* **2017**, *11*, 102–111. [CrossRef] [PubMed]
23. Di Gregorio, J.; Robuffo, I.; Spalletta, S.; Giambuzzi, G.; De Iuliis, V.; Toniato, E.; Martinotti, S.; Conti, P.; Flati, V. The Epithelial-to-Mesenchymal Transition as a Possible Therapeutic Target in Fibrotic Disorders. *Front. Cell Dev. Biol.* **2020**, *8*, 607483. [CrossRef] [PubMed]
24. Rowe, R.G.; Lin, Y.; Shimizu-Hirota, R.; Hanada, S.; Neilson, E.G.; Greenson, J.K.; Weiss, S.J. Hepatocyte-derived Snail1 propagates liver fibrosis progression. *Mol. Cell Biol.* **2011**, *31*, 2392–2403. [CrossRef]
25. Zhang, J.; Zhang, H.; Liu, J.; Tu, X.; Zang, Y.; Zhu, J.; Chen, J.; Dong, L.; Zhang, J. miR-30 inhibits TGF-β1-induced epithelial-to-mesenchymal transition in hepatocyte by targeting Snail1. *Biochem. Biophys. Res. Commun.* **2012**, *417*, 1100–1105. [CrossRef]
26. Zhan, J.; Liu, S.; Meng, Y.; Yang, Q.; Wang, Z.; Zhang, S.; Ge, L.; Zhao, L.; Xu, X.; Zhao, Y.; et al. Systematic review of the mechanism and assessment of liver fibrosis in biliary atresia. *Pediatr. Surg. Int.* **2024**, *40*, 205. [CrossRef]
27. Rygiel, K.A.; Robertson, H.; Marshall, H.L.; Pekalski, M.; Zhao, L.; Booth, T.A.; Jones, D.E.; Burt, A.D.; Kirby, J.A. Epithelial-mesenchymal transition contributes to portal tract fibrogenesis during human chronic liver disease. *Lab. Investig.* **2008**, *88*, 112–123. [CrossRef]
28. Harada, K.; Sato, Y.; Ikeda, H.; Isse, K.; Ozaki, S.; Enomae, M.; Ohama, K.; Katayanagi, K.; Kurumaya, H.; Matsui, A.; et al. Epithelial-mesenchymal transition induced by biliary innate immunity contributes to the sclerosing cholangiopathy of biliary atresia. *J. Pathol.* **2009**, *217*, 654–664. [CrossRef]
29. Zhang, J.; Yao, H.; Song, G.; Liao, X.; Xian, Y.; Li, W. Regulation of epithelial-mesenchymal transition by tumor-associated macrophages in cancer. *Am. J. Transl. Res.* **2015**, *7*, 1699–1711.
30. Yang, M.; Ma, B.; Shao, H.; Clark, A.M.; Wells, A. Macrophage phenotypic subtypes diametrically regulate epithelial-mesenchymal plasticity in breast cancer cells. *BMC Cancer.* **2016**, *16*, 419. [CrossRef]
31. Tsuchida, T.; Friedman, S.L. Mechanisms of hepatic stellate cell activation. *Nat. Rev. Gastroenterol. Hepatol.* **2017**, *14*, 397–411. [CrossRef] [PubMed]
32. Herrera, J.; Henke, C.A.; Bitterman, P.B. Extracellular matrix as a driver of progressive fibrosis. *J. Clin. Investig.* **2018**, *128*, 45–53. [CrossRef] [PubMed]
33. Xu, F.; Liu, C.; Zhou, D.; Zhang, L. TGF-β/SMAD Pathway and Its Regulation in Hepatic Fibrosis. *J. Histochem. Cytochem.* **2016**, *64*, 157–167. [CrossRef] [PubMed]
34. Murakami, Y.; Toyoda, H.; Tanaka, M.; Kuroda, M.; Harada, Y.; Matsuda, F.; Tajima, A.; Kosaka, N.; Ochiya, T.; Shimotohno, K. The progression of liver fibrosis is related with overexpression of the miR-199 and 200 families. *PLoS ONE* **2011**, *6*, 16081. [CrossRef]
35. Li, Q.; Li, Z.; Lin, Y.; Che, H.; Hu, Y.; Kang, X.; Zhang, Y.; Wang, L.; Zhang, Y. High glucose promotes hepatic fibrosis via miR-32/MTA3-mediated epithelial-to-mesenchymal transition. *Mol. Med. Rep.* **2019**, *19*, 3190–3200. [CrossRef]
36. Gao, Y.; Li, L.; Zhang, S.N.; Mang, Y.Y.; Zhang, X.B.; Feng, S.M. HepG2.2.15-derived exosomes facilitate the activation and fibrosis of hepatic stellate cells. *World J. Gastroenterol.* **2024**, *30*, 2553–2563. [CrossRef]
37. Ezhilarasan, D. MicroRNA interplay between hepatic stellate cell quiescence and activation. *Eur. J. Pharmacol.* **2020**, *885*, 173507. [CrossRef]
38. Zheng, J.; Wang, W.; Yu, F.; Dong, P.; Chen, B.; Zhou, M.T. MicroRNA-30a Suppresses the Activation of Hepatic Stellate Cells by Inhibiting Epithelial-to-Mesenchymal Transition. *Cell Physiol. Biochem.* **2018**, *46*, 82–92. [CrossRef]
39. Chen, J.; Yu, Y.; Li, S.; Liu, Y.; Zhou, S.; Cao, S.; Yin, J.; Li, G. MicroRNA-30a ameliorates hepatic fibrosis by inhibiting Beclin1-mediated autophagy. *J. Cell Mol. Med.* **2017**, *21*, 3679–3692. [CrossRef]

40. Xu, W.; Mo, W.; Han, D.; Dai, W.; Xu, X.; Li, J.; Xu, X. Hepatocyte-derived exosomes deliver the lncRNA CYTOR to hepatic stellate cells and promote liver fibrosis. *J. Cell Mol. Med.* **2024**, *28*, 18234. [CrossRef]
41. Dong, Z.; Li, S.; Wang, X.; Si, L.; Ma, R.; Bao, L.; Bo, A. lncRNA GAS5 restrains CCl4-induced hepatic fibrosis by targeting miR-23a through the PTEN/PI3K/Akt signaling pathway. *Am. J. Physiol. Gastrointest. Liver Physiol.* **2019**, *316*, 539–550. [CrossRef] [PubMed]
42. Chen, T.; Lin, H.; Chen, X.; Li, G.; Zhao, Y.; Zheng, L.; Shi, Z.; Zhang, K.; Hong, W.; Han, T. LncRNA Meg8 suppresses activation of hepatic stellate cells and epithelial-mesenchymal transition of hepatocytes via the Notch pathway. *Biochem. Biophys. Res. Commun.* **2020**, *521*, 921–927. [CrossRef] [PubMed]
43. Ou, Q.; Zhao, Y.; Zhou, J.; Wu, X. Comprehensive circular RNA expression profiles in a mouse model of nonalcoholic steatohepatitis. *Mol. Med. Rep.* **2019**, *19*, 2636–2648. [CrossRef] [PubMed]
44. Zhao, Q.; Liu, J.; Deng, H.; Ma, R.; Liao, J.Y.; Liang, H.; Hu, J.; Li, J.; Guo, Z.; Cai, J.; et al. Targeting Mitochondria-Located circRNA SCAR Alleviates NASH via Reducing mROS Output. *Cell* **2020**, *183*, 76–93. [CrossRef]
45. Zollner, G.; Trauner, M. Nuclear receptors as therapeutic targets in cholestatic liver diseases. *Br. J. Pharmacol.* **2009**, *156*, 7–27. [CrossRef]
46. Wang, Y.D.; Chen, W.D.; Wang, M.; Yu, D.; Forman, B.M.; Huang, W. Farnesoid X receptor antagonizes nuclear factor kappaB in hepatic inflammatory response. *Hepatology* **2008**, *48*, 1632–1643. [CrossRef]
47. Wagner, M.; Zollner, G.; Trauner, M. Nuclear bile acid receptor farnesoid X receptor meets nuclear factor-kappaB: New insights into hepatic inflammation. *Hepatology* **2008**, *48*, 1383–1386. [CrossRef]
48. Tran, M.; Liu, Y.; Huang, W.; Wang, L. Nuclear receptors and liver disease: Summary of the 2017 basic research symposium. *Hepatol Commun.* **2018**, *2*, 765–777. [CrossRef]
49. Jin, L.; Li, Y. Structural and functional insights into nuclear receptor signaling. *Adv. Drug Deliv. Rev.* **2010**, *62*, 1218–1226. [CrossRef]
50. Wu, W.B.; Chen, Y.Y.; Zhu, B.; Peng, X.M.; Zhang, S.W.; Zhou, M.L. Excessive bile acid activated NF-kappa B and promoted the development of alcoholic steatohepatitis in farnesoid X receptor deficient mice. *Biochimie* **2015**, *115*, 86–92. [CrossRef]
51. Kong, B.; Luyendyk, J.P.; Tawfik, O.; Guo, G.L. Farnesoid X receptor deficiency induces nonalcoholic steatohepatitis in low-density lipoprotein receptor-knockout mice fed a high-fat diet. *J. Pharmacol. Exp. Ther.* **2009**, *328*, 116–122. [CrossRef] [PubMed]
52. Baghdasaryan, A.; Claudel, T.; Gumhold, J.; Silbert, D.; Adorini, L.; Roda, A.; Vecchiotti, S.; Gonzalez, F.J.; Schoonjans, K.; Strazzabosco, M.; et al. Dual farnesoid X receptor/TGR5 agonist INT-767 reduces liver injury in the Mdr2-/- (Abcb4-/-) mouse cholangiopathy model by promoting biliary HCO^{-}_{3} output. *Hepatology* **2011**, *54*, 1303–1312. [CrossRef] [PubMed]
53. Sinha, R.A. Targeting nuclear receptors for NASH/MASH: From bench to bedside. *Liver Res.* **2024**, *8*, 34–45. [CrossRef] [PubMed]
54. Königshofer, P.; Brusilovskaya, K.; Petrenko, O.; Hofer, B.S.; Schwabl, P.; Trauner, M.; Reiberger, T. Nuclear receptors in liver fibrosis. *Biochim. Biophys. Acta Mol. Basis Dis.* **2021**, *1867*, 166235. [CrossRef]
55. Wang, X.C.; Song, K.; Tu, B.; Sun, H.; Zhou, Y.; Xu, S.S.; Lu, D.; Sha, J.M.; Tao, H. New aspects of the epigenetic regulation of EMT related to pulmonary fibrosis. *Eur. J. Pharmacol.* **2023**, *956*, 175959. [CrossRef]
56. Sisto, M.; Lisi, S. Epigenetic Regulation of EMP/EMT-Dependent Fibrosis. *Int. J. Mol. Sci.* **2024**, *25*, 2775. [CrossRef]
57. Liu, Y.; Wen, D.; Ho, C.; Yu, L.; Zheng, D.; O'Reilly, S.; Gao, Y.; Li, Q.; Zhang, Y. Epigenetics as a versatile regulator of fibrosis. *J. Transl. Med.* **2023**, *21*, 164. [CrossRef]
58. Liu, R.; Li, Y.; Zheng, Q.; Ding, M.; Zhou, H.; Li, X. Epigenetic modification in liver fibrosis: Promising therapeutic direction with significant challenges ahead. *Acta Pharm. Sin. B* **2024**, *14*, 1009–1029. [CrossRef]
59. Tao, S.; Duan, R.; Xu, T.; Hong, J.; Gu, W.; Lin, A.; Lian, L.; Huang, H.; Lu, J.; Li, T. Salvianolic acid B inhibits the progression of liver fibrosis in rats via modulation of the Hedgehog signaling pathway. *Exp. Ther. Med.* **2022**, *23*, 116. [CrossRef]
60. Yu, F.; Lu, Z.; Chen, B.; Wu, X.; Dong, P.; Zheng, J. Salvianolic acid B-induced microRNA-152 inhibits liver fibrosis by attenuating DNMT1-mediated Patched1 methylation. *J. Cell Mol. Med.* **2015**, *19*, 2617–2632. [CrossRef]
61. Guillot, A.; Tacke, F. Liver Macrophages: Old Dogmas and New Insights. *Hepatol. Commun.* **2019**, *3*, 730–743. [CrossRef] [PubMed]
62. Hoeffel, G.; Chen, J.; Lavin, Y.; Low, D.; Almeida, F.F.; See, P.; Beaudin, A.E.; Lum, J.; Low, I.; Forsberg, E.C.; et al. C-Myb(+) erythro-myeloid progenitor-derived fetal monocytes give rise to adult tissue-resident macrophages. *Immunity* **2015**, *42*, 665–678. [CrossRef] [PubMed]
63. Gomez Perdiguero, E.; Klapproth, K.; Schulz, C.; Busch, K.; Azzoni, E.; Crozet, L.; Garner, H.; Trouillet, C.; de Bruijn, M.F.; Geissmann, F.; et al. Tissue-resident macrophages originate from yolk-sac-derived erythro-myeloid progenitors. *Nature* **2015**, *518*, 547–551. [CrossRef]
64. Li, W.; Chang, N.; Li, L. Heterogeneity and Function of Kupffer Cells in Liver Injury. *Front. Immunol.* **2022**, *13*, 940867. [CrossRef]
65. Scott, C.L.; Zheng, F.; De Baetselier, P.; Martens, L.; Saeys, Y.; De Prijck, S.; Lippens, S.; Abels, C.; Schoonooghe, S.; Raes, G.; et al. Bone marrow-derived monocytes give rise to self-renewing and fully differentiated Kupffer cells. *Nat. Commun.* **2016**, *7*, 10321. [CrossRef]

66. Park, M.D.; Silvin, A.; Ginhoux, F.; Merad, M. Macrophages in health and disease. *Cell* **2022**, *185*, 4259–4279. [CrossRef]
67. Martrus, G.; Goebels, H.; Langeneckert, A.E.; Kah, J.; Flomm, F.; Ziegler, A.E.; Niehrs, A.; Löbl, S.M.; Russu, K.; Hess, L.U.; et al. CD49a Expression Identifies a Subset of Intrahepatic Macrophages in Humans. *Front. Immunol.* **2019**, *10*, 1247. [CrossRef]
68. Heymann, F.; Tacke, F. Immunology in the liver--from homeostasis to disease. *Nat. Rev. Gastroenterol. Hepatol.* **2016**, *13*, 88–110. [CrossRef]
69. Fogg, D.K.; Sibon, C.; Miled, C.; Jung, S.; Aucouturier, P.; Littman, D.R.; Cumano, A.; Geissmann, F. A clonogenic bone marrow progenitor specific for macrophages and dendritic cells. *Science* **2006**, *311*, 83–87. [CrossRef]
70. Tacke, F.; Zimmermann, H.W. Macrophage heterogeneity in liver injury and fibrosis. *J. Hepatol.* **2014**, *60*, 1090–1096. [CrossRef]
71. Pradere, J.P.; Kluwe, J.; De Minicis, S.; Jiao, J.J.; Gwak, G.Y.; Dapito, D.H.; Jang, M.K.; Guenther, N.D.; Mederacke, I.; Friedman, R.; et al. Hepatic macrophages but not dendritic cells contribute to liver fibrosis by promoting the survival of activated hepatic stellate cells in mice. *Hepatology* **2013**, *58*, 1461–1473. [CrossRef] [PubMed]
72. Ramachandran, P.; Pellicoro, A.; Vernon, M.A.; Boulter, L.; Aucott, R.L.; Ali, A.; Hartland, S.N.; Snowdon, V.K.; Cappon, A.; Gordon-Walker, T.T.; et al. Differential Ly-6C expression identifies the recruited macrophage phenotype, which orchestrates the regression of murine liver fibrosis. *Proc. Natl. Acad. Sci. USA* **2012**, *109*, 3186–3195. [CrossRef]
73. Traber, P.G.; Chou, H.; Zomer, E.; Hong, F.; Klyosov, A.; Fiel, M.I.; Friedman, S.L. Regression of fibrosis and reversal of cirrhosis in rats by galectin inhibitors in thioacetamide-induced liver disease. *PLoS ONE* **2013**, *8*, 75361. [CrossRef] [PubMed]
74. Khambu, B.; Yan, S.; Huda, N.; Yin, X.M. Role of High-Mobility Group Box-1 in Liver Pathogenesis. *Int. J. Mol. Sci.* **2019**, *20*, 5314. [CrossRef] [PubMed]
75. Tian, Z.; Hou, X.; Liu, W.; Han, Z.; Wei, L. Macrophages and hepatocellular carcinoma. *Cell Biosci.* **2019**, *9*, 79. [CrossRef]
76. Wan, J.; Benkdane, M.; Teixeira-Clerc, F.; Bonnafous, S.; Louvet, A.; Lafdil, F.; Pecker, F.; Tran, A.; Gual, P.; Mallat, A.; et al. M2 Kupffer cells promote M1 Kupffer cell apoptosis: A protective mechanism against alcoholic and nonalcoholic fatty liver disease. *Hepatology* **2014**, *59*, 130–142. [CrossRef]
77. Shapouri-Moghaddam, A.; Mohammadian, S.; Vazini, H.; Taghadosi, M.; Esmaeili, S.A.; Mardani, F.; Seifi, B.; Mohammadi, A.; Afshari, J.T.; Sahebkar, A. Macrophage plasticity, polarization, and function in health and disease. *J. Cell Physiol.* **2018**, *233*, 6425–6440. [CrossRef]
78. Spiller, K.L.; Wrona, E.A.; Romero-Torres, S.; Pallotta, I.; Graney, P.L.; Witherel, C.E.; Panicker, L.M.; Feldman, R.A.; Urbanska, A.M.; Santambrogio, L.; et al. Differential gene expression in human, murine, and cell line-derived macrophages upon polarization. *Exp. Cell Res.* **2016**, *347*, 1–13. [CrossRef]
79. Braga, T.T.; Agudelo, J.S.; Camara, N.O. Macrophages During the Fibrotic Process: M2 as Friend and Foe. *Front. Immunol.* **2015**, *6*, 602. [CrossRef]
80. Xue, J.; Schmidt, S.V.; Sander, J.; Draffehn, A.; Krebs, W.; Quester, I.; De Nardo, D.; Gohel, T.D.; Emde, M.; Schmidleithner, L.; et al. Transcriptome-based network analysis reveals a spectrum model of human macrophage activation. *Immunity* **2014**, *40*, 274–288. [CrossRef]
81. Murray, P.J.; Allen, J.E.; Biswas, S.K.; Fisher, E.A.; Gilroy, D.W.; Goerdt, S.; Gordon, S.; Hamilton, J.A.; Ivashkiv, L.B.; Lawrence, T.; et al. Macrophage activation and polarization: Nomenclature and experimental guidelines. *Immunity* **2014**, *41*, 14–20. [CrossRef] [PubMed]
82. Tacke, F. Targeting hepatic macrophages to treat liver diseases. *J. Hepatol.* **2017**, *66*, 1300–1312. [CrossRef] [PubMed]
83. Krenkel, O.; Tacke, F. Liver macrophages in tissue homeostasis and disease. *Nat. Rev. Immunol.* **2017**, *17*, 306–321. [CrossRef]
84. Ritz, T.; Krenkel, O.; Tacke, F. Dynamic plasticity of macrophage functions in diseased liver. *Cell Immunol.* **2018**, *330*, 175–182. [CrossRef]
85. Trus, E.; Basta, S.; Gee, K. Who's in charge here? Macrophage colony stimulating factor and granulocyte macrophage colony stimulating factor: Competing factors in macrophage polarization. *Cytokine* **2020**, *127*, 154939. [CrossRef]
86. Petrina, M.; Alothaimeen, T.; Bouzeineddine, N.Z.; Trus, E.; Banete, A.; Gee, K.; Basta, S. Granulocyte macrophage colony stimulating factor exerts dominant effects over macrophage colony stimulating factor during macrophage differentiation in vitro to induce an inflammatory phenotype. *Inflamm. Res.* **2024**, *73*, 253–262. [CrossRef]
87. Zheng, S.; Zhang, P.; Chen, Y.; Zheng, S.; Zheng, L.; Weng, Z. Inhibition of Notch Signaling Attenuates Schistosomiasis Hepatic Fibrosis via Blocking Macrophage M2 Polarization. *PLoS ONE* **2016**, *11*, e0166808. [CrossRef]
88. Bansal, R.; van Baarlen, J.; Storm, G.; Prakash, J. The interplay of the Notch signaling in hepatic stellate cells and macrophages determines the fate of liver fibrogenesis. *Sci. Rep.* **2015**, *5*, 18272. [CrossRef]
89. Krenkel, O.; Hundertmark, J.; Abdallah, A.T.; Kohlhepp, M.; Puengel, T.; Roth, T.; Branco, D.P.P.; Mossanen, J.C.; Luedde, T.; Trautwein, C.; et al. Myeloid cells in liver and bone marrow acquire a functionally distinct inflammatory phenotype during obesity-related steatohepatitis. *Gut* **2020**, *69*, 551–563. [CrossRef]
90. Xiong, X.; Kuang, H.; Ansari, S.; Liu, T.; Gong, J.; Wang, S.; Zhao, X.Y.; Ji, Y.; Li, C.; Guo, L.; et al. Landscape of Intercellular Crosstalk in Healthy and NASH Liver Revealed by Single-Cell Secretome Gene Analysis. *Mol. Cell.* **2019**, *75*, 644–660. [CrossRef]

91. Ramachandran, P.; Dobie, R.; Wilson-Kanamori, J.R.; Dora, E.F.; Henderson, B.E.P.; Luu, N.T.; Portman, J.R.; Matchett, K.P.; Brice, M.; Marwick, J.A.; et al. Resolving the fibrotic niche of human liver cirrhosis at single-cell level. *Nature* **2019**, *575*, 512–518. [CrossRef] [PubMed]
92. Xu, W.; Wu, M.; Chen, B.; Wang, H. Myeloid cells in alcoholic liver diseases: Mechanism and prospect. *Front. Immunol.* **2022**, *13*, 971346. [CrossRef] [PubMed]
93. Zhou, L.; Shen, H.; Li, X.; Wang, H. Endoplasmic reticulum stress in innate immune cells—A significant contribution to non-alcoholic fatty liver disease. *Front. Immunol.* **2022**, *13*, 951406. [CrossRef]
94. Mentink-Kane, M.M.; Cheever, A.W.; Wilson, M.S.; Madala, S.K.; Beers, L.M.; Ramalingam, T.R.; Wynn, T.A. Accelerated and progressive and lethal liver fibrosis in mice that lack interleukin (IL)-10, IL-12p40, and IL-13Rα2. *Gastroenterology* **2011**, *141*, 2200–2209. [CrossRef]
95. Li, F.; Li, Q.H.; Wang, J.Y.; Zhan, C.Y.; Xie, C.; Lu, W.Y. Effects of interferon-gamma liposomes targeted to platelet-derived growth factor receptor-beta on hepatic fibrosis in rats. *J. Control Release.* **2012**, *159*, 261–270. [CrossRef]
96. Naim, A.; Pan, Q.; Baig, M.S. Matrix Metalloproteinases (MMPs) in Liver Diseases. *J. Clin. Exp. Hepatol.* **2017**, *7*, 367–372. [CrossRef]
97. Robert, S.; Gicquel, T.; Bodin, A.; Lagente, V.; Boichot, E. Characterization of the MMP/TIMP Imbalance and Collagen Production Induced by IL-1β or TNF-α Release from Human Hepatic Stellate Cells. *PLoS ONE* **2016**, *11*, 0153118. [CrossRef]
98. Mederacke, I.; Hsu, C.C.; Troeger, J.S.; Huebener, P.; Mu, X.; Dapito, D.H.; Pradere, J.P.; Schwabe, R.F. Fate tracing reveals hepatic stellate cells as dominant contributors to liver fibrosis independent of its aetiology. *Nat. Commun.* **2013**, *4*, 2823. [CrossRef]
99. Hernandez-Gea, V.; Friedman, S.L. Pathogenesis of liver fibrosis. *Annu. Rev. Pathol.* **2011**, *6*, 425–456. [CrossRef]
100. Pinzani, M. Epithelial-mesenchymal transition in chronic liver disease: Fibrogenesis or escape from death? *J. Hepatol.* **2011**, *55*, 459–465. [CrossRef]
101. Chen, Y.; Fan, Y.; Guo, D.Y.; Xu, B.; Shi, X.Y.; Li, J.T.; Duan, L.F. Study on the relationship between hepatic fibrosis and epithelial-mesenchymal transition in intrahepatic cells. *Biomed. Pharmacother.* **2020**, *129*, 110413. [CrossRef] [PubMed]
102. Ribera, J.; Pauta, M.; Melgar-Lesmes, P.; Córdoba, B.; Bosch, A.; Calvo, M.; Rodrigo-Torres, D.; Sancho-Bru, P.; Mira, A.; Jiménez, W.; et al. A small population of liver endothelial cells undergoes endothelial-to-mesenchymal transition in response to chronic liver injury. *Am. J. Physiol. Gastrointest. Liver Physiol.* **2017**, *313*, 492–504. [CrossRef]
103. Piera-Velazquez, S.; Li, Z.; Jimenez, S.A. Role of endothelial-mesenchymal transition (EndoMT) in the pathogenesis of fibrotic disorders. *Am. J. Pathol.* **2011**, *179*, 1074–1080. [CrossRef] [PubMed]
104. Parola, M.; Pinzani, M. Liver fibrosis: Pathophysiology, pathogenetic targets and clinical issues. *Mol. Aspects Med.* **2019**, *65*, 37–55. [CrossRef] [PubMed]
105. Novo, E.; Bocca, C.; Foglia, B.; Protopapa, F.; Maggiora, M.; Parola, M.; Cannito, S. Liver fibrogenesis: Un update on established and emerging basic concepts. *Arch. Biochem. Biophys.* **2020**, *689*, 108445. [CrossRef]
106. Thoen, L.F.; Guimarães, E.L.; Dollé, L.; Mannaerts, I.; Najimi, M.; Sokal, E.; van Grunsven, L.A. A role for autophagy during hepatic stellate cell activation. *J. Hepatol.* **2011**, *55*, 1353–1360. [CrossRef]
107. Ni, H.M.; Woolbright, B.L.; Williams, J.; Copple, B.; Cui, W.; Luyendyk, J.P.; Jaeschke, H.; Ding, W.X. Nrf2 promotes the development of fibrosis and tumorigenesis in mice with defective hepatic autophagy. *J. Hepatol.* **2014**, *61*, 617–625. [CrossRef]
108. Hernández-Gea, V.; Ghiassi-Nejad, Z.; Rozenfeld, R.; Gordon, R.; Fiel, M.I.; Yue, Z.; Czaja, M.J.; Friedman, S.L. Autophagy releases lipid that promotes fibrogenesis by activated hepatic stellate cells in mice and in human tissues. *Gastroenterology* **2012**, *142*, 938–946. [CrossRef]
109. Mullan, L.A.; Mularczyk, E.J.; Kung, L.H.; Forouhan, M.; Wragg, J.M.; Goodacre, R.; Bateman, J.F.; Swanton, E.; Briggs, M.D.; Boot-Handford, R.P. Increased intracellular proteolysis reduces disease severity in an ER stress-associated dwarfism. *J. Clin. Investig.* **2017**, *127*, 3861–3865. [CrossRef]
110. Hidvegi, T.; Ewing, M.; Hale, P.; Dippold, C.; Beckett, C.; Kemp, C.; Maurice, N.; Mukherjee, A.; Goldbach, C.; Watkins, S.; et al. An autophagy-enhancing drug promotes degradation of mutant alpha1-antitrypsin Z and reduces hepatic fibrosis. *Science.* **2010**, *329*, 229–232. [CrossRef]
111. González-Rodríguez, A.; Mayoral, R.; Agra, N.; Valdecantos, M.P.; Pardo, V.; Miquilena-Colina, M.E.; Vargas-Castrillón, J.; Lo Iacono, O.; Corazzari, M.; Fimia, G.M.; et al. Impaired autophagic flux is associated with increased endoplasmic reticulum stress during the development of NAFLD. *Cell Death Dis.* **2014**, *5*, 1179. [CrossRef] [PubMed]
112. Bridle, K.R.; Popa, C.; Morgan, M.L.; Sobbe, A.L.; Clouston, A.D.; Fletcher, L.M.; Crawford, D.H. Rapamycin inhibits hepatic fibrosis in rats by attenuating multiple profibrogenic pathways. *Liver Transpl.* **2009**, *15*, 1315–1324. [CrossRef] [PubMed]
113. Gao, J.; Wei, B.; de Assuncao, T.M.; Liu, Z.; Hu, X.; Ibrahim, S.; Cooper, S.A.; Cao, S.; Shah, V.H.; Kostallari, E. Hepatic stellate cell autophagy inhibits extracellular vesicle release to attenuate liver fibrosis. *J. Hepatol.* **2020**, *73*, 1144–1154. [CrossRef]
114. Dobie, R.; Wilson-Kanamori, J.R.; Henderson, B.E.P.; Smith, J.R.; Matchett, K.P.; Portman, J.R.; Wallenborg, K.; Picelli, S.; Zagorska, A.; Pendem, S.V.; et al. Single-Cell Transcriptomics Uncovers Zonation of Function in the Mesenchyme during Liver Fibrosis. *Cell Rep.* **2019**, *29*, 1832–1847. [CrossRef]

115. Khan, M.A.; Fischer, J.; Harrer, L.; Schwiering, F.; Groneberg, D.; Friebe, A. Hepatic stellate cells in zone 1 engage in capillarization rather than myofibroblast formation in murine liver fibrosis. *Sci. Rep.* **2024**, *14*, 18840. [CrossRef]
116. Du, K.; Jun, J.H.; Dutta, R.K.; Diehl, A.M. Plasticity, heterogeneity, and multifunctionality of hepatic stellate cells in liver pathophysiology. *Hepatol. Commun.* **2024**, *8*, 0411. [CrossRef]
117. Zhang, W.J.; Chen, S.J.; Zhou, S.C.; Wu, S.Z.; Wang, H. Inflammasomes and Fibrosis. *Front. Immunol.* **2021**, *12*, 643149. [CrossRef]
118. Ramos-Tovar, E.; Muriel, P. Molecular Mechanisms That Link Oxidative Stress, Inflammation, and Fibrosis in the Liver. *Antioxidants* **2020**, *9*, 1279. [CrossRef]
119. Knorr, J.; Wree, A.; Tacke, F.; Feldstein, A.E. The NLRP3 Inflammasome in Alcoholic and Nonalcoholic Steatohepatitis. *Semin. Liver Dis.* **2020**, *40*, 298–306. [CrossRef]
120. Liu, C.; Chen, X.; Yang, L.; Kisseleva, T.; Brenner, D.A.; Seki, E. Transcriptional repression of the transforming growth factor β (TGF-β) Pseudoreceptor BMP and activin membrane-bound inhibitor (BAMBI) by Nuclear Factor κB (NF-κB) p50 enhances TGF-β signaling in hepatic stellate cells. *J. Biol. Chem.* **2014**, *289*, 7082–7091. [CrossRef]
121. Bartneck, M.; Koppe, C.; Fech, V.; Warzecha, K.T.; Kohlhepp, M.; Huss, S.; Weiskirchen, R.; Trautwein, C.; Luedde, T.; Tacke, F. Roles of CCR2 and CCR5 for Hepatic Macrophage Polarization in Mice With Liver Parenchymal Cell-Specific NEMO Deletion. *Cell Mol. Gastroenterol. Hepatol.* **2021**, *11*, 327–347. [CrossRef] [PubMed]
122. Iredale, J.P.; Thompson, A.; Henderson, N.C. Extracellular matrix degradation in liver fibrosis: Biochemistry and regulation. *Biochim. Biophys. Acta* **2013**, *1832*, 876–883. [CrossRef] [PubMed]
123. Seki, E.; de Minicis, S.; Inokuchi, S.; Taura, K.; Miyai, K.; van Rooijen, N.; Schwabe, R.F.; Brenner, D.A. CCR2 promotes hepatic fibrosis in mice. *Hepatology* **2009**, *50*, 185–197. [CrossRef]
124. Baeck, C.; Wehr, A.; Karlmark, K.R.; Heymann, F.; Vucur, M.; Gassler, N.; Huss, S.; Klussmann, S.; Eulberg, D.; Luedde, T.; et al. Pharmacological inhibition of the chemokine CCL2 (MCP-1) diminishes liver macrophage infiltration and steatohepatitis in chronic hepatic injury. *Gut* **2012**, *61*, 416–426. [CrossRef]
125. Cai, X.; Li, Z.; Zhang, Q.; Qu, Y.; Xu, M.; Wan, X.; Lu, L. CXCL6-EGFR-induced Kupffer cells secrete TGF-β1 promoting hepatic stellate cell activation via the SMAD2/BRD4/C-MYC/EZH2 pathway in liver fibrosis. *J. Cell Mol. Med.* **2018**, *22*, 5050–5061. [CrossRef]
126. Roehlen, N.; Crouchet, E.; Baumert, T.F. Liver Fibrosis: Mechanistic Concepts and Therapeutic Perspectives. *Cells* **2020**, *9*, 875. [CrossRef]
127. Sasaki, R.; Devhare, P.B.; Steele, R.; Ray, R.; Ray, R.B. Hepatitis C virus-induced CCL5 secretion from macrophages activates hepatic stellate cells. *Hepatology* **2017**, *66*, 746–757. [CrossRef]
128. Roh, Y.S.; Seki, E. Chemokines and Chemokine Receptors in the Development of NAFLD. *Adv. Exp. Med. Biol.* **2018**, *1061*, 45–53.
129. Matsuda, M.; Seki, E. Hepatic Stellate Cell-Macrophage Crosstalk in Liver Fibrosis and Carcinogenesis. *Semin. Liver Dis.* **2020**, *40*, 307–320. [CrossRef]
130. Kocabayoglu, P.; Lade, A.; Lee, Y.A.; Dragomir, A.C.; Sun, X.; Fiel, M.I.; Thung, S.; Aloman, C.; Soriano, P.; Hoshida, Y.; et al. β-PDGF receptor expressed by hepatic stellate cells regulates fibrosis in murine liver injury, but not carcinogenesis. *J. Hepatol.* **2015**, *63*, 141–147. [CrossRef]
131. Hedger, M.P.; de Kretser, D.M. The activins and their binding protein, follistatin-Diagnostic and therapeutic targets in inflammatory disease and fibrosis. *Cytokine Growth Factor. Rev.* **2013**, *24*, 285–295. [CrossRef] [PubMed]
132. Youssef, S.S.; Mostafa, A.; Saad, A.; Omran, M.H.; El Zanaty, T.; Mohamed Seif, S. Impact of IL12B gene rs 3212227 polymorphism on fibrosis, liver inflammation, and response to treatment in genotype 4 Egyptian hepatitis C patients. *Dis. Markers* **2013**, *35*, 431–437. [CrossRef] [PubMed]
133. Minutti, C.M.; Modak, R.V.; Macdonald, F.; Li, F.; Smyth, D.J.; Dorward, D.A.; Blair, N.; Husovsky, C.; Muir, A.; Giampazolias, E.; et al. A Macrophage-Pericyte Axis Directs Tissue Restoration via Amphiregulin-Induced Transforming Growth Factor Beta Activation. *Immunity* **2019**, *50*, 645–654. [CrossRef] [PubMed]
134. Qu, J.; Wang, L.; Li, Y.; Li, X. Liver sinusoidal endothelial cell: An important yet often overlooked player in the liver fibrosis. *Clin. Mol. Hepatol.* **2024**, *30*, 303–325. [CrossRef] [PubMed]
135. Schildberg, F.A.; Wojtalla, A.; Siegmund, S.V.; Endl, E.; Diehl, L.; Abdullah, Z.; Kurts, C.; Knolle, P.A. Murine hepatic stellate cells veto CD8 T cell activation by a CD54-dependent mechanism. *Hepatology* **2011**, *54*, 262–272. [CrossRef]
136. Géraud, C.; Evdokimov, K.; Straub, B.K.; Peitsch, W.K.; Demory, A.; Dörflinger, Y.; Schledzewski, K.; Schmieder, A.; Schemmer, P.; Augustin, H.G.; et al. Unique cell type-specific junctional complexes in vascular endothelium of human and rat liver sinusoids. *PLoS ONE* **2012**, *7*, 34206. [CrossRef]
137. Jophlin, L.L.; Cao, S.; Shah, V.H. The Transcriptome of Hepatic Fibrosis Revealed by Single-Cell RNA Sequencing. *Hepatology* **2020**, *71*, 1865–1867. [CrossRef]
138. Liu, D.; Fu, X.; Wang, Y.; Wang, X.; Wang, H.; Wen, J.; Kang, N. Protein diaphanous homolog 1 (Diaph1) promotes myofibroblastic activation of hepatic stellate cells by regulating Rab5a activity and TGFβ receptor endocytosis. *FASEB J.* **2020**, *34*, 7345–7359. [CrossRef]

139. Hammoutene, A.; Biquard, L.; Lasselin, J.; Kheloufi, M.; Tanguy, M.; Vion, A.C.; Mérian, J.; Colnot, N.; Loyer, X.; Tedgui, A.; et al. A defect in endothelial autophagy occurs in patients with non-alcoholic steatohepatitis and promotes inflammation and fibrosis. *J. Hepatol.* **2020**, *72*, 528–538. [CrossRef]
140. Li, Z.; Chen, B.; Dong, W.; Kong, M.; Fan, Z.; Yu, L.; Wu, D.; Lu, J.; Xu, Y. MKL1 promotes endothelial-to-mesenchymal transition and liver fibrosis by activating TWIST1 transcription. *Cell Death Dis.* **2019**, *10*, 899. [CrossRef]
141. Derynck, R.; Budi, E.H. Specificity, versatility, and control of TGF-β family signaling. *Sci. Signal.* **2019**, *12*, eaav5183. [CrossRef] [PubMed]
142. Fabregat, I.; Moreno-Càceres, J.; Sánchez, A.; Dooley, S.; Dewidar, B.; Giannelli, G.; Ten Dijke, P.; IT-LIVER Consortium. TGF-β signalling and liver disease. *FEBS J.* **2016**, *283*, 2219–2232. [CrossRef] [PubMed]
143. Wang, X.L.; Yang, M.; Wang, Y. Roles of transforming growth factor-β signaling in liver disease. *World J. Hepatol.* **2024**, *16*, 973–979. [CrossRef]
144. Carter, J.K.; Friedman, S.L. Hepatic Stellate Cell-Immune Interactions in NASH. *Front. Endocrinol.* **2022**, *13*, 867940. [CrossRef]
145. Xiang, D.M.; Sun, W.; Ning, B.F.; Zhou, T.F.; Li, X.F.; Zhong, W.; Cheng, Z.; Xia, M.Y.; Wang, X.; Deng, X.; et al. The HLF/IL-6/STAT3 feedforward circuit drives hepatic stellate cell activation to promote liver fibrosis. *Gut* **2018**, *67*, 1704–1715. [CrossRef]
146. Kou, K.; Li, S.; Qiu, W.; Fan, Z.; Li, M.; Lv, G. Hypoxia-inducible factor 1α/IL-6 axis in activated hepatic stellate cells aggravates liver fibrosis. *Biochem. Biophys. Res. Commun.* **2023**, *653*, 21–30. [CrossRef]
147. Eguchi, A.; Yan, R.; Pan, S.Q.; Wu, R.; Kim, J.; Chen, Y.; Ansong, C.; Smith, R.D.; Tempaku, M.; Ohno-Machado, L.; et al. Comprehensive characterization of hepatocyte-derived extracellular vesicles identifies direct miRNA-based regulation of hepatic stellate cells and DAMP-based hepatic macrophage IL-1β and IL-17 upregulation in alcoholic hepatitis mice. *J. Mol. Med.* **2020**, *98*, 1021–1034. [CrossRef]
148. Lodyga, M.; Cambridge, E.; Karvonen, H.M.; Pakshir, P.; Wu, B.; Boo, S.; Kiebalo, M.; Kaarteenaho, R.; Glogauer, M.; Kapoor, M.; et al. Cadherin-11-mediated adhesion of macrophages to myofibroblasts establishes a profibrotic niche of active TGF-β. *Sci Signal.* **2019**, *12*, eaao3469. [CrossRef]
149. Poisson, J.; Lemoinne, S.; Boulanger, C.; Durand, F.; Moreau, R.; Valla, D.; Rautou, P.E. Liver sinusoidal endothelial cells: Physiology and role in liver diseases. *J. Hepatol.* **2017**, *66*, 212–227. [CrossRef]
150. McConnell, M.J.; Kostallari, E.; Ibrahim, S.H.; Iwakiri, Y. The evolving role of liver sinusoidal endothelial cells in liver health and disease. *Hepatology* **2023**, *78*, 649–669. [CrossRef]
151. Du, W.; Wang, L. The Crosstalk Between Liver Sinusoidal Endothelial Cells and Hepatic Microenvironment in NASH Related Liver Fibrosis. *Front. Immunol.* **2022**, *13*, 936196. [CrossRef] [PubMed]
152. Guo, Q.; Furuta, K.; Islam, S.; Caporarello, N.; Kostallari, E.; Dielis, K.; Tschumperlin, D.J.; Hirsova, P.; Ibrahim, S.H. Liver sinusoidal endothelial cell expressed vascular cell adhesion molecule 1 promotes liver fibrosis. *Front. Immunol.* **2022**, *13*, 983255. [CrossRef] [PubMed]
153. Strauss, O.; Phillips, A.; Ruggiero, K.; Bartlett, A.; Dunbar, P.R. Immunofluorescence identifies distinct subsets of endothelial cells in the human liver. *Sci. Rep.* **2017**, *7*, 44356. [CrossRef]
154. Wei, M.; Zhang, Y.; Zhang, H.; Huang, Z.; Miao, H.; Zhang, T.; Lu, B.; Ji, L. HMGB1 induced endothelial to mesenchymal transition in liver fibrosis: The key regulation of early growth response factor 1. *Biochim. Biophys. Acta Gen. Subj.* **2022**, *1866*, 130202. [CrossRef]
155. Ruan, B.; Duan, J.L.; Xu, H.; Tao, K.S.; Han, H.; Dou, G.R.; Wang, L. Capillarized liver sinusoidal endothelial cells undergo partial endothelial-mesenchymal transition to actively deposit sinusoidal ECM in liver fibrosis. *Front. Cell Dev. Biol.* **2021**, *9*, 671081. [CrossRef]
156. Dewidar, B.; Meyer, C.; Dooley, S.; Meindl-Beinker, A.N. TGF-β in Hepatic Stellate Cell Activation and Liver Fibrogenesis-Updated 2019. *Cells* **2019**, *8*, 1419. [CrossRef]
157. de Gouville, A.C.; Boullay, V.; Krysa, G.; Pilot, J.; Brusq, J.M.; Loriolle, F.; Gauthier, J.M.; Papworth, S.A.; Laroze, A.; Gellibert, F.; et al. Inhibition of TGF-beta signaling by an ALK5 inhibitor protects rats from dimethylnitrosamine-induced liver fibrosis. *Br. J. Pharmacol.* **2005**, *145*, 166–177. [CrossRef]
158. Chen, Y.; Li, Q.; Tu, K.; Wang, Y.; Wang, X.; Liu, D.; Chen, C.; Liu, D.; Yang, R.; Qiu, W.; et al. Focal Adhesion Kinase Promotes Hepatic Stellate Cell Activation by Regulating Plasma Membrane Localization of TGFβ Receptor 2. *Hepatol Commun.* **2019**, *4*, 268–283. [CrossRef]
159. Robertson, I.B.; Rifkin, D.B. Regulation of the Bioavailability of TGF-β and TGF-β-Related Proteins. *Cold Spring Harb. Perspect. Biol.* **2016**, *8*, a021907. [CrossRef]
160. Dong, X.; Zhao, B.; Iacob, R.E.; Zhu, J.; Koksal, A.C.; Lu, C.; Engen, J.R.; Springer, T.A. Force interacts with macromolecular structure in activation of TGF-β. *Nature* **2017**, *542*, 55–59. [CrossRef]
161. Reed, N.I.; Jo, H.; Chen, C.; Tsujino, K.; Arnold, T.D.; DeGrado, W.F.; Sheppard, D. The αvβ1 integrin plays a critical in vivo role in tissue fibrosis. *Sci. Transl. Med.* **2015**, *7*, 288ra79. [CrossRef] [PubMed]

162. Wipff, P.J.; Rifkin, D.B.; Meister, J.J.; Hinz, B. Myofibroblast contraction activates latent TGF-beta1 from the extracellular matrix. *J. Cell Biol.* **2007**, *179*, 1311–1323. [CrossRef]
163. Peng, Z.W.; Ikenaga, N.; Liu, S.B.; Sverdlov, D.Y.; Vaid, K.A.; Dixit, R.; Weinreb, P.H.; Violette, S.; Sheppard, D.; Schuppan, D.; et al. Integrin αvβ6 critically regulates hepatic progenitor cell function and promotes ductular reaction, fibrosis, and tumorigenesis. *Hepatology* **2016**, *63*, 217–232. [CrossRef] [PubMed]
164. Wang, B.; Dolinski, B.M.; Kikuchi, N.; Leone, D.R.; Peters, M.G.; Weinreb, P.H.; Violette, S.M.; Bissell, D.M. Role of alphavbeta6 integrin in acute biliary fibrosis. *Hepatology* **2007**, *46*, 1404–1412. [CrossRef] [PubMed]
165. Henderson, N.C.; Arnold, T.D.; Katamura, Y.; Giacomini, M.M.; Rodriguez, J.D.; McCarty, J.H.; Pellicoro, A.; Raschperger, E.; Betsholtz, C.; Ruminski, P.G.; et al. Targeting of αv integrin identifies a core molecular pathway that regulates fibrosis in several organs. *Nat. Med.* **2013**, *19*, 1617–1624. [CrossRef]
166. Braunersreuther, V.; Viviani, G.L.; Mach, F.; Montecucco, F. Role of cytokines and chemokines in non-alcoholic fatty liver disease. *World J. Gastroenterol.* **2012**, *18*, 727–735. [CrossRef]
167. Ahmed, H.; Umar, M.I.; Imran, S.; Javaid, F.; Syed, S.K.; Riaz, R.; Hassan, W. TGF-β1 signaling can worsen NAFLD with liver fibrosis backdrop. *Exp. Mol. Pathol.* **2022**, *124*, 104733. [CrossRef]
168. Wang, B.; Koh, P.; Winbanks, C.; Coughlan, M.T.; McClelland, A.; Watson, A.; Jandeleit-Dahm, K.; Burns, W.C.; Thomas, M.C.; Cooper, M.E.; et al. *miR*-200a Prevents renal fibrogenesis through repression of TGF-β2 expression. *Diabetes* **2011**, *60*, 280–287. [CrossRef]
169. Voumvouraki, A.; Koulentaki, M.; Tzardi, M.; Sfakianaki, O.; Manousou, P.; Notas, G.; Kouroumalis, E. Increased TGF-β3 in primary biliary cirrhosis: An abnormality related to pathogenesis? *World J. Gastroenterol.* **2010**, *16*, 5057–5064. [CrossRef]
170. McLane, L.M.; Abdel-Hakeem, M.S.; Wherry, E.J. CD8 T Cell Exhaustion During Chronic Viral Infection and Cancer. *Annu. Rev. Immunol.* **2019**, *37*, 457–495. [CrossRef]
171. Kurachi, M. CD8+ T cell exhaustion. *Semin. Immunopathol.* **2019**, *41*, 327–337. [CrossRef] [PubMed]
172. Li, T.Y.; Yang, Y.; Zhou, G.; Tu, Z.K. Immune suppression in chronic hepatitis B infection associated liver disease: A review. *World J. Gastroenterol.* **2019**, *25*, 3527–3537. [CrossRef] [PubMed]
173. Li, H.; Zhai, N.; Wang, Z.; Song, H.; Yang, Y.; Cui, A.; Li, T.; Wang, G.; Niu, J.; Crispe, I.N.; et al. Regulatory NK cells mediated between immunosuppressive monocytes and dysfunctional T cells in chronic HBV infection. *Gut* **2018**, *67*, 2035–2044. [CrossRef]
174. Kiagiadaki, F.; Kampa, M.; Voumvouraki, A.; Castanas, E.; Kouroumalis, E.; Notas, G. Activin-A causes Hepatic stellate cell activation via the induction of TNFα and TGFβ in Kupffer cells. *Biochim. Biophys. Acta Mol. Basis Dis.* **2018**, *1864*, 891–899. [CrossRef]
175. Tsuda, M.; Zhang, W.; Yang, G.X.; Tsuneyama, K.; Ando, Y.; Kawata, K.; Park, O.; Leung, P.S.; Coppel, R.L.; Ansari, A.A.; et al. Deletion of interleukin (IL)-12p35 induces liver fibrosis in dominant-negative TGFβ receptor type II mice. *Hepatology* **2013**, *57*, 806–816. [CrossRef]
176. Masola, V.; Carraro, A.; Granata, S.; Signorini, L.; Bellin, G.; Violi, P.; Lupo, A.; Tedeschi, U.; Onisto, M.; Gambaro, G.; et al. In vitro effects of interleukin (IL)-1 beta inhibition on the epithelial-to-mesenchymal transition (EMT) of renal tubular and hepatic stellate cells. *J. Transl. Med.* **2019**, *17*, 12. [CrossRef]
177. Sudo, K.; Yamada, Y.; Moriwaki, H.; Saito, K.; Seishima, M. Lack of tumor necrosis factor receptor type 1 inhibits liver fibrosis induced by carbon tetrachloride in mice. *Cytokine* **2005**, *29*, 236–244. [CrossRef]
178. Seki, E.; De Minicis, S.; Osterreicher, C.H.; Kluwe, J.; Osawa, Y.; Brenner, D.A.; Schwabe, R.F. TLR4 enhances TGF-beta signaling and hepatic fibrosis. *Nat. Med.* **2007**, *13*, 1324–1332. [CrossRef]
179. Miura, K.; Kodama, Y.; Inokuchi, S.; Schnabl, B.; Aoyama, T.; Ohnishi, H.; Olefsky, J.M.; Brenner, D.A.; Seki, E. Toll-like receptor 9 promotes steatohepatitis by induction of interleukin-1beta in mice. *Gastroenterology* **2010**, *139*, 323–334. [CrossRef]
180. Kulkarni, A.B.; Karlsson, S. Inflammation and TGF beta 1: Lessons from the TGF beta 1 null mouse. *Res. Immunol.* **1997**, *148*, 453–456. [CrossRef]
181. Tsomidis, I.; Notas, G.; Xidakis, C.; Voumvouraki, A.; Samonakis, D.N.; Koulentaki, M.; Kouroumalis, E. Enzymes of Fibrosis in Chronic Liver Disease. *Biomedicines* **2022**, *10*, 3179. [CrossRef] [PubMed]
182. Akkız, H.; Gieseler, R.K.; Canbay, A. Liver Fibrosis: From Basic Science towards Clinical Progress, Focusing on the Central Role of Hepatic Stellate Cells. *Int. J. Mol. Sci.* **2024**, *25*, 7873. [CrossRef] [PubMed]
183. Hammerich, L.; Tacke, F. Hepatic inflammatory responses in liver fibrosis. *Nat. Rev. Gastroenterol. Hepatol.* **2023**, *20*, 633–646. [CrossRef] [PubMed]
184. Jeong, W.I.; Park, O.; Suh, Y.G.; Byun, J.S.; Park, S.Y.; Choi, E.; Kim, J.K.; Ko, H.; Wang, H.; Miller, A.M.; et al. Suppression of innate immunity (natural killer cell/interferon-γ) in the advanced stages of liver fibrosis in mice. *Hepatology* **2011**, *53*, 1342–1351. [CrossRef]
185. Glässner, A.; Eisenhardt, M.; Krämer, B.; Körner, C.; Coenen, M.; Sauerbruch, T.; Spengler, U.; Nattermann, J. NK cells from HCV-infected patients effectively induce apoptosis of activated primary human hepatic stellate cells in a TRAIL-, FasL- and NKG2D-dependent manner. *Lab. Investig.* **2012**, *92*, 967–977. [CrossRef]

186. Krizhanovsky, V.; Yon, M.; Dickins, R.A.; Hearn, S.; Simon, J.; Miething, C.; Yee, H.; Zender, L.; Lowe, S.W. Senescence of activated stellate cells limits liver fibrosis. *Cell* **2008**, *134*, 657–667. [CrossRef]
187. Wang, H.; Yin, S. Natural killer T cells in liver injury, inflammation and cancer. *Expert. Rev. Gastroenterol. Hepatol.* **2015**, *9*, 1077–1085. [CrossRef]
188. Wang, Y.; Li, Y.; Qiu, Y.; Shen, M.; Wang, L.; Shao, J.; Zhang, F.; Xu, X.; Zhang, Z.; Guo, M.; et al. Artesunate Induces Ferroptosis in Hepatic Stellate Cells and Alleviates Liver Fibrosis via the ROCK1/ATF3 Axis. *J. Clin. Transl. Hepatol.* **2024**, *12*, 36–51. [CrossRef]
189. Kisseleva, T.; Brenner, D. Molecular and cellular mechanisms of liver fibrosis and its regression. *Nat. Rev. Gastroenterol. Hepatol.* **2021**, *18*, 151–166. [CrossRef]
190. Campana, L.; Esser, H.; Huch, M.; Forbes, S. Liver regeneration and inflammation: From fundamental science to clinical applications. *Nat. Rev. Mol. Cell Biol.* **2021**, *22*, 608–624. [CrossRef]
191. Vonderlin, J.; Chavakis, T.; Sieweke, M.; Tacke, F. The Multifaceted Roles of Macrophages in NAFLD Pathogenesis. *Cell Mol. Gastroenterol. Hepatol.* **2023**, *15*, 1311–1324. [CrossRef] [PubMed]
192. Tacke, F.; Puengel, T.; Loomba, R.; Friedman, S.L. An integrated view of anti-inflammatory and antifibrotic targets for the treatment of NASH. *J. Hepatol.* **2023**, *79*, 552–566. [CrossRef] [PubMed]
193. Campana, L.; Iredale, J.P. Regression of Liver Fibrosis. *Semin. Liver Dis.* **2017**, *37*, 1–10.
194. Zhang, L.; Schuppan, D. Traditional Chinese Medicine (TCM) for fibrotic liver disease: Hope and hype. *J. Hepatol.* **2014**, *61*, 166–168. [CrossRef]
195. Li, Z.; Zhu, J.F.; Ouyang, H. Progress on traditional Chinese medicine in improving hepatic fibrosis through inhibiting oxidative stress. *World J. Hepatol.* **2023**, *15*, 1091–1108. [CrossRef]
196. Dai, Z.; Liao, X.; Wieland, L.S.; Hu, J.; Wang, Y.; Kim, T.H.; Liu, J.P.; Zhan, S.; Robinson, N. Cochrane systematic reviews on traditional Chinese medicine: What matters-the quantity or quality of evidence? *Phytomedicine* **2022**, *98*, 153921. [CrossRef]
197. Schulze, R.J.; Schott, M.B.; Casey, C.A.; Tuma, P.L.; McNiven, M.A. The cell biology of the hepatocyte: A membrane trafficking machine. *J. Cell Biol.* **2019**, *218*, 2096–2112. [CrossRef]
198. Kubes, P.; Jenne, C. Immune Responses in the Liver. *Annu. Rev. Immunol.* **2018**, *36*, 247–277. [CrossRef]
199. Gong, J.; Tu, W.; Liu, J.; Tian, D. Hepatocytes: A key role in liver inflammation. *Front. Immunol.* **2023**, *13*, 1083780. [CrossRef]
200. Shetty, S.; Lalor, P.F.; Adams, D.H. Liver sinusoidal endothelial cells—Gatekeepers of hepatic immunity. *Nat. Rev. Gastroenterol. Hepatol.* **2018**, *15*, 555–567. [CrossRef]
201. Schildberg, F.A.; Hegenbarth, S.I.; Schumak, B.; Scholz, K.; Limmer, A.; Knolle, P.A. Liver sinusoidal endothelial cells veto CD8 T cell activation by antigen-presenting dendritic cells. *Eur. J. Immunol.* **2008**, *38*, 957–967. [CrossRef] [PubMed]
202. Diehl, L.; Schurich, A.; Grochtmann, R.; Hegenbarth, S.; Chen, L.; Knolle, P.A. Tolerogenic maturation of liver sinusoidal endothelial cells promotes B7-homolog 1-dependent CD8+ T cell tolerance. *Hepatology* **2008**, *47*, 296–305. [CrossRef] [PubMed]
203. Crispe, I.N.; Giannandrea, M.; Klein, I.; John, B.; Sampson, B.; Wuensch, S. Cellular and molecular mechanisms of liver tolerance. *Immunol. Rev.* **2006**, *213*, 101–118. [CrossRef] [PubMed]
204. Harada, K.; Isse, K.; Sato, Y.; Ozaki, S.; Nakanuma, Y. Endotoxin tolerance in human intrahepatic biliary epithelial cells is induced by upregulation of IRAK-M. *Liver Int.* **2006**, *26*, 935–942. [CrossRef]
205. Zheng, M.; Tian, Z. Liver-Mediated Adaptive Immune Tolerance. *Front. Immunol.* **2019**, *10*, 2525. [CrossRef]
206. Jenne, C.N.; Kubes, P. Immune surveillance by the liver. *Nat. Immunol.* **2013**, *14*, 996–1006. [CrossRef]
207. Horst, A.K.; Neumann, K.; Diehl, L.; Tiegs, G. Modulation of liver tolerance by conventional and nonconventional antigen-presenting cells and regulatory immune cells. *Cell Mol. Immunol.* **2016**, *13*, 277–292. [CrossRef]
208. Yu, J.; Chen, Y.; Wu, Y.; Ye, L.; Lian, Z.; Wei, H.; Sun, R.; Tian, Z. The differential organogenesis and functionality of two liver-draining lymph nodes in mice. *J. Autoimmun.* **2017**, *84*, 109–121. [CrossRef]
209. Michalek, R.D.; Gerriets, V.A.; Jacobs, S.R.; Macintyre, A.N.; MacIver, N.J.; Mason, E.F.; Sullivan, S.A.; Nichols, A.G.; Rathmell, J.C. Cutting edge: Distinct glycolytic and lipid oxidative metabolic programs are essential for effector and regulatory CD4+ T cell subsets. *J. Immunol.* **2011**, *186*, 3299–3303. [CrossRef]
210. Vats, D.; Mukundan, L.; Odegaard, J.I.; Zhang, L.; Smith, K.L.; Morel, C.R.; Wagner, R.A.; Greaves, D.R.; Murray, P.J.; Chawla, A. Oxidative metabolism and PGC-1beta attenuate macrophage-mediated inflammation. *Cell Metab.* **2006**, *4*, 13–24. [CrossRef]
211. Jung, J.; Zeng, H.; Horng, T. Metabolism as a guiding force for immunity. *Nat. Cell Biol.* **2019**, *21*, 85–93. [CrossRef] [PubMed]
212. Cramer, T.; Yamanishi, Y.; Clausen, B.E.; Förster, I.; Pawlinski, R.; Mackman, N.; Haase, V.H.; Jaenisch, R.; Corr, M.; Nizet, V.; et al. HIF-1alpha is essential for myeloid cell-mediated inflammation. *Cell* **2003**, *112*, 645–657. [CrossRef] [PubMed]
213. Zhou, Y.; Zhang, H.; Yao, Y.; Zhang, X.; Guan, Y.; Zheng, F. CD4+ T cell activation and inflammation in NASH-related fibrosis. *Front. Immunol.* **2022**, *13*, 967410. [CrossRef]
214. Alegre, F.; Pelegrin, P.; Feldstein, A.E. Inflammasomes in Liver Fibrosis. *Semin. Liver Dis.* **2017**, *37*, 119–127. [CrossRef]
215. Zhou, Y.; Wu, R.; Wang, X.; Bao, X.; Lu, C. Roles of necroptosis in alcoholic liver disease and hepatic pathogenesis. *Cell Prolif.* **2022**, *55*, 13193. [CrossRef]
216. Bataller, R.; Arab, J.P.; Shah, V.H. Alcohol-Associated Hepatitis. *N. Engl. J. Med.* **2022**, *387*, 2436–2448. [CrossRef]

217. Arab, J.P.; Arrese, M.; Shah, V.H. Gut microbiota in non-alcoholic fatty liver disease and alcohol-related liver disease: Current concepts and perspectives. *Hepatol. Res.* **2020**, *50*, 407–418. [CrossRef]
218. Albillos, A.; Martin-Mateos, R.; Van der Merwe, S.; Wiest, R.; Jalan, R.; Álvarez-Mon, M. Cirrhosis-associated immune dysfunction. *Nat. Rev. Gastroenterol. Hepatol.* **2022**, *19*, 112–134. [CrossRef]
219. Wiering, L.; Subramanian, P.; Hammerich, L. Hepatic Stellate Cells: Dictating Outcome in Nonalcoholic Fatty Liver Disease. *Cell Mol. Gastroenterol. Hepatol.* **2023**, *15*, 1277–1292. [CrossRef]
220. Zhangdi, H.J.; Su, S.B.; Wang, F.; Liang, Z.Y.; Yan, Y.D.; Qin, S.Y.; Jiang, H.X. Crosstalk network among multiple inflammatory mediators in liver fibrosis. *World J. Gastroenterol.* **2019**, *25*, 4835–4849. [CrossRef]
221. Berumen, J.; Baglieri, J.; Kisseleva, T.; Mekeel, K. Liver fibrosis: Pathophysiology and clinical implications. *WIREs Mech. Dis.* **2021**, *13*, 1499. [CrossRef] [PubMed]
222. Nakamoto, N.; Kanai, T. Role of toll-like receptors in immune activation and tolerance in the liver. *Front. Immunol.* **2014**, *5*, 221. [CrossRef] [PubMed]
223. Torre, P.; Motta, B.M.; Sciorio, R.; Masarone, M.; Persico, M. Inflammation and Fibrogenesis in MAFLD: Role of the Hepatic Immune System. *Front. Med.* **2021**, *8*, 781567. [CrossRef]
224. Liu, Y.; Dong, Y.; Wu, X.; Wang, X.; Niu, J. Identification of Immune Microenvironment Changes and the Expression of Immune-Related Genes in Liver Cirrhosis. *Front. Immunol.* **2022**, *13*, 918445. [CrossRef]
225. Khanam, A.; Chua, J.V.; Kottilil, S. Immunopathology of Chronic Hepatitis B Infection: Role of Innate and Adaptive Immune Response in Disease Progression. *Int. J. Mol. Sci.* **2021**, *22*, 5497. [CrossRef]
226. Martinon, F. Detection of immune danger signals by NALP3. *J. Leukoc. Biol.* **2008**, *83*, 507–511. [CrossRef]
227. Swanson, K.V.; Deng, M.; Ting, J.P. The NLRP3 inflammasome: Molecular activation and regulation to therapeutics. *Nat. Rev. Immunol.* **2019**, *19*, 477–489. [CrossRef]
228. Gaul, S.; Leszczynska, A.; Alegre, F.; Kaufmann, B.; Johnson, C.D.; Adams, L.A.; Wree, A.; Damm, G.; Seehofer, D.; Calvente, C.J.; et al. Hepatocyte pyroptosis and release of inflammasome particles induce stellate cell activation and liver fibrosis. *J. Hepatol.* **2021**, *74*, 156–167. [CrossRef]
229. Kong, F.; You, H.; Zheng, K.; Tang, R.; Zheng, C. The crosstalk between pattern-recognition receptor signaling and calcium signaling. *Int. J. Biol. Macromol.* **2021**, *192*, 745–756. [CrossRef]
230. Wree, A.; Holtmann, T.M.; Inzaugarat, M.E.; Feldstein, A.E. Novel Drivers of the Inflammatory Response in Liver Injury and Fibrosis. *Semin. Liver Dis.* **2019**, *39*, 275–282. [CrossRef]
231. Jiang, Y.; Que, W.; Zhu, P.; Li, X.K. The Role of Diverse Liver Cells in Liver Transplantation Tolerance. *Front. Immunol.* **2020**, *11*, 1203. [CrossRef] [PubMed]
232. Mühlbauer, M.; Fleck, M.; Schütz, C.; Weiss, T.; Froh, M.; Blank, C.; Schölmerich, J.; Hellerbrand, C. PD-L1 is induced in hepatocytes by viral infection and by interferon-alpha and -gamma and mediates T cell apoptosis. *J. Hepatol.* **2006**, *45*, 520–528. [CrossRef] [PubMed]
233. Mooring, M.; Fowl, B.H.; Lum, S.Z.C.; Liu, Y.; Yao, K.; Softic, S.; Kirchner, R.; Bernstein, A.; Singhi, A.D.; Jay, D.G.; et al. Hepatocyte Stress Increases Expression of Yes-Associated Protein and Transcriptional Coactivator With PDZ-Binding Motif in Hepatocytes to Promote Parenchymal Inflammation and Fibrosis. *Hepatology* **2020**, *71*, 1813–1830. [CrossRef] [PubMed]
234. Futakuchi, A.; Inoue, T.; Wei, F.Y.; Inoue-Mochita, M.; Fujimoto, T.; Tomizawa, K.; Tanihara, H. YAP/TAZ Are Essential for TGF-β2-Mediated Conjunctival Fibrosis. *Investig. Ophthalmol. Vis. Sci.* **2018**, *59*, 3069–3078. [CrossRef] [PubMed]
235. Filliol, A.; Schwabe, R.F. FoxM1 Induces CCl2 Secretion From Hepatocytes Triggering Hepatic Inflammation, Injury, Fibrosis, and Liver Cancer. *Cell Mol. Gastroenterol. Hepatol.* **2020**, *9*, 555–556. [CrossRef]
236. Kurahashi, T.; Yoshida, Y.; Ogura, S.; Egawa, M.; Furuta, K.; Hikita, H.; Kodama, T.; Sakamori, R.; Kiso, S.; Kamada, Y.; et al. Forkhead Box M1 Transcription Factor Drives Liver Inflammation Linking to Hepatocarcinogenesis in Mice. *Cell Mol. Gastroenterol. Hepatol.* **2020**, *9*, 425–446. [CrossRef]
237. Lu, J.G.; Iyasu, A.; French, B.; Tillman, B.; French, S.W. Overexpression of MHCII by hepatocytes in alcoholic hepatitis (AH) compared to non-alcoholic steatohepatitis (NASH) and normal controls. *Alcohol* **2020**, *84*, 27–32. [CrossRef]
238. Huby, T.; Gautier, E.L. Immune cell-mediated features of non-alcoholic steatohepatitis. *Nat. Rev. Immunol.* **2022**, *22*, 429–443. [CrossRef]
239. Zhang, Q.; Qu, Y.; Zhang, Q.; Li, F.; Li, B.; Li, Z.; Dong, Y.; Lu, L.; Cai, X. Exosomes derived from hepatitis B virus-infected hepatocytes promote liver fibrosis via miR-222/TFRC axis. *Cell Biol. Toxicol.* **2023**, *39*, 467–481. [CrossRef]
240. Francis, H.; Wu, N.; Alpini, G.; Meng, F. Hepatocyte Autophagy: Maintaining a Toxic-Free Environment. *Hepatology* **2020**, *72*, 371–374. [CrossRef]
241. Kim, Y.S.; Kim, S.G. Endoplasmic reticulum stress and autophagy dysregulation in alcoholic and non-alcoholic liver diseases. *Clin. Mol. Hepatol.* **2020**, *26*, 715–727. [CrossRef] [PubMed]
242. Kouroumalis, E.; Voumvouraki, A.; Augoustaki, A.; Samonakis, D.N. Autophagy in liver diseases. *World J. Hepatol.* **2021**, *13*, 6–65. [CrossRef]

243. Shiode, Y.; Hikita, H.; Tanaka, S.; Shirai, K.; Doi, A.; Sakane, S.; Kai, Y.; Nakabori, T.; Yamada, R.; Kodama, T.; et al. Hepatitis C virus enhances Rubicon expression, leading to autophagy inhibition and intracellular innate immune activation. *Sci. Rep.* **2020**, *10*, 15290. [CrossRef] [PubMed]
244. Sir, D.; Tian, Y.; Chen, W.L.; Ann, D.K.; Yen, T.S.; Ou, J.H. The early autophagic pathway is activated by hepatitis B virus and required for viral DNA replication. *Proc. Natl. Acad. Sci. USA* **2010**, *107*, 4383–4388. [CrossRef]
245. Tavera-Mendoza, L.E.; Westerling, T.; Libby, E.; Marusyk, A.; Cato, L.; Cassani, R.; Cameron, L.A.; Ficarro, S.B.; Marto, J.A.; Klawitter, J.; et al. Vitamin D receptor regulates autophagy in the normal mammary gland and in luminal breast cancer cells. *Proc. Natl. Acad. Sci. USA* **2017**, *114*, 2186–2194. [CrossRef]
246. Barchetta, I.; Carotti, S.; Labbadia, G.; Gentilucci, U.V.; Muda, A.O.; Angelico, F.; Silecchia, G.; Leonetti, F.; Fraioli, A.; Picardi, A.; et al. Liver vitamin D receptor, CYP2R1, and CYP27A1 expression: Relationship with liver histology and vitamin D3 levels in patients with nonalcoholic steatohepatitis or hepatitis C virus. *Hepatology* **2012**, *56*, 2180–2187. [CrossRef]
247. He, W.; Ni, W.; Zhao, L.; Wang, X.; Liu, L.; Fan, Z. MicroRNA-125a/VDR axis impaired autophagic flux and contributed to fibrosis in a CCL4-induced mouse model and patients with liver cirrhosis. *Life Sci.* **2021**, *264*, 118666. [CrossRef]
248. Malhi, H.; Kaufman, R.J. Endoplasmic reticulum stress in liver disease. *J. Hepatol.* **2011**, *54*, 795–809. [CrossRef]
249. Mollica, M.P.; Lionetti, L.; Putti, R.; Cavaliere, G.; Gaita, M.; Barletta, A. From chronic overfeeding to hepatic injury: Role of endoplasmic reticulum stress and inflammation. *Nutr. Metab. Cardiovasc. Dis.* **2011**, *21*, 222–230. [CrossRef]
250. Aravinthan, A.; Pietrosi, G.; Hoare, M.; Jupp, J.; Marshall, A.; Verrill, C.; Davies, S.; Bateman, A.; Sheron, N.; Allison, M.; et al. Hepatocyte expression of the senescence marker p21 is linked to fibrosis and an adverse liver-related outcome in alcohol-related liver disease. *PLoS ONE* **2013**, *8*, 72904. [CrossRef]
251. Aravinthan, A.; Scarpini, C.; Tachtatzis, P.; Verma, S.; Penrhyn-Lowe, S.; Harvey, R.; Davies, S.E.; Allison, M.; Coleman, N.; Alexander, G. Hepatocyte senescence predicts progression in non-alcohol-related fatty liver disease. *J. Hepatol.* **2013**, *58*, 549–556. [CrossRef] [PubMed]
252. Barnard, A.; Moch, A.; Saab, S. Relationship between Telomere Maintenance and Liver Disease. *Gut Liver.* **2019**, *13*, 11–15. [CrossRef] [PubMed]
253. Nault, J.C.; Ningarhari, M.; Rebouissou, S.; Zucman-Rossi, J. The role of telomeres and telomerase in cirrhosis and liver cancer. *Nat. Rev. Gastroenterol. Hepatol.* **2019**, *16*, 544–558. [CrossRef]
254. Wijayasiri, P.; Astbury, S.; Kaye, P.; Oakley, F.; Alexander, G.J.; Kendall, T.J.; Aravinthan, A.D. Role of Hepatocyte Senescence in the Activation of Hepatic Stellate Cells and Liver Fibrosis Progression. *Cells* **2022**, *11*, 2221. [CrossRef]
255. Cai, J.; Zhang, X.J.; Li, H. The Role of Innate Immune Cells in Nonalcoholic Steatohepatitis. *Hepatology* **2019**, *70*, 1026–1037. [CrossRef] [PubMed]
256. Krenkel, O.; Puengel, T.; Govaere, O.; Abdallah, A.T.; Mossanen, J.C.; Kohlhepp, M.; Liepelt, A.; Lefebvre, E.; Luedde, T.; Hellerbrand, C.; et al. Therapeutic inhibition of inflammatory monocyte recruitment reduces steatohepatitis and liver fibrosis. *Hepatology* **2018**, *67*, 1270–1283. [CrossRef]
257. Lee, Y.S.; Seki, E. In Vivo and In Vitro Models to Study Liver Fibrosis: Mechanisms and Limitations. *Cell Mol. Gastroenterol. Hepatol.* **2023**, *16*, 355–367. [CrossRef]
258. David, B.A.; Rezende, R.M.; Antunes, M.M.; Santos, M.M.; Freitas Lopes, M.A.; Diniz, A.B.; Sousa Pereira, R.V.; Marchesi, S.C.; Alvarenga, D.M.; Nakagaki, B.N.; et al. Combination of Mass Cytometry and Imaging Analysis Reveals Origin, Location, and Functional Repopulation of Liver Myeloid Cells in Mice. *Gastroenterology* **2016**, *15*, 1176–1191. [CrossRef]
259. Devisscher, L.; Scott, C.L.; Lefere, S.; Raevens, S.; Bogaerts, E.; Paridaens, A.; Verhelst, X.; Geerts, A.; Guilliams, M.; Van Vlierberghe, H. Non-alcoholic steatohepatitis induces transient changes within the liver macrophage pool. *Cell Immunol.* **2017**, *322*, 74–83. [CrossRef]
260. Ait Ahmed, Y.; Lafdil, F.; Tacke, F. Ambiguous Pathogenic Roles of Macrophages in Alcohol-Associated Liver Diseases. *Hepat. Med.* **2023**, *15*, 113–127. [CrossRef]
261. Wang, Z.; Du, K.; Jin, N.; Tang, B.; Zhang, W. Macrophage in liver Fibrosis: Identities and mechanisms. *Int. Immunopharmacol.* **2023**, *120*, 110357. [CrossRef] [PubMed]
262. An, S.Y.; Petrescu, A.D.; DeMorrow, S. Targeting Certain Interleukins as Novel Treatment Options for Liver Fibrosis. *Front. Pharmacol.* **2021**, *12*, 645703. [CrossRef] [PubMed]
263. Liu, J.; Yu, Q.; Wu, W.; Huang, X.; Broering, R.; Werner, M.; Roggendorf, M.; Yang, D.; Lu, M. TLR2 Stimulation Strengthens Intrahepatic Myeloid-Derived Cell-Mediated T Cell Tolerance through Inducing Kupffer Cell Expansion and IL-10 Production. *J. Immunol.* **2018**, *200*, 2341–2351. [CrossRef]
264. Wang, Q.; Zhang, H.; Chen, Z.; Chen, L.; Pan, F.; Zhou, Q. Proliferation of CD11b+ myeloid cells induced by TLR4 signaling promotes hepatitis B virus clearance. *Cytokine* **2022**, *153*, 155867. [CrossRef]
265. Li, Y.; He, M.; Wang, Z.; Duan, Z.; Guo, Z.; Wang, Z.; Gong, R.; Chu, T.; Cai, J.; Gao, B. STING signaling activation inhibits HBV replication and attenuates the severity of liver injury and HBV-induced fibrosis. *Cell Mol. Immunol.* **2022**, *19*, 92–107. [CrossRef]

266. Yang, Y.; Zhao, X.; Wang, Z.; Shu, W.; Li, L.; Li, Y.; Guo, Z.; Gao, B.; Xiong, S. Nuclear Sensor Interferon-Inducible Protein 16 Inhibits the Function of Hepatitis B Virus Covalently Closed Circular DNA by Integrating Innate Immune Activation and Epigenetic Suppression. *Hepatology* **2020**, *71*, 1154–1169. [CrossRef]
267. Pose, E.; Coll, M.; Martínez-Sánchez, C.; Zeng, Z.; Surewaard, B.G.J.; Català, C.; Velasco-de Andrés, M.; Lozano, J.J.; Ariño, S.; Fuster, D.; et al. Programmed Death Ligand 1 Is Overexpressed in Liver Macrophages in Chronic Liver Diseases, and Its Blockade Improves the Antibacterial Activity Against Infections. *Hepatology* **2021**, *74*, 296–311. [CrossRef]
268. Lough, J.; Rosenthall, L.; Arzoumanian, A.; Goresky, C.A. Kupffer cell depletion associated with capillarization of liver sinusoids in carbon tetrachloride-induced rat liver cirrhosis. *J. Hepatol.* **1987**, *5*, 190–198. [CrossRef]
269. Buonomo, E.L.; Mei, S.; Guinn, S.R.; Leo, I.R.; Peluso, M.J.; Nolan, M.A.; Schildberg, F.A.; Zhao, L.; Lian, C.; Xu, S.; et al. Liver stromal cells restrict macrophage maturation and stromal IL-6 limits the differentiation of cirrhosis-linked macrophages. *J. Hepatol.* **2022**, *76*, 1127–1137. [CrossRef]
270. Li, X.; Hollingshead, N.; Lampert, S.; Truong, C.D.; Li, W.; Niu, J.; Crispe, I.N.; Soysa, R. A conserved pathway of transdifferentiation in murine Kupffer cells. *Eur. J. Immunol.* **2021**, *51*, 2452–2463. [CrossRef]
271. Vadasz, Z.; Kessler, O.; Akiri, G.; Gengrinovitch, S.; Kagan, H.M.; Baruch, Y.; Izhak, O.B.; Neufeld, G. Abnormal deposition of collagen around hepatocytes in Wilson's disease is associated with hepatocyte specific expression of lysyl oxidase and lysyl oxidase like protein-2. *J. Hepatol.* **2005**, *43*, 499–507. [CrossRef] [PubMed]
272. Feng, M.; Ding, J.; Wang, M.; Zhang, J.; Zhu, X.; Guan, W. Kupffer-derived matrix metalloproteinase-9 contributes to liver fibrosis resolution. *Int. J. Biol. Sci.* **2018**, *14*, 1033–1040. [CrossRef] [PubMed]
273. Li, W.; He, F. Infusion of Kupffer Cells Expanded in Vitro Ameliorated Liver Fibrosis in a Murine Model of Liver Injury. *Cell Transplant.* **2021**, *30*, 9636897211004090. [CrossRef]
274. Wu, H.; Chen, G.; Wang, J.; Deng, M.; Yuan, F.; Gong, J. TIM-4 interference in Kupffer cells against CCL4-induced liver fibrosis by mediating Akt1/Mitophagy signalling pathway. *Cell Prolif.* **2020**, *53*, 12731. [CrossRef] [PubMed]
275. Tu, Z.; Bozorgzadeh, A.; Pierce, R.H.; Kurtis, J.; Crispe, I.N.; Orloff, M.S. TLR-dependent cross talk between human Kupffer cells and NK cells. *J. Exp. Med.* **2008**, *205*, 233–244. [CrossRef] [PubMed]
276. Boltjes, A.; van Montfoort, N.; Biesta, P.J.; Op den Brouw, M.L.; Kwekkeboom, J.; van der Laan, L.J.; Janssen, H.L.; Boonstra, A.; Woltman, A.M. Kupffer cells interact with hepatitis B surface antigen in vivo and in vitro, leading to proinflammatory cytokine production and natural killer cell function. *J. Infect. Dis.* **2015**, *211*, 1268–1278. [CrossRef]
277. Hosomura, N.; Kono, H.; Tsuchiya, M.; Ishii, K.; Ogiku, M.; Matsuda, M.; Fujii, H. HCV-related proteins activate Kupffer cells isolated from human liver tissues. *Dig. Dis. Sci.* **2011**, *56*, 1057–1064. [CrossRef]
278. Chang, S.; Dolganiuc, A.; Szabo, G. Toll-like receptors 1 and 6 are involved in TLR2-mediated macrophage activation by hepatitis C virus core and NS3 proteins. *J. Leukoc. Biol.* **2007**, *82*, 479–487. [CrossRef]
279. Ju, C.; Tacke, F. Hepatic macrophages in homeostasis and liver diseases: From pathogenesis to novel therapeutic strategies. *Cell Mol. Immunol.* **2016**, *13*, 316–327. [CrossRef]
280. Jindal, A.; Bruzzì, S.; Sutti, S.; Locatelli, I.; Bozzola, C.; Paternostro, C.; Parola, M.; Albano, E. Fat-laden macrophages modulate lobular inflammation in nonalcoholic steatohepatitis (NASH). *Exp. Mol. Pathol.* **2015**, *99*, 155–162. [CrossRef]
281. Hirsova, P.; Ibrahim, S.H.; Krishnan, A.; Verma, V.K.; Bronk, S.F.; Werneburg, N.W.; Charlton, M.R.; Shah, V.H.; Malhi, H.; Gores, G.J. Lipid-Induced Signaling Causes Release of Inflammatory Extracellular Vesicles From Hepatocytes. *Gastroenterology* **2016**, *150*, 956–967. [CrossRef] [PubMed]
282. Cannito, S.; Morello, E.; Bocca, C.; Foglia, B.; Benetti, E.; Novo, E.; Chiazza, F.; Rogazzo, M.; Fantozzi, R.; Povero, D.; et al. Microvesicles released from fat-laden cells promote activation of hepatocellular NLRP3 inflammasome: A pro-inflammatory link between lipotoxicity and non-alcoholic steatohepatitis. *PLoS ONE* **2017**, *12*, e0172575. [CrossRef] [PubMed]
283. Morello, E.; Sutti, S.; Foglia, B.; Novo, E.; Cannito, S.; Bocca, C.; Rajsky, M.; Bruzzì, S.; Abate, M.L.; Rosso, C.; et al. Hypoxia-inducible factor 2α drives nonalcoholic fatty liver progression by triggering hepatocyte release of histidine-rich glycoprotein. *Hepatology* **2018**, *67*, 2196–2214. [CrossRef]
284. Bartneck, M.; Fech, V.; Ehling, J.; Govaere, O.; Warzecha, K.T.; Hittatiya, K.; Vucur, M.; Gautheron, J.; Luedde, T.; Trautwein, C.; et al. Histidine-rich glycoprotein promotes macrophage activation and inflammation in chronic liver disease. *Hepatology* **2016**, *63*, 1310–1324. [CrossRef]
285. Suraweera, D.B.; Weeratunga, A.N.; Hu, R.W.; Pandol, S.J.; Hu, R. Alcoholic hepatitis: The pivotal role of Kupffer cells. *World J. Gastrointest. Pathophysiol.* **2015**, *6*, 90–98. [CrossRef]
286. Ju, C.; Mandrekar, P. Macrophages and Alcohol-Related Liver Inflammation. *Alcohol Res.* **2015**, *37*, 251–262.
287. Wang, M.; You, Q.; Lor, K.; Chen, F.; Gao, B.; Ju, C. Chronic alcohol ingestion modulates hepatic macrophage populations and functions in mice. *J. Leukoc. Biol.* **2014**, *96*, 657–665. [CrossRef]
288. Petrasek, J.; Bala, S.; Csak, T.; Lippai, D.; Kodys, K.; Menashy, V.; Barrieau, M.; Min, S.Y.; Kurt-Jones, E.A.; Szabo, G. IL-1 receptor antagonist ameliorates inflammasome-dependent alcoholic steatohepatitis in mice. *J. Clin. Investig.* **2012**, *122*, 3476–3489. [CrossRef]

289. Calmus, Y.; Poupon, R. Shaping macrophages function and innate immunity by bile acids: Mechanisms and implication in cholestatic liver diseases. *Clin. Res. Hepatol. Gastroenterol.* **2014**, *38*, 550–556. [CrossRef]
290. Gong, Z.; Zhou, J.; Zhao, S.; Tian, C.; Wang, P.; Xu, C.; Chen, Y.; Cai, W.; Wu, J. Chenodeoxycholic acid activates NLRP3 inflammasome and contributes to cholestatic liver fibrosis. *Oncotarget* **2016**, *7*, 83951–83963. [CrossRef]
291. Guo, C.; Xie, S.; Chi, Z.; Zhang, J.; Liu, Y.; Zhang, L.; Zheng, M.; Zhang, X.; Xia, D.; Ke, Y.; et al. Bile Acids Control Inflammation and Metabolic Disorder through Inhibition of NLRP3 Inflammasome. *Immunity* **2016**, *45*, 802–816. [CrossRef] [PubMed]
292. Keitel, V.; Donner, M.; Winandy, S.; Kubitz, R.; Häussinger, D. Expression and function of the bile acid receptor TGR5 in Kupffer cells. *Biochem. Biophys. Res. Commun.* **2008**, *372*, 78–84. [CrossRef] [PubMed]
293. Duwaerts, C.C.; Gehring, S.; Cheng, C.W.; van Rooijen, N.; Gregory, S.H. Contrasting responses of Kupffer cells and inflammatory mononuclear phagocytes to biliary obstruction in a mouse model of cholestatic liver injury. *Liver Int.* **2013**, *33*, 255–265. [CrossRef] [PubMed]
294. Chang, J.; Hisamatsu, T.; Shimamura, K.; Yoneno, K.; Adachi, M.; Naruse, H.; Igarashi, T.; Higuchi, H.; Matsuoka, K.; Kitazume, M.T.; et al. Activated hepatic stellate cells mediate the differentiation of macrophages. *Hepatol. Res.* **2013**, *43*, 658–669. [CrossRef]
295. Xiao, C.; Ghosh, S. NF-kappaB, an evolutionarily conserved mediator of immune and inflammatory responses. *Adv. Exp. Med. Biol.* **2005**, *560*, 41–45.
296. Pahl, H.L. Activators and target genes of Rel/NF-kappaB transcription factors. *Oncogene* **1999**, *18*, 6853–6866. [CrossRef]
297. Luedde, T.; Schwabe, R.F. NF-κB in the liver--linking injury, fibrosis and hepatocellular carcinoma. *Nat. Rev. Gastroenterol. Hepatol.* **2011**, *8*, 108–118. [CrossRef]
298. Twu, Y.C.; Lee, T.S.; Lin, Y.L.; Hsu, S.M.; Wang, Y.H.; Liao, C.Y.; Wang, C.K.; Liang, Y.C.; Liao, Y.J. Niemann-Pick Type C2 Protein Mediates Hepatic Stellate Cells Activation by Regulating Free Cholesterol Accumulation. *Int. J. Mol. Sci.* **2016**, *17*, 1122. [CrossRef]
299. Tomita, K.; Teratani, T.; Suzuki, T.; Shimizu, M.; Sato, H.; Narimatsu, K.; Usui, S.; Furuhashi, H.; Kimura, A.; Nishiyama, K.; et al. Acyl-CoA:cholesterol acyltransferase 1 mediates liver fibrosis by regulating free cholesterol accumulation in hepatic stellate cells. *J. Hepatol.* **2014**, *61*, 98–106. [CrossRef]
300. Tomita, K.; Teratani, T.; Suzuki, T.; Shimizu, M.; Sato, H.; Narimatsu, K.; Okada, Y.; Kurihara, C.; Irie, R.; Yokoyama, H.; et al. Free cholesterol accumulation in hepatic stellate cells: Mechanism of liver fibrosis aggravation in nonalcoholic steatohepatitis in mice. *Hepatology* **2014**, *59*, 154–169. [CrossRef]
301. Teratani, T.; Tomita, K.; Suzuki, T.; Oshikawa, T.; Yokoyama, H.; Shimamura, K.; Tominaga, S.; Hiroi, S.; Irie, R.; Okada, Y.; et al. A high-cholesterol diet exacerbates liver fibrosis in mice via accumulation of free cholesterol in hepatic stellate cells. *Gastroenterology* **2012**, *142*, 152–164. [CrossRef] [PubMed]
302. Wang, X.; Cai, B.; Yang, X.; Sonubi, O.O.; Zheng, Z.; Ramakrishnan, R.; Shi, H.; Valenti, L.; Pajvani, U.B.; Sandhu, J.; et al. Cholesterol Stabilizes TAZ in Hepatocytes to Promote Experimental Non-alcoholic Steatohepatitis. *Cell Metab.* **2020**, *31*, 969–986. [CrossRef] [PubMed]
303. Zhang, H.; Yan, X.; Yang, C.; Zhan, Q.; Fu, Y.; Luo, H.; Luo, H. Intrahepatic T helper 17 cells recruited by hepatitis B virus X antigen-activated hepatic stellate cells exacerbate the progression of chronic hepatitis B virus infection. *J. Viral Hepat.* **2020**, *27*, 1138–1149. [CrossRef]
304. Chou, H.S.; Hsieh, C.C.; Yang, H.R.; Wang, L.; Arakawa, Y.; Brown, K.; Wu, Q.; Lin, F.; Peters, M.; Fung, J.J.; et al. Hepatic stellate cells regulate immune response by way of induction of myeloid suppressor cells in mice. *Hepatology* **2011**, *53*, 1007–1019. [CrossRef]
305. Jiang, G.; Yang, H.R.; Wang, L.; Wildey, G.M.; Fung, J.; Qian, S.; Lu, L. Hepatic stellate cells preferentially expand allogeneic CD4+ CD25+ FoxP3+ regulatory T cells in an IL-2-dependent manner. *Transplantation* **2008**, *86*, 1492–1502. [CrossRef]
306. Li, Y.; Lu, L.; Qian, S.; Fung, J.J.; Lin, F. Hepatic Stellate Cells Directly Inhibit B Cells via Programmed Death-Ligand 1. *J. Immunol.* **2016**, *196*, 1617–1625. [CrossRef]
307. Ding, X.; Saxena, N.K.; Lin, S.; Xu, A.; Srinivasan, S.; Anania, F.A. The roles of leptin and adiponectin: A novel paradigm in adipocytokine regulation of liver fibrosis and stellate cell biology. *Am. J. Pathol.* **2005**, *166*, 1655–1669. [CrossRef]
308. Ouchi, N.; Parker, J.L.; Lugus, J.J.; Walsh, K. Adipokines in inflammation and metabolic disease. *Nat. Rev. Immunol.* **2011**, *11*, 85–97. [CrossRef]
309. Saxena, N.K.; Anania, F.A. Adipocytokines and hepatic fibrosis. *Trends Endocrinol. Metab.* **2015**, *26*, 153–161. [CrossRef]
310. Zhai, X.; Yan, K.; Fan, J.; Niu, M.; Zhou, Q.; Zhou, Y.; Chen, H.; Zhou, Y. The β-catenin pathway contributes to the effects of leptin on SREBP-1c expression in rat hepatic stellate cells and liver fibrosis. *Br. J. Pharmacol.* **2013**, *169*, 197–212. [CrossRef]
311. Dong, Z.; Su, L.; Esmaili, S.; Iseli, T.J.; Ramezani-Moghadam, M.; Hu, L.; Xu, A.; George, J.; Wang, J. Adiponectin attenuates liver fibrosis by inducing nitric oxide production of hepatic stellate cells. *J. Mol. Med.* **2015**, *93*, 1327–1339. [CrossRef] [PubMed]
312. Kumar, P.; Smith, T.; Rahman, K.; Mells, J.E.; Thorn, N.E.; Saxena, N.K.; Anania, F.A. Adiponectin modulates focal adhesion disassembly in activated hepatic stellate cells: Implication for reversing hepatic fibrosis. *FASEB J.* **2014**, *28*, 5172–5183. [CrossRef] [PubMed]

313. Ramezani-Moghadam, M.; Wang, J.; Ho, V.; Iseli, T.J.; Alzahrani, B.; Xu, A.; Van der Poorten, D.; Qiao, L.; George, J.; Hebbard, L. Adiponectin reduces hepatic stellate cell migration by promoting tissue inhibitor of metalloproteinase-1 (TIMP-1) secretion. *J. Biol. Chem.* **2015**, *290*, 5533–5542. [CrossRef]
314. Tardelli, M.; Moreno-Viedma, V.; Zeyda, M.; Itariu, B.K.; Langer, F.B.; Prager, G.; Stulnig, T.M. Adiponectin regulates aquaglyceroporin expression in hepatic stellate cells altering their functional state. *J. Gastroenterol. Hepatol.* **2017**, *32*, 253–260. [CrossRef] [PubMed]
315. Wang, H.; Zhang, H.; Zhang, Z.; Huang, B.; Cheng, X.; Wang, D.; la Gahu, Z.; Xue, Z.; Da, Y.; Li, D.; et al. Adiponectin-derived active peptide ADP355 exerts anti-inflammatory and anti-fibrotic activities in thioacetamide-induced liver injury. *Sci. Rep.* **2016**, *6*, 19445. [CrossRef]
316. Carambia, A.; Freund, B.; Schwinge, D.; Heine, M.; Laschtowitz, A.; Huber, S.; Wraith, D.C.; Korn, T.; Schramm, C.; Lohse, A.W.; et al. TGF-β-dependent induction of $CD4^{+}CD25^{+}Foxp3^{+}$ Tregs by liver sinusoidal endothelial cells. *J. Hepatol.* **2014**, *61*, 594–599. [CrossRef]
317. Yang, M.; Zhang, C. The role of liver sinusoidal endothelial cells in cancer liver metastasis. *Am. J. Cancer Res.* **2021**, *11*, 1845–1860.
318. Ishikawa, T.; Yokoyama, H.; Matsuura, T.; Fujiwara, Y. Fc gamma RIIb expression levels in human liver sinusoidal endothelial cells during progression of non-alcoholic fatty liver disease. *PLoS ONE* **2019**, *14*, 0211543. [CrossRef]
319. Baiocchini, A.; Del Nonno, F.; Taibi, C.; Visco-Comandini, U.; D'Offizi, G.; Piacentini, M.; Falasca, L. Liver sinusoidal endothelial cells (LSECs) modifications in patients with chronic hepatitis C. *Sci. Rep.* **2019**, *9*, 8760, Erratum in: *Sci. Rep.* **2020**, *10*, 1420. [CrossRef]
320. Maretti-Mira, A.C.; Wang, X.; Wang, L.; DeLeve, L.D. Incomplete Differentiation of Engrafted Bone Marrow Endothelial Progenitor Cells Initiates Hepatic Fibrosis in the Rat. *Hepatology* **2019**, *69*, 1259–1272. [CrossRef]
321. Desroches-Castan, A.; Tillet, E.; Ricard, N.; Ouarné, M.; Mallet, C.; Belmudes, L.; Couté, Y.; Boillot, O.; Scoazec, J.Y.; Bailly, S.; et al. Bone Morphogenetic Protein 9 Is a Paracrine Factor Controlling Liver Sinusoidal Endothelial Cell Fenestration and Protecting Against Hepatic Fibrosis. *Hepatology* **2019**, *70*, 1392–1408. [CrossRef] [PubMed]
322. Desroches-Castan, A.; Tillet, E.; Ricard, N.; Ouarné, M.; Mallet, C.; Feige, J.J.; Bailly, S. Differential Consequences of Bmp9 Deletion on Sinusoidal Endothelial Cell Differentiation and Liver Fibrosis in 129/Ola and C57BL/6 Mice. *Cells* **2019**, *8*, 1079. [CrossRef] [PubMed]
323. Li, P.; Li, Y.; Zhu, L.; Yang, Z.; He, J.; Wang, L.; Shang, Q.; Pan, H.; Wang, H.; Ma, X.; et al. Targeting secreted cytokine BMP9 gates the attenuation of hepatic fibrosis. *Biochim. Biophys. Acta Mol. Basis Dis.* **2018**, *1864*, 709–720. [CrossRef] [PubMed]
324. Chen, H.; Li, Y.Y.; Nio, K.; Tang, H. Unveiling the Impact of BMP9 in Liver Diseases: Insights into Pathogenesis and Therapeutic Potential. *Biomolecules* **2024**, *14*, 1013. [CrossRef]
325. Wang, L.; Feng, Y.; Xie, X.; Wu, H.; Su, X.N.; Qi, J.; Xin, W.; Gao, L.; Zhang, Y.; Shah, V.H.; et al. Neuropilin-1 aggravates liver cirrhosis by promoting angiogenesis via VEGFR2-dependent PI3K/Akt pathway in hepatic sinusoidal endothelial cells. *EBioMedicine* **2019**, *43*, 525–536. [CrossRef]
326. Kong, L.J.; Li, H.; Du, Y.J.; Pei, F.H.; Hu, Y.; Zhao, L.L.; Chen, J. Vatalanib, a tyrosine kinase inhibitor, decreases hepatic fibrosis and sinusoidal capillarization in CCl4-induced fibrotic mice. *Mol. Med. Rep.* **2017**, *15*, 2604–2610. [CrossRef]
327. Ogawa, H.; Kaji, K.; Nishimura, N.; Takagi, H.; Ishida, K.; Takaya, H.; Kawaratani, H.; Moriya, K.; Namisaki, T.; Akahane, T.; et al. Lenvatinib prevents liver fibrosis by inhibiting hepatic stellate cell activation and sinusoidal capillarization in experimental liver fibrosis. *J. Cell Mol. Med.* **2021**, *25*, 4001–4013. [CrossRef]
328. Wu, Y.; Li, Z.; Xiu, A.Y.; Meng, D.X.; Wang, S.N.; Zhang, C.Q. Carvedilol attenuates carbon tetrachloride-induced liver fibrosis and hepatic sinusoidal capillarization in mice. *Drug Des. Devel Ther.* **2019**, *13*, 2667–2676. [CrossRef]
329. Wang, Q.; Zhang, F.; Lei, Y.; Liu, P.; Liu, C.; Tao, Y. microRNA-322/424 promotes liver fibrosis by regulating angiogenesis through targeting CUL2/HIF-1α pathway. *Life Sci.* **2021**, *266*, 118819. [CrossRef]
330. Meyer, J.; Balaphas, A.; Fontana, P.; Morel, P.; Robson, S.C.; Sadoul, K.; Gonelle-Gispert, C.; Bühler, L. Platelet Interactions with Liver Sinusoidal Endothelial Cells and Hepatic Stellate Cells Lead to Hepatocyte Proliferation. *Cells* **2020**, *9*, 1243. [CrossRef]
331. Zheng, Y.; Wang, J.; Zhao, T.; Wang, L.; Wang, J. Modulation of the VEGF/AKT/eNOS signaling pathway to regulate liver angiogenesis to explore the anti-hepatic fibrosis mechanism of curcumol. *J. Ethnopharmacol.* **2021**, *280*, 114480. [CrossRef] [PubMed]
332. Ruart, M.; Chavarria, L.; Campreciós, G.; Suárez-Herrera, N.; Montironi, C.; Guixé-Muntet, S.; Bosch, J.; Friedman, S.L.; Garcia-Pagán, J.C.; Hernández-Gea, V. Impaired endothelial autophagy promotes liver fibrosis by aggravating the oxidative stress response during acute liver injury. *J. Hepatol.* **2019**, *70*, 458–469. [CrossRef] [PubMed]
333. Li, Y.; Liu, R.; Wu, J.; Li, X. Self-eating: Friend or foe? The emerging role of autophagy in fibrotic diseases. *Theranostics* **2020**, *10*, 7993–8017. [CrossRef]
334. Luo, X.; Wang, D.; Zhu, X.; Wang, G.; You, Y.; Ning, Z.; Li, Y.; Jin, S.; Huang, Y.; Hu, Y.; et al. Autophagic degradation of caveolin-1 promotes liver sinusoidal endothelial cells defenestration. *Cell Death Dis.* **2018**, *9*, 576. [CrossRef]

335. Kohara, S.; Ogawa, K. Eph/Ephrin Promotes the Adhesion of Liver Tissue-Resident Macrophages to a Mimicked Surface of Liver Sinusoidal Endothelial Cells. *Biomedicines* **2022**, *10*, 3234. [CrossRef]
336. Sakai, M.; Troutman, T.D.; Seidman, J.S.; Ouyang, Z.; Spann, N.J.; Abe, Y.; Ego, K.M.; Bruni, C.M.; Deng, Z.; Schlachetzki, J.C.M.; et al. Liver-Derived Signals Sequentially Reprogram Myeloid Enhancers to Initiate and Maintain Kupffer Cell Identity. *Immunity* **2019**, *51*, 655–670. [CrossRef]
337. Ganesan, L.P.; Mohanty, S.; Kim, J.; Clark, K.R.; Robinson, J.M.; Anderson, C.L. Rapid and efficient clearance of blood-borne virus by liver sinusoidal endothelium. *PLoS Pathog.* **2011**, *7*, 1002281. [CrossRef]
338. Mates, J.M.; Yao, Z.; Cheplowitz, A.M.; Suer, O.; Phillips, G.S.; Kwiek, J.J.; Rajaram, M.V.; Kim, J.; Robinson, J.M.; Ganesan, L.P.; et al. Mouse Liver Sinusoidal Endothelium Eliminates HIV-Like Particles from Blood at a Rate of 100 Million per Minute by a Second-Order Kinetic Process. *Front. Immunol.* **2017**, *8*, 35. [CrossRef]
339. Breiner, K.M.; Schaller, H.; Knolle, P.A. Endothelial cell-mediated uptake of a hepatitis B virus: A new concept of liver targeting of hepatotropic microorganisms. *Hepatology* **2001**, *34*, 803–808. [CrossRef]
340. Cormier, E.G.; Tsamis, F.; Kajumo, F.; Durso, R.J.; Gardner, J.P.; Dragic, T. CD81 is an entry coreceptor for hepatitis C virus. *Proc. Natl. Acad. Sci. USA* **2004**, *101*, 7270–7274. [CrossRef]
341. Rowe, I.A.; Galsinh, S.K.; Wilson, G.K.; Parker, R.; Durant, S.; Lazar, C.; Branza-Nichita, N.; Bicknell, R.; Adams, D.H.; Balfe, P.; et al. Paracrine signals from liver sinusoidal endothelium regulate hepatitis C virus replication. *Hepatology* **2014**, *59*, 375–384. [CrossRef] [PubMed]
342. Giugliano, S.; Kriss, M.; Golden-Mason, L.; Dobrinskikh, E.; Stone, A.E.; Soto-Gutierrez, A.; Mitchell, A.; Khetani, S.R.; Yamane, D.; Stoddard, M.; et al. Hepatitis C virus infection induces autocrine interferon signaling by human liver endothelial cells and release of exosomes, which inhibits viral replication. *Gastroenterology* **2015**, *148*, 392–402. [CrossRef] [PubMed]
343. Gao, F.; Chiu, S.M.; Motan, D.A.; Zhang, Z.; Chen, L.; Ji, H.L.; Tse, H.F.; Fu, Q.L.; Lian, Q. Mesenchymal stem cells and immunomodulation: Current status and future prospects. *Cell Death Dis.* **2016**, *7*, 2062. [CrossRef] [PubMed]
344. Lee, K.D.; Kuo, T.K.; Whang-Peng, J.; Chung, Y.F.; Lin, C.T.; Chou, S.H.; Chen, J.R.; Chen, Y.P.; Lee, O.K. In vitro hepatic differentiation of human mesenchymal stem cells. *Hepatology* **2004**, *40*, 1275–1284. [CrossRef]
345. Li, W.; Ren, G.; Huang, Y.; Su, J.; Han, Y.; Li, J.; Chen, X.; Cao, K.; Chen, Q.; Shou, P.; et al. Mesenchymal stem cells: A double-edged sword in regulating immune responses. *Cell Death Differ.* **2012**, *19*, 1505–1513. [CrossRef]
346. Shi, Y.; Wang, Y.; Li, Q.; Liu, K.; Hou, J.; Shao, C.; Wang, Y. Immunoregulatory mechanisms of mesenchymal stem and stromal cells in inflammatory diseases. *Nat. Rev. Nephrol.* **2018**, *14*, 493–507. [CrossRef]
347. Viswanathan, S.; Shi, Y.; Galipeau, J.; Krampera, M.; Leblanc, K.; Martin, I.; Nolta, J.; Phinney, D.G.; Sensebe, L. Mesenchymal stem versus stromal cells: International Society for Cell & Gene Therapy (ISCT®) Mesenchymal Stromal Cell committee position statement on nomenclature. *Cytotherapy* **2019**, *21*, 1019–1024.
348. Costa, L.A.; Eiro, N.; Fraile, M.; Gonzalez, L.O.; Saá, J.; Garcia-Portabella, P.; Vega, B.; Schneider, J.; Vizoso, F.J. Functional heterogeneity of mesenchymal stem cells from natural niches to culture conditions: Implications for further clinical uses. *Cell Mol. Life Sci.* **2021**, *78*, 447–467. [CrossRef]
349. Han, Y.; Yang, J.; Fang, J.; Zhou, Y.; Candi, E.; Wang, J.; Hua, D.; Shao, C.; Shi, Y. The secretion profile of mesenchymal stem cells and potential applications in treating human diseases. *Signal Transduct. Target. Ther.* **2022**, *7*, 92. [CrossRef]
350. Murakami, J.; Ishii, M.; Suehiro, F.; Ishihata, K.; Nakamura, N.; Nishimura, M. Vascular endothelial growth factor-C induces osteogenic differentiation of human mesenchymal stem cells through the ERK and RUNX2 pathway. *Biochem. Biophys. Res. Commun.* **2017**, *484*, 710–718. [CrossRef]
351. Deng, Y.; Zhang, Y.; Ye, L.; Zhang, T.; Cheng, J.; Chen, G.; Zhang, Q.; Yang, Y. Umbilical Cord-derived Mesenchymal Stem Cells Instruct Monocytes Towards an IL10-producing Phenotype by Secreting IL6 and HGF. *Sci. Rep.* **2016**, *6*, 37566. [CrossRef] [PubMed]
352. Prockop, D.J. Concise review: Two negative feedback loops place mesenchymal stem/stromal cells at the center of early regulators of inflammation. *Stem Cells* **2013**, *31*, 2042–2046. [CrossRef] [PubMed]
353. Ezquer, F.; Ezquer, M.; Contador, D.; Ricca, M.; Simon, V.; Conget, P. The antidiabetic effect of mesenchymal stem cells is unrelated to their transdifferentiation potential but to their capability to restore Th1/Th2 balance and to modify the pancreatic microenvironment. *Stem Cells* **2012**, *30*, 1664–1674. [CrossRef]
354. Tao, H.; Liu, Q.; Zeng, A.; Song, L. Unlocking the potential of Mesenchymal stem cells in liver Fibrosis: Insights into the impact of autophagy and aging. *Int. Immunopharmacol.* **2023**, *21*, 110497. [CrossRef]
355. Giacomini, C.; Granéli, C.; Hicks, R.; Dazzi, F. The critical role of apoptosis in mesenchymal stromal cell therapeutics and implications in homeostasis and normal tissue repair. *Cell Mol. Immunol.* **2023**, *20*, 570–582. [CrossRef]
356. Li, P.; Ou, Q.; Shi, S.; Shao, C. Immunomodulatory properties of mesenchymal stem cells/dental stem cells and their therapeutic applications. *Cell Mol. Immunol.* **2023**, *20*, 558–569. [CrossRef]
357. Zhou, J.; Shi, Y. Mesenchymal stem/stromal cells (MSCs): Origin, immune regulation, and clinical applications. *Cell Mol. Immunol.* **2023**, *20*, 555–557. [CrossRef]

358. Abel, A.M.; Yang, C.; Thakar, M.S.; Malarkannan, S. Natural Killer Cells: Development, Maturation, and Clinical Utilization. *Front. Immunol.* **2018**, *9*, 1869. [CrossRef]
359. Melhem, A.; Muhanna, N.; Bishara, A.; Alvarez, C.E.; Ilan, Y.; Bishara, T.; Horani, A.; Nassar, M.; Friedman, S.L.; Safadi, R. Anti-fibrotic activity of NK cells in experimental liver injury through killing of activated HSC. *J. Hepatol.* **2006**, *45*, 60–71. [CrossRef]
360. Radaeva, S.; Sun, R.; Jaruga, B.; Nguyen, V.T.; Tian, Z.; Gao, B. Natural killer cells ameliorate liver fibrosis by killing activated stellate cells in NKG2D-dependent and tumor necrosis factor-related apoptosis-inducing ligand-dependent manners. *Gastroenterology* **2006**, *130*, 435–452. [CrossRef]
361. Baroni, G.S.; D'Ambrosio, L.; Curto, P.; Casini, A.; Mancini, R.; Jezequel, A.M.; Benedetti, A. Interferon gamma decreases hepatic stellate cell activation and extracellular matrix deposition in rat liver fibrosis. *Hepatology* **1996**, *23*, 1189–1199. [CrossRef] [PubMed]
362. Jeong, W.I.; Park, O.; Radaeva, S.; Gao, B. STAT1 inhibits liver fibrosis in mice by inhibiting stellate cell proliferation and stimulating NK cell cytotoxicity. *Hepatology* **2006**, *44*, 1441–1451. [CrossRef] [PubMed]
363. Choi, W.M.; Ryu, T.; Lee, J.H.; Shim, Y.R.; Kim, M.H.; Kim, H.H.; Kim, Y.E.; Yang, K.; Kim, K.; Choi, S.E.; et al. Metabotropic Glutamate Receptor 5 in Natural Killer Cells Attenuates Liver Fibrosis by Exerting Cytotoxicity to Activated Stellate Cells. *Hepatology* **2021**, *74*, 2170–2185. [CrossRef] [PubMed]
364. Kawarabayashi, N.; Seki, S.; Hatsuse, K.; Ohkawa, T.; Koike, Y.; Aihara, T.; Habu, Y.; Nakagawa, R.; Ami, K.; Hiraide, H.; et al. Decrease of CD56(+)T cells and natural killer cells in cirrhotic livers with hepatitis C may be involved in their susceptibility to hepatocellular carcinoma. *Hepatology* **2000**, *32*, 962–969. [CrossRef]
365. Morishima, C.; Paschal, D.M.; Wang, C.C.; Yoshihara, C.S.; Wood, B.L.; Yeo, A.E.; Emerson, S.S.; Shuhart, M.C.; Gretch, D.R. Decreased NK cell frequency in chronic hepatitis C does not affect ex vivo cytolytic killing. *Hepatology* **2006**, *43*, 573–580. [CrossRef]
366. Muhanna, N.; Doron, S.; Wald, O.; Horani, A.; Eid, A.; Pappo, O.; Friedman, S.L.; Safadi, R. Activation of hepatic stellate cells after phagocytosis of lymphocytes: A novel pathway of fibrogenesis. *Hepatology* **2008**, *48*, 963–977. [CrossRef]
367. Gan, J.; Mao, X.R.; Zheng, S.J.; Li, J.F. Invariant natural killer T cells: Not to be ignored in liver disease. *J. Dig. Dis.* **2021**, *22*, 136–142. [CrossRef]
368. Sajid, M.; Liu, L.; Sun, C. The Dynamic Role of NK Cells in Liver Cancers: Role in HCC and HBV Associated HCC and Its Therapeutic Implications. *Front. Immunol.* **2022**, *13*, 887186. [CrossRef]
369. Ma, Q.; Dong, X.; Liu, S.; Zhong, T.; Sun, D.; Zong, L.; Zhao, C.; Lu, Q.; Zhang, M.; Gao, Y.; et al. Hepatitis B e Antigen Induces NKG2A+ Natural Killer Cell Dysfunction via Regulatory T Cell-Derived Interleukin 10 in Chronic Hepatitis B Virus Infection. *Front. Cell Dev. Biol.* **2020**, *8*, 421. [CrossRef]
370. Diedrich, T.; Kummer, S.; Galante, A.; Drolz, A.; Schlicker, V.; Lohse, A.W.; Kluwe, J.; Eberhard, J.M.; Schulze Zur Wiesch, J. Characterization of the immune cell landscape of patients with NAFLD. *PLoS ONE* **2020**, *15*, 0230307. [CrossRef]
371. Gu, M.; Zhang, Y.; Lin, Z.; Hu, X.; Zhu, Y.; Xiao, W.; Jia, X.; Chen, W.; Lu, G.; Gong, W. Decrease in UCP1 by sustained high lipid promotes NK cell necroptosis to exacerbate nonalcoholic liver fibrosis. *Cell Death Dis.* **2024**, *15*, 518. [CrossRef] [PubMed]
372. Ravichandran, G.; Neumann, K.; Berkhout, L.K.; Weidemann, S.; Langeneckert, A.E.; Schwinge, D.; Poch, T.; Huber, S.; Schiller, B.; Hess, L.U.; et al. Interferon-γ-dependent immune responses contribute to the pathogenesis of sclerosing cholangitis in mice. *J. Hepatol.* **2019**, *71*, 773–782. [CrossRef] [PubMed]
373. Siwicki, M.; Kubes, P. Neutrophils in host defense, healing, and hypersensitivity: Dynamic cells within a dynamic host. *J. Allergy Clin. Immunol.* **2023**, *151*, 634–655. [CrossRef] [PubMed]
374. Brinkmann, V.; Reichard, U.; Goosmann, C.; Fauler, B.; Uhlemann, Y.; Weiss, D.S.; Weinrauch, Y.; Zychlinsky, A. Neutrophil extracellular traps kill bacteria. *Science* **2004**, *303*, 1532–1535. [CrossRef]
375. Koyama, Y.; Wang, P.; Liang, S.; Iwaisako, K.; Liu, X.; Xu, J.; Zhang, M.; Sun, M.; Cong, M.; Karin, D.; et al. Mesothelin/mucin 16 signaling in activated portal fibroblasts regulates cholestatic liver fibrosis. *J. Clin. Investig.* **2017**, *127*, 1254–1270. [CrossRef]
376. Mridha, A.R.; Wree, A.; Robertson, A.A.B.; Yeh, M.M.; Johnson, C.D.; Van Rooyen, D.M.; Haczeyni, F.; Teoh, N.C.; Savard, C.; Ioannou, G.N.; et al. NLRP3 inflammasome blockade reduces liver inflammation and fibrosis in experimental NASH in mice. *J. Hepatol.* **2017**, *66*, 1037–1046. [CrossRef]
377. Moles, A.; Murphy, L.; Wilson, C.L.; Chakraborty, J.B.; Fox, C.; Park, E.J.; Mann, J.; Oakley, F.; Howarth, R.; Brain, J.; et al. A TLR2/S100A9/CXCL-2 signaling network is necessary for neutrophil recruitment in acute and chronic liver injury in the mouse. *J. Hepatol.* **2014**, *60*, 782–791. [CrossRef]
378. Peiseler, M.; Kubes, P. More friend than foe: The emerging role of neutrophils in tissue repair. *J. Clin. Investig.* **2019**, *129*, 2629–2639. [CrossRef]
379. Peiseler, M.; Schwabe, R.; Hampe, J.; Kubes, P.; Heikenwälder, M.; Tacke, F. Immune mechanisms linking metabolic injury to inflammation and fibrosis in fatty liver disease—Novel insights into cellular communication circuits. *J. Hepatol.* **2022**, *77*, 1136–1160. [CrossRef]

380. Wan, Y.; Li, X.; Slevin, E.; Harrison, K.; Li, T.; Zhang, Y.; Klaunig, J.E.; Wu, C.; Shetty, A.K.; Dong, X.C.; et al. Endothelial dysfunction in pathological processes of chronic liver disease during aging. *FASEB J.* **2022**, *36*, e22125. [CrossRef]
381. Inverso, D.; Iannacone, M. Spatiotemporal dynamics of effector CD8+ T cell responses within the liver. *J. Leukoc. Biol.* **2016**, *99*, 51–55. [CrossRef] [PubMed]
382. Wohlleber, D.; Knolle, P.A. The role of liver sinusoidal cells in local hepatic immune surveillance. *Clin. Transl. Immunol.* **2016**, *5*, 117. [CrossRef] [PubMed]
383. Pennington, D.J.; Vermijlen, D.; Wise, E.L.; Clarke, S.L.; Tigelaar, R.E.; Hayday, A.C. The integration of conventional and unconventional T cells that characterizes cell-mediated responses. *Adv. Immunol.* **2005**, *87*, 27–59. [PubMed]
384. Godfrey, D.I.; Uldrich, A.P.; McCluskey, J.; Rossjohn, J.; Moody, D.B. The burgeoning family of unconventional T cells. *Nat. Immunol.* **2015**, *16*, 1114–1123. [CrossRef]
385. Nguyen, Q.P.; Deng, T.Z.; Witherden, D.A.; Goldrath, A.W. Origins of CD4+ circulating and tissue-resident memory T-cells. *Immunology* **2019**, *157*, 3–12. [CrossRef]
386. Zhang, M.; Zhang, S. T Cells in Fibrosis and Fibrotic Diseases. *Front. Immunol.* **2020**, *11*, 1142. [CrossRef]
387. Wang, H.; Luo, H.; Wan, X.; Fu, X.; Mao, Q.; Xiang, X.; Zhou, Y.; He, W.; Zhang, J.; Guo, Y.; et al. TNF-α/IFN-γ profile of HBV-specific CD4 T cells is associated with liver damage and viral clearance in chronic HBV infection. *J. Hepatol.* **2020**, *72*, 45–56. [CrossRef]
388. Li, Y.; You, Z.; Tang, R.; Ma, X. Tissue-resident memory T cells in chronic liver diseases: Phenotype, development and function. *Front. Immunol.* **2022**, *13*, 967055. [CrossRef]
389. Herkel, J.; Jagemann, B.; Wiegard, C.; Lazaro, J.F.; Lueth, S.; Kanzler, S.; Blessing, M.; Schmitt, E.; Lohse, A.W. MHC class II-expressing hepatocytes function as antigen-presenting cells and activate specific CD4 T lymphocyutes. *Hepatology* **2003**, *37*, 1079–1085. [CrossRef]
390. Koch, K.S.; Leffert, H.L. Hypothesis: Targeted Ikkβ deletion upregulates MIF signaling responsiveness and MHC class II expression in mouse hepatocytes. *Hepat. Med.* **2010**, *2010*, 39–47. [CrossRef]
391. Cabeza-Cabrerizo, M.; Cardoso, A.; Minutti, C.M.; Pereira da Costa, M.; Reis e Sousa, C. Dendritic Cells Revisited. *Annu. Rev. Immunol.* **2021**, *39*, 131–166. [CrossRef] [PubMed]
392. Eckert, C.; Klein, N.; Kornek, M.; Lukacs-Kornek, V. The complex myeloid network of the liver with diverse functional capacity at steady state and in inflammation. *Front. Immunol.* **2015**, *6*, 179. [CrossRef] [PubMed]
393. Rahman, A.H.; Aloman, C. Dendritic cells and liver fibrosis. *Biochim. Biophys. Acta* **2013**, *1832*, 998–1004. [CrossRef] [PubMed]
394. Doherty, D.G. Immunity, tolerance and autoimmunity in the liver: A comprehensive review. *J. Autoimmun.* **2016**, *66*, 60–75. [CrossRef]
395. Guilliams, M.; Bonnardel, J.; Haest, B.; Vanderborght, B.; Wagner, C.; Remmerie, A.; Bujko, A.; Martens, L.; Thoné, T.; Browaeys, R.; et al. Spatial proteogenomics reveals distinct and evolutionarily conserved hepatic macrophage niches. *Cell* **2022**, *185*, 379–396. [CrossRef]
396. Haas, J.T.; Vonghia, L.; Mogilenko, D.A.; Verrijken, A.; Molendi-Coste, O.; Fleury, S.; Deprince, A.; Nikitin, A.; Woitrain, E.; Ducrocq-Geoffroym, L.; et al. Transcriptional Network Analysis Implicates Altered Hepatic Immune Function in NASH development and resolution. *Nat. Metab.* **2019**, *1*, 604–614. [CrossRef]
397. Kambayashi, T.; Laufer, T.M. Atypical MHC class II-expressing antigen-presenting cells: Can anything replace a dendritic cell? *Nat. Rev. Immunol.* **2014**, *14*, 719–730. [CrossRef]
398. Alcover, A.; Alarcón, B.; Di Bartolo, V. Cell Biology of T Cell Receptor Expression and Regulation. *Annu. Rev. Immunol.* **2018**, *36*, 103–125. [CrossRef]
399. Elhai, M.; Avouac, J.; Hoffmann-Vold, A.M.; Ruzehaji, N.; Amiar, O.; Ruiz, B.; Brahiti, H.; Ponsoye, M.; Fréchet, M.; Burgevin, A.; et al. OX40L blockade protects against inflammation-driven fibrosis. *Proc. Natl. Acad. Sci. USA* **2016**, *113*, 3901–3910. [CrossRef]
400. Sun, G.; Jin, H.; Zhang, C.; Meng, H.; Zhao, X.; Wei, D.; Ou, X.; Wang, Q.; Li, S.; Wang, T.; et al. OX40 Regulates Both Innate and Adaptive Immunity and Promotes Nonalcoholic Steatohepatitis. *Cell Rep.* **2018**, *25*, 3786–3799. [CrossRef]
401. Webb, G.J.; Hirschfield, G.M.; Lane, P.J. OX40, OX40L and Autoimmunity: A Comprehensive Review. *Clin. Rev. Allergy Immunol.* **2016**, *50*, 312–332. [CrossRef] [PubMed]
402. Shah, K.; Al-Haidari, A.; Sun, J.; Kazi, J.U. T cell receptor (TCR) signaling in health and disease. *Signal Transduct. Target. Ther.* **2021**, *6*, 412. [CrossRef] [PubMed]
403. Liang, Q.; Hu, Y.; Zhang, M.; Lin, C.; Zhang, W.; Li, Y.; Zhu, P.; Xue, P.; Chen, Y.; Li, Q.; et al. The T Cell Receptor Immune Repertoire Protects the Liver From Reconsitution. *Front. Immunol.* **2020**, *11*, 584979. [CrossRef] [PubMed]
404. Safadi, R.; Ohta, M.; Alvarez, C.E.; Fiel, M.I.; Bansal, M.; Mehal, W.Z.; Friedman, S.L. Immune stimulation of hepatic fibrogenesis by CD8 cells and attenuation by transgenic interleukin-10 from hepatocytes. *Gastroenterology* **2004**, *127*, 870–882. [CrossRef]
405. Tang, L.; Chen, C.; Gao, X.; Zhang, W.; Yan, X.; Zhou, Y.; Guo, L.; Zheng, X.; Wang, W.; Yang, F.; et al. Interleukin 21 Reinvigorates the Antiviral Activity of Hepatitis B Virus (HBV)-Specific CD8+ T Cells in Chronic HBV Infection. *J. Infect. Dis.* **2019**, *219*, 750–759. [CrossRef]

406. Liu, H.; Hu, B.; Huang, J.; Wang, Q.; Wang, F.; Pan, F.; Chen, L. Endoplasmic Reticulum Aminopeptidase 1 Is Involved in Anti-viral Immune Response of Hepatitis B Virus by Trimming Hepatitis B Core Antigen to Generate 9-Mers Peptides. *Front. Microbiol.* **2022**, *13*, 829241. [CrossRef]
407. Li, C.; Yu, T.; Shi, X.; Yu, J. Interleukin-33 Reinvigorates Antiviral Function of Viral-Specific CD8+ T Cells in Chronic Hepatitis B Virus Infection. *Viral Immunol.* **2022**, *35*, 41–49. [CrossRef]
408. Roger, P.M.; Chaillou, S.; Breittmayer, J.P.; Dahman, M.; St Paul, M.C.; Chevallier, P.; Benzaken, S.; Ticchioni, M.; Bernard, A.; Dellamonica, P.; et al. Intrahepatic CD4 T-Cell apoptosis is related to METAVIR score in patients with chronic hepatitis C virus. *Scand. J. Immunol.* **2005**, *62*, 168–175. [CrossRef]
409. Glässner, A.; Eisenhardt, M.; Kokordelis, P.; Krämer, B.; Wolter, F.; Nischalke, H.D.; Boesecke, C.; Sauerbruch, T.; Rockstroh, J.K.; Spengler, U.; et al. Impaired CD4$^+$ T cell stimulation of NK cell anti-fibrotic activity may contribute to accelerated liver fibrosis progression in HIV/HCV patients. *J. Hepatol.* **2013**, *59*, 427–433. [CrossRef]
410. Her, Z.; Tan, J.H.L.; Lim, Y.S.; Tan, S.Y.; Chan, X.Y.; Tan, W.W.S.; Liu, M.; Yong, K.S.M.; Lai, F.; Ceccarello, E.; et al. CD4+ T Cells Mediate the Development of Liver Fibrosis in High Fat Diet-Induced NAFLD in Humanized Mice. *Front. Immunol.* **2020**, *11*, 580968. [CrossRef]
411. Rau, M.; Schilling, A.K.; Meertens, J.; Hering, I.; Weiss, J.; Jurowich, C.; Kudlich, T.; Hermanns, H.M.; Bantel, H.; Beyersdorf, N.; et al. Progression from Nonalcoholic Fatty Liver to Nonalcoholic Steatohepatitis Is Marked by a Higher Frequency of Th17 Cells in the Liver and an Increased Th17/Resting Regulatory T Cell Ratio in Peripheral Blood and in the Liver. *J. Immunol.* **2016**, *196*, 97–105. [CrossRef] [PubMed]
412. Sutti, S.; Albano, E. Adaptive immunity: An emerging player in the progression of NAFLD. *Nat. Rev. Gastroenterol. Hepatol.* **2020**, *17*, 81–92. [CrossRef] [PubMed]
413. O'Garra, A.; Robinson, D. Development and function of T helper 1 cells. *Adv. Immunol.* **2004**, *83*, 133–162. [PubMed]
414. Luo, X.Y.; Takahara, T.; Kawai, K.; Fujino, M.; Sugiyama, T.; Tsuneyama, K.; Tsukada, K.; Nakae, S.; Zhong, L.; Li, X.K. IFN-γ deficiency attenuates hepatic inflammation and fibrosis in a steatohepatitis model induced by a methionine- and choline-deficient high-fat diet. *Am. J. Physiol. Gastrointest. Liver Physiol.* **2013**, *305*, 891–899. [CrossRef]
415. Ferreyra Solari, N.E.; Inzaugarat, M.E.; Baz, P.; De Matteo, E.; Lezama, C.; Galoppo, M.; Galoppo, C.; Cherñavsky, A.C. The role of innate cells is coupled to a Th1-polarized immune response in pediatric nonalcoholic steatohepatitis. *J. Clin. Immunol.* **2012**, *32*, 611–621. [CrossRef]
416. Inzaugarat, M.E.; Ferreyra Solari, N.E.; Billordo, L.A.; Abecasis, R.; Gadano, A.C.; Cherñavsky, A.C. Altered phenotype and functionality of circulating immune cells characterize adult patients with nonalcoholic steatohepatitis. *J. Clin. Immunol.* **2011**, *31*, 1120–1130. [CrossRef]
417. Rolla, S.; Alchera, E.; Imarisio, C.; Bardina, V.; Valente, G.; Cappello, P.; Mombello, C.; Follenzi, A.; Novelli, F.; Carini, R. The balance between IL-17 and IL-22 produced by liver-infiltrating T-helper cells critically controls NASH development in mice. *Clin. Sci.* **2016**, *130*, 193–203. [CrossRef]
418. Nakayama, T.; Hirahara, K.; Onodera, A.; Endo, Y.; Hosokawa, H.; Shinoda, K.; Tumes, D.J.; Okamoto, Y. Th2 Cells in Health and Disease. *Annu. Rev. Immunol.* **2017**, *35*, 53–84. [CrossRef]
419. Zhang, C.; Li, L.; Feng, K.; Fan, D.; Xue, W.; Lu, J. 'Repair' Treg Cells in Tissue Injury. *Cell Physiol. Biochem.* **2017**, *43*, 2155–2169. [CrossRef]
420. Shimamura, T.; Fujisawa, T.; Husain, S.R.; Kioi, M.; Nakajima, A.; Puri, R.K. Novel role of IL-13 in fibrosis induced by nonalcoholic steatohepatitis and its amelioration by IL-13R-directed cytotoxin in a rat model. *J. Immunol.* **2008**, *181*, 4656–4665. [CrossRef]
421. Gao, Y.; Liu, Y.; Yang, M.; Guo, X.; Zhang, M.; Li, H.; Li, J.; Zhao, J. IL-33 treatment attenuated diet-induced hepatic steatosis but aggravated hepatic fibrosis. *Oncotarget* **2016**, *7*, 33649–33661. [CrossRef] [PubMed]
422. Lafoz, E.; Ruart, M.; Anton, A.; Oncins, A.; Hernández-Gea, V. The Endothelium as a Driver of Liver Fibrosis and Regeneration. *Cells* **2020**, *9*, 929. [CrossRef] [PubMed]
423. Zhong, Y.; Xu, M.; Hu, J.; Huang, X.; Lin, N.; Deng, M. Inhibiting Th1/2 cells influences hepatic capillarization by adjusting sinusoidal endothelial fenestrae through Rho-ROCK-myosin pathway. *Aging* **2021**, *13*, 5069–5086. [CrossRef] [PubMed]
424. Kremer, M.; Hines, I.N.; Milton, R.J.; Wheeler, M.D. Favored T helper 1 response in a mouse model of hepatosteatosis is associated with enhanced T cell-mediated hepatitis. *Hepatology* **2006**, *44*, 216–227. [CrossRef]
425. Molina, M.F.; Abdelnabi, M.N.; Fabre, T.; Shoukry, N.H. Type 3 cytokines in liver fibrosis and liver cancer. *Cytokine* **2019**, *124*, 154497. [CrossRef]
426. Fabre, T.; Kared, H.; Friedman, S.L.; Shoukry, N.H. IL-17A enhances the expression of profibrotic genes through upregulation of the TGF-β receptor on hepatic stellate cells in a JNK-dependent manner. *J. Immunol.* **2014**, *193*, 3925–3933. [CrossRef]
427. Meng, F.; Wang, K.; Aoyama, T.; Grivennikov, S.I.; Paik, Y.; Scholten, D.; Cong, M.; Iwaisako, K.; Liu, X.; Zhang, M.; et al. Interleukin-17 signaling in inflammatory, Kupffer cells, and hepatic stellate cells exacerbates liver fibrosis in mice. *Gastroenterology* **2012**, *143*, 765–776. [CrossRef]

428. Tan, Z.; Qian, X.; Jiang, R.; Liu, Q.; Wang, Y.; Chen, C.; Wang, X.; Ryffel, B.; Sun, B. IL-17A plays a critical role in the pathogenesis of liver fibrosis through hepatic stellate cell activation. *J. Immunol.* **2013**, *191*, 1835–1844. [CrossRef]
429. Giles, D.A.; Moreno-Fernandez, M.E.; Stankiewicz, T.E.; Cappelletti, M.; Huppert, S.S.; Iwakura, Y.; Dong, C.; Shanmukhappa, S.K.; Divanovic, S. Regulation of Inflammation by IL-17A and IL-17F Modulates Non-Alcoholic Fatty Liver Disease Pathogenesis. *PLoS ONE* **2016**, *11*, 0149783. [CrossRef]
430. Van Herck, M.A.; Weyler, J.; Kwanten, W.J.; Dirinck, E.L.; De Winter, B.Y.; Francque, S.M.; Vonghia, L. The Differential Roles of T Cells in Non-alcoholic Fatty Liver Disease and Obesity. *Front. Immunol.* **2019**, *10*, 82. [CrossRef]
431. Gomes, A.L.; Teijeiro, A.; Burén, S.; Tummala, K.S.; Yilmaz, M.; Waisman, A.; Theurillat, J.P.; Perna, C.; Djouder, N. Metabolic Inflammation-Associated IL-17A Causes Non-alcoholic Steatohepatitis and Hepatocellular Carcinoma. *Cancer Cell.* **2016**, *30*, 161–175. [CrossRef] [PubMed]
432. Tang, Y.; Bian, Z.; Zhao, L.; Liu, Y.; Liang, S.; Wang, Q.; Han, X.; Peng, Y.; Chen, X.; Shen, L.; et al. Interleukin-17 exacerbates hepatic steatosis and inflammation in non-alcoholic fatty liver disease. *Clin. Exp. Immunol.* **2011**, *166*, 281–290. [CrossRef] [PubMed]
433. Xu, R.; Tao, A.; Zhang, S.; Zhang, M. Neutralization of interleukin-17 attenuates high fat diet-induced non-alcoholic fatty liver disease in mice. *Acta Biochim. Biophys. Sin.* **2013**, *45*, 726–733. [CrossRef]
434. Harley, I.T.; Stankiewicz, T.E.; Giles, D.A.; Softic, S.; Flick, L.M.; Cappelletti, M.; Sheridan, R.; Xanthakos, S.A.; Steinbrecher, K.A.; Sartor, R.B.; et al. IL-17 signaling accelerates the progression of nonalcoholic fatty liver disease in mice. *Hepatology* **2014**, *59*, 1830–1839. [CrossRef] [PubMed]
435. Zhong, S.; Zhang, T.; Tang, L.; Li, Y. Cytokines and Chemokines in HBV Infection. *Front. Mol. Biosci.* **2021**, *8*, 805625. [CrossRef]
436. Ge, D.; You, Z. Expression of interleukin-17RC protein in normal human tissues. *Int. Arch. Med.* **2008**, *1*, 19. [CrossRef]
437. Lemmers, A.; Moreno, C.; Gustot, T.; Maréchal, R.; Degré, D.; Demetter, P.; de Nadai, P.; Geerts, A.; Quertinmont, E.; Vercruysse, V.; et al. The interleukin-17 pathway is involved in human alcoholic liver disease. *Hepatology* **2009**, *49*, 646–657. [CrossRef]
438. Paquissi, F.C. Immunity and Fibrogenesis: The Role of Th17/IL-17 Axis in HBV and HCV-induced Chronic Hepatitis and Progression to Cirrhosis. *Front. Immunol.* **2017**, *8*, 1195. [CrossRef]
439. Buschow, S.I.; Jansen, D.T.S.L. CD4+ T Cells in Chronic Hepatitis B and T Cell-Directed Immunotherapy. *Cells* **2021**, *10*, 1114. [CrossRef]
440. Zhu, L.; Li, J.; Xu, J.; Chen, F.; Wu, X.; Zhu, C. Significance of T-Cell Subsets for Clinical Response to Peginterferon Alfa-2a Therapy in HBeAg-Positive Chronic Hepatitis B Patients. *Int. J. Gen. Med.* **2022**, *15*, 4441–4451. [CrossRef] [PubMed]
441. Liu, B.; Gao, W.; Zhang, L.; Wang, J.; Chen, M.; Peng, M.; Ren, H.; Hu, P. Th17/Treg imbalance and increased interleukin-21 are associated with liver injury in patients with chronic severe hepatitis B. *Int. Immunopharmacol.* **2017**, *46*, 48–55. [CrossRef] [PubMed]
442. Jiang, Q.; Yang, G.; Xiao, F.; Xie, J.; Wang, S.; Lu, L.; Cui, D. Role of Th22 Cells in the Pathogenesis of Autoimmune Diseases. *Front. Immunol.* **2021**, *12*, 688066. [CrossRef] [PubMed]
443. Wang, X.; Ota, N.; Manzanillo, P.; Kates, L.; Zavala-Solorio, J.; Eidenschenk, C.; Zhang, J.; Lesch, J.; Lee, W.P.; Ross, J.; et al. Interleukin-22 alleviates metabolic disorders and restores mucosal immunity in diabetes. *Nature* **2014**, *514*, 237–241. [CrossRef]
444. Yang, L.; Zhang, Y.; Wang, L.; Fan, F.; Zhu, L.; Li, Z.; Ruan, X.; Huang, H.; Wang, Z.; Huang, Z.; et al. Amelioration of high fat diet induced liver lipogenesis and hepatic steatosis by interleukin-22. *J. Hepatol.* **2010**, *53*, 339–347. [CrossRef]
445. Jiang, R.; Tan, Z.; Deng, L.; Chen, Y.; Xia, Y.; Gao, Y.; Wang, X.; Sun, B. Interleukin-22 promotes human hepatocellular carcinoma by activation of STAT3. *Hepatology.* **2011**, *54*, 900–909. [CrossRef]
446. Barron, L.; Wynn, T.A. Fibrosis is regulated by Th2 and Th17 responses and by dynamic interactions between fibroblasts and macrophages. *Am. J. Physiol. Gastrointest. Liver Physiol.* **2011**, *300*, 723–728. [CrossRef]
447. Fabre, T.; Molina, M.F.; Soucy, G.; Goulet, J.P.; Willems, B.; Villeneuve, J.P.; Bilodeau, M.; Shoukry, N.H. Type 3 cytokines IL-17A and IL-22 drive TGF-β-dependent liver fibrosis. *Sci. Immunol.* **2018**, *3*, 7754. [CrossRef]
448. Zhang, S.; Huang, D.; Weng, J.; Huang, Y.; Liu, S.; Zhang, Q.; Li, N.; Wen, M.; Zhu, G.; Lin, F.; et al. Neutralization of Interleukin-17 Attenuates Cholestatic Liver Fibrosis in Mice. *Scand. J. Immunol.* **2016**, *83*, 102–108. [CrossRef]
449. Hara, M.; Kono, H.; Furuya, S.; Hirayama, K.; Tsuchiya, M.; Fujii, H. Interleukin-17A plays a pivotal role in cholestatic liver fibrosis in mice. *J. Surg. Res.* **2013**, *183*, 574–582. [CrossRef]
450. Wree, A.; McGeough, M.D.; Inzaugarat, M.E.; Eguchi, A.; Schuster, S.; Johnson, C.D.; Peña, C.A.; Geisler, L.J.; Papouchado, B.G.; Hoffman, H.M.; et al. NLRP3 inflammasome driven liver injury and fibrosis: Roles of IL-17 and TNF in mice. *Hepatology* **2018**, *67*, 736–749. [CrossRef]
451. Gieseck, R.L., 3rd; Wilson, M.S.; Wynn, T.A. Type 2 immunity in tissue repair and fibrosis. *Nat. Rev. Immunol.* **2018**, *18*, 62–76. [CrossRef] [PubMed]
452. Lee, C.G.; Homer, R.J.; Zhu, Z.; Lanone, S.; Wang, X.; Koteliansky, V.; Shipley, J.M.; Gotwals, P.; Noble, P.; Chen, Q.; et al. Interleukin-13 induces tissue fibrosis by selectively stimulating and activating transforming growth factor beta(1). *J. Exp. Med.* **2001**, *194*, 809–821. [CrossRef] [PubMed]

453. Kaviratne, M.; Hesse, M.; Leusink, M.; Cheever, A.W.; Davies, S.J.; McKerrow, J.H.; Wakefield, L.M.; Letterio, J.J.; Wynn, T.A. IL-13 activates a mechanism of tissue fibrosis that is completely TGF-beta independent. *J. Immunol.* **2004**, *173*, 4020–4029. [CrossRef]
454. Gieseck, R.L., 3rd; Ramalingam, T.R.; Hart, K.M.; Vannella, K.M.; Cantu, D.A.; Lu, W.Y.; Ferreira-González, S.; Forbes, S.J.; Vallier, L.; Wynn, T.A. Interleukin-13 Activates Distinct Cellular Pathways Leading to Ductular Reaction, Steatosis, and Fibrosis. *Immunity* **2016**, *45*, 145–158. [CrossRef]
455. Fan, Y.; Zhang, W.; Wei, H.; Sun, R.; Tian, Z.; Chen, Y. Hepatic NK Cells Attenuate Fibrosis Progression of Non-Alcoholic Steatohepatitis in Dependent of CXCL10-Mediated Recruitment. *Liver Int.* **2020**, *40*, 598–608. [CrossRef]
456. Hart, K.M.; Fabre, T.; Sciurba, J.C.; Gieseck, R.L., 3rd; Borthwick, L.A.; Vannella, K.M.; Acciani, T.H.; de Queiroz Prado, R.; Thompson, R.W.; White, S.; et al. Type 2 immunity is protective in metabolic disease but exacerbates NAFLD collaboratively with TGF-β. *Sci. Transl. Med.* **2017**, *9*, 3694.
457. Tosello-Trampont, A.C.; Krueger, P.; Narayanan, S.; Landes, S.G.; Leitinger, N.; Hahn, Y.S. NKp46(+) natural killer cells attenuate metabolism-induced hepatic fibrosis by regulating macrophage activation in mice. *Hepatology* **2016**, *63*, 799–812. [CrossRef]
458. Zhang, H.; Meadows, G.G. Chronic alcohol consumption in mice increases the proportion of peripheral memory T cells by homeostatic proliferation. *J. Leukoc. Biol.* **2005**, *78*, 1070–1080. [CrossRef]
459. Zuluaga, P.; Sanvisens, A.; Teniente-Serra, A.; El Ars, O.; Fuster, D.; Quirant-Sánchez, B.; Martínez-Cáceres, E.; Muga, R. Loss of naive T lymphocytes is associated with advanced liver fibrosis in alcohol use disorder. *Drug Alcohol Depend.* **2020**, *213*, 108046. [CrossRef]
460. Kita, H.; Matsumura, S.; He, X.S.; Ansari, A.A.; Lian, Z.X.; Van de Water, J.; Coppel, R.L.; Kaplan, M.M.; Gershwin, M.E. Quantitative and functional analysis of PDC-E2-specific autoreactive cytotoxic T lymphocytes in primary biliary cirrhosis. *J. Clin. Investig.* **2002**, *109*, 1231–1240. [CrossRef]
461. Zhang, W.; Ono, Y.; Miyamura, Y.; Bowlus, C.L.; Gershwin, M.E.; Maverakis, E. T cell clonal expansions detected in patients with primary biliary cirrhosis express CX3CR1. *J. Autoimmun.* **2011**, *37*, 71–78. [CrossRef] [PubMed]
462. Crispe, I.N. Immune tolerance in liver disease. *Hepatology* **2014**, *60*, 2109–2117. [CrossRef] [PubMed]
463. Zhu, J.; Paul, W.E. CD4 T cells: Fates, functions, and faults. *Blood* **2008**, *112*, 1557–1569. [CrossRef] [PubMed]
464. Ma, X.; Hua, J.; Mohamood, A.R.; Hamad, A.R.; Ravi, R.; Li, Z. A high-fat diet and regulatory T cells influence susceptibility to endotoxin-induced liver injury. *Hepatology* **2007**, *46*, 1519–1529. [CrossRef]
465. He, B.; Wu, L.; Xie, W.; Shao, Y.; Jiang, J.; Zhao, Z.; Yan, M.; Chen, Z.; Cui, D. The imbalance of Th17/Treg cells is involved in the progression of nonalcoholic fatty liver disease in mice. *BMC Immunol.* **2017**, *18*, 33. [CrossRef]
466. Ma, C.; Kesarwala, A.H.; Eggert, T.; Medina-Echeverz, J.; Kleiner, D.E.; Jin, P.; Stroncek, D.F.; Terabe, M.; Kapoor, V.; ElGindi, M.; et al. NAFLD causes selective CD4(+) T lymphocyte loss and promotes hepatocarcinogenesis. *Nature* **2016**, *531*, 253–257. [CrossRef]
467. Francisco, V.; Pino, J.; Campos-Cabaleiro, V.; Ruiz-Fernández, C.; Mera, A.; Gonzalez-Gay, M.A.; Gómez, R.; Gualillo, O. Obesity, Fat Mass and Immune System: Role for Leptin. *Front. Physiol.* **2018**, *9*, 640. [CrossRef]
468. Wang, H.; Zhang, H.; Wang, Y.; Brown, Z.J.; Xia, Y.; Huang, Z.; Shen, C.; Hu, Z.; Beane, J.; Ansa-Addo, E.A.; et al. Regulatory T-cell and neutrophil extracellular trap interaction contributes to carcinogenesis in non-alcoholic steatohepatitis. *J. Hepatol.* **2021**, *75*, 1271–1283. [CrossRef]
469. Dywicki, J.; Buitrago-Molina, L.E.; Noyan, F.; Davalos-Misslitz, A.C.; Hupa-Breier, K.L.; Lieber, M.; Hapke, M.; Schlue, J.; Falk, C.S.; Raha, S.; et al. The Detrimental Role of Regulatory T Cells in Nonalcoholic Steatohepatitis. *Hepatol. Commun.* **2022**, *6*, 320–333. [CrossRef]
470. Katz, S.C.; Ryan, K.; Ahmed, N.; Plitas, G.; Chaudhry, U.I.; Kingham, T.P.; Naheed, S.; Nguyen, C.; Somasundar, P.; Espat, N.J.; et al. Obstructive jaundice expands intrahepatic regulatory T cells, which impair liver T lymphocyte function but modulate liver cholestasis and fibrosis. *J. Immunol.* **2011**, *187*, 1150–1156. [CrossRef]
471. Claassen, M.A.; de Knegt, R.J.; Tilanus, H.W.; Janssen, H.L.; Boonstra, A. Abundant numbers of regulatory T cells localize to the liver of chronic hepatitis C infected patients and limit the extent of fibrosis. *J. Hepatol.* **2010**, *52*, 315–321. [CrossRef] [PubMed]
472. Langhans, B.; Krämer, B.; Louis, M.; Nischalke, H.D.; Hüneburg, R.; Staratschek-Jox, A.; Odenthal, M.; Manekeller, S.; Schepke, M.; Kalff, J.; et al. Intrahepatic IL-8 producing Foxp3$^+$CD4$^+$ regulatory T cells and fibrogenesis in chronic hepatitis C. *J. Hepatol.* **2013**, *59*, 229–235. [CrossRef] [PubMed]
473. Li, J.; Qiu, S.J.; She, W.M.; Wang, F.P.; Gao, H.; Li, L.; Tu, C.T.; Wang, J.Y.; Shen, X.Z.; Jiang, W. Significance of the balance between regulatory T (Treg) and T helper 17 (Th17) cells during hepatitis B virus related liver fibrosis. *PLoS ONE* **2012**, *7*, 39307. [CrossRef]
474. Liu, C.; Zeng, X.; Yu, S.; Ren, L.; Sun, X.; Long, Y.; Wang, X.; Lu, S.; Song, Y.; Sun, X.H.; et al. Up-regulated DNA-binding inhibitor Id3 promotes differentiation of regulatory T cell to influence antiviral immunity in chronic hepatitis B virus infection. *Life Sci.* **2021**, *285*, 119991. [CrossRef]
475. Trehanpati, N.; Vyas, A.K. Immune Regulation by T Regulatory Cells in Hepatitis B Virus-Related Inflammation and Cancer. *Scand. J. Immunol.* **2017**, *85*, 175–181. [CrossRef]

476. Zeng, X.; Bahabayi, A.; Tuerhanbayi, B.; Zheng, M.; Liu, T.; Xu, L.; Long, Y.; Xia, C.; Lu, S.; Song, Y.; et al. The altered HLA-DQ expression in peripheral blood T cells of chronic hepatitis B patients characterizes the function of T cells. *J. Viral Hepat.* **2022**, *29*, 340–351. [CrossRef]
477. Liu, F.; Zhang, S.; Wong, D.K.; Huang, F.Y.; Cheung, K.S.; Mak, L.Y.; Fung, J.; Yuen, M.F.; Seto, W.K. Phenotypic Changes of PD-1 and GITR in T Cells Are Associated With Hepatitis B Surface Antigen Seroclearance. *J. Clin. Gastroenterol.* **2022**, *56*, e31–e37. [CrossRef]
478. Wang, X.; Dong, Q.; Li, Q.; Li, Y.; Zhao, D.; Sun, J.; Fu, J.; Meng, F.; Lin, H.; Luan, J.; et al. Dysregulated Response of Follicular Helper T Cells to Hepatitis B Surface Antigen Promotes HBV Persistence in Mice and Associates With Outcomes of Patients. *Gastroenterology* **2018**, *154*, 2222–2236. [CrossRef]
479. Tangye, S.G.; Ma, C.S. Regulation of the germinal center and humoral immunity by interleukin-21. *J. Exp. Med.* **2020**, *217*, e20191638. [CrossRef]
480. Liu, Y.; Cheng, L.S.; Wu, S.D.; Wang, S.Q.; Li, L.; She, W.M.; Li, J.; Wang, J.Y.; Jiang, W. IL-10-producing regulatory B-cells suppressed effector T-cells but enhanced regulatory T-cells in chronic HBV infection. *Clin. Sci.* **2016**, *130*, 907–919. [CrossRef]
481. Yang, L.; Shao, X.; Jia, S.; Zhang, Q.; Jin, Z. Interleukin-35 Dampens CD8+ T Cells Activity in Patients With Non-viral Hepatitis-Related Hepatocellular Carcinoma. *Front. Immunol.* **2019**, *10*, 1032. [CrossRef]
482. Zhang, Q.; Yang, L.; Liu, S.; Zhang, M.; Jin, Z. Interleukin-35 Suppresses Interleukin-9-Secreting CD4+ T Cell Activity in Patients With Hepatitis B-Related Hepatocellular Carcinoma. *Front. Immunol.* **2021**, *12*, 645835. [CrossRef]
483. Tang, Y.; Ma, T.; Jia, S.; Zhang, Q.; Liu, S.; Qi, L.; Yang, L. The Mechanism of Interleukin-35 in Chronic Hepatitis B. *Semin. Liver Dis.* **2021**, *41*, 516–524. [CrossRef] [PubMed]
484. Huang, E.; Peng, N.; Xiao, F.; Hu, D.; Wang, X.; Lu, L. The Roles of Immune Cells in the Pathogenesis of Fibrosis. *Int. J. Mol. Sci.* **2020**, *21*, 5203. [CrossRef] [PubMed]
485. Fillatreau, S. B cells and their cytokine activities implications in human diseases. *Clin. Immunol.* **2018**, *186*, 26–31. [CrossRef] [PubMed]
486. Novobrantseva, T.I.; Majeau, G.R.; Amatucci, A.; Kogan, S.; Brenner, I.; Casola, S.; Shlomchik, M.J.; Koteliansky, V.; Hochman, P.S.; Ibraghimov, A. Attenuated liver fibrosis in the absence of B cells. *J. Clin. Investig.* **2005**, *115*, 3072–3082. [CrossRef]
487. Bruzzì, S.; Sutti, S.; Giudici, G.; Burlone, M.E.; Ramavath, N.N.; Toscani, A.; Bozzola, C.; Schneider, P.; Morello, E.; Parola, M.; et al. B2-Lymphocyte responses to oxidative stress-derived antigens contribute to the evolution of nonalcoholic fatty liver disease (NAFLD). *Free Radic. Biol. Med.* **2018**, *124*, 249–259. [CrossRef]
488. Gong, Y.; Zhao, C.; Zhao, P.; Wang, M.; Zhou, G.; Han, F.; Cui, Y.; Qian, J.; Zhang, H.; Xiong, H.; et al. Role of IL-10-Producing Regulatory B Cells in Chronic Hepatitis B Virus Infection. *Dig. Dis. Sci.* **2015**, *60*, 1308–1314. [CrossRef]
489. Jin, X.; Yan, Z.H.; Lu, L.; Lu, S.; Zhang, G.; Lin, W. Peripheral Immune Cells Exhaustion and Functional Impairment in Patients With Chronic Hepatitis B. *Front. Med.* **2021**, *8*, 759292. [CrossRef]
490. Liu, Y.; Luo, Y.; Zhu, T.; Jiang, M.; Tian, Z.; Tang, G.; Liang, X. Regulatory B Cells Dysregulated T Cell Function in an IL-35-Dependent Way in Patients With Chronic Hepatitis B. *Front. Immunol.* **2021**, *12*, 653198. [CrossRef]
491. Zheng, P.; Dou, Y.; Wang, Q. Immune response and treatment targets of chronic hepatitis B virus infection: Innate and adaptive immunity. *Front. Cell Infect. Microbiol.* **2023**, *13*, 1206720. [CrossRef] [PubMed]
492. Jia, H.; Chen, J.; Zhang, X.; Bi, K.; Zhou, H.; Liu, T.; Xu, J.; Diao, H. IL-17A produced by invariant natural killer T cells and CD3+ CD56+ αGalcer-CD1d tetramer- T cells promote liver fibrosis in patients with primary biliary cholangitis. *J. Leukoc. Biol.* **2022**, *112*, 1079–1087. [CrossRef]
493. Hammerich, L.; Tacke, F. Role of gamma-delta T cells in liver inflammation and fibrosis. *World J. Gastrointest. Pathophysiol.* **2014**, *5*, 107–113. [CrossRef] [PubMed]
494. Bartish, M.; Del Rincón, S.V.; Rudd, C.E.; Saragovi, H.U. Aiming for the Sweet Spot: Glyco-Immune Checkpoints and γδ T Cells in Targeted Immunotherapy. *Front. Immunol.* **2020**, *11*, 564499. [CrossRef]
495. Pellicci, D.G.; Koay, H.F.; Berzins, S.P. Thymic development of unconventional T cells: How NKT cells, MAIT cells and γδ T cells emerge. *Nat. Rev. Immunol.* **2020**, *20*, 756–770. [CrossRef]
496. Kurioka, A.; Walker, L.J.; Klenerman, P.; Willberg, C.B. MAIT cells: New guardians of the liver. *Clin. Transl. Immunology.* **2016**, *5*, 98. [CrossRef]
497. Bandyopadhyay, K.; Marrero, I.; Kumar, V. NKT cell subsets as key participants in liver physiology and pathology. *Cell Mol. Immunol.* **2016**, *13*, 337–346. [CrossRef]
498. Ibidapo-Obe, O.; Bruns, T. Tissue-resident and innate-like T cells in patients with advanced chronic liver disease. *JHEP Rep.* **2023**, *5*, 100812. [CrossRef]
499. Wei, X.; Qian, J.; Yao, W.; Chen, L.; Guan, H.; Chen, Y.; Xie, Y.; Lu, H.; Zhang, Z.; Shi, L.; et al. Hyperactivated peripheral invariant natural killer T cells correlate with the progression of HBV-relative liver cirrhosis. *Scand. J. Immunol.* **2019**, *90*, 12775. [CrossRef]

500. Tang, W.; Zhou, J.; Yang, W.; Feng, Y.; Wu, H.; Mok, M.T.S.; Zhang, L.; Liang, Z.; Liu, X.; Xiong, Z.; et al. Aberrant cholesterol metabolic signaling impairs antitumor immunosurveillance through natural killer T cell dysfunction in obese liver. *Cell Mol. Immunol.* **2022**, *19*, 834–847. [CrossRef]
501. Zheng, S.; Yang, W.; Yao, D.; Tang, S.; Hou, J.; Chang, X. A comparative study on roles of natural killer T cells in two diet-induced non-alcoholic steatohepatitis-related fibrosis in mice. *Ann. Med.* **2022**, *54*, 2233–2245. [CrossRef] [PubMed]
502. Chan, C.W.; Chen, H.W.; Wang, Y.W.; Lin, C.I.; Chuang, Y.H. IL-21, not IL-17A, exacerbates murine primary biliary cholangitis. *Clin. Exp. Immunol.* **2024**, *215*, 137–147. [CrossRef] [PubMed]
503. Chen, Y.; Tian, Z. Roles of Hepatic Innate and Innate-Like Lymphocytes in Nonalcoholic Steatohepatitis. *Front. Immunol.* **2020**, *11*, 1500. [CrossRef]
504. Torres-Hernandez, A.; Wang, W.; Nikiforov, Y.; Tejada, K.; Torres, L.; Kalabin, A.; Adam, S.; Wu, J.; Lu, L.; Chen, R.; et al. $\gamma\delta$ T Cells Promote Steatohepatitis by Orchestrating Innate and Adaptive Immune Programming. *Hepatology* **2020**, *71*, 477–494. [CrossRef] [PubMed]
505. Wang, X.; Gao, B. $\gamma\delta$T Cells and CD1d, Novel Immune Players in Alcoholic and Nonalcoholic Steatohepatitis? *Hepatology* **2020**, *71*, 408–410. [CrossRef] [PubMed]
506. Li, F.; Hao, X.; Chen, Y.; Bai, L.; Gao, X.; Lian, Z.; Wei, H.; Sun, R.; Tian, Z. The microbiota maintain homeostasis of liver-resident $\gamma\delta$T-17 cells in a lipid antigen/CD1d-dependent manner. *Nat. Commun.* **2017**, *7*, 13839. [CrossRef]
507. Hammerich, L.; Bangen, J.M.; Govaere, O.; Zimmermann, H.W.; Gassler, N.; Huss, S.; Liedtke, C.; Prinz, I.; Lira, S.A.; Luedde, T.; et al. Chemokine receptor CCR6-dependent accumulation of $\gamma\delta$ T cells in injured liver restricts hepatic inflammation and fibrosis. *Hepatology* **2014**, *59*, 630–642. [CrossRef]
508. Spits, H.; Artis, D.; Colonna, M.; Diefenbach, A.; Di Santo, J.P.; Eberl, G.; Koyasu, S.; Locksley, R.M.; McKenzie, A.N.; Mebius, R.E.; et al. Innate lymphoid cells—A proposal for uniform nomenclature. *Nat. Rev. Immunol.* **2013**, *13*, 145–149. [CrossRef]
509. Vivier, E.; Artis, D.; Colonna, M.; Diefenbach, A.; Di Santo, J.P.; Eberl, G.; Koyasu, S.; Locksley, R.M.; McKenzie, A.N.J.; Mebius, R.E.; et al. Innate Lymphoid Cells: 10 Years On. *Cell* **2018**, *174*, 1054–1066. [CrossRef]
510. Wang, S.; Li, J.; Wu, S.; Cheng, L.; Shen, Y.; Ma, W.; She, W.; Yang, C.; Wang, J.; Jiang, W. Type 3 innate lymphoid cell: A new player in liver fibrosis progression. *Clin. Sci.* **2018**, *132*, 2565–2582. [CrossRef]
511. Wang, Y.; Zhang, C. The Roles of Liver-Resident Lymphocytes in Liver Diseases. *Front. Immunol.* **2019**, *10*, 1582. [CrossRef] [PubMed]
512. Liedtke, C.; Nevzorova, Y.A.; Luedde, T.; Zimmermann, H.; Kroy, D.; Strnad, P.; Berres, M.L.; Bernhagen, J.; Tacke, F.; Nattermann, J.; et al. Liver Fibrosis-From Mechanisms of Injury to Modulation of Disease. *Front. Med.* **2022**, *8*, 814496. [CrossRef] [PubMed]
513. Seillet, C.; Brossay, L.; Vivier, E. Natural killers or ILC1s? That is the question. *Curr. Opin. Immunol.* **2021**, *68*, 48–53. [CrossRef] [PubMed]
514. Ebbo, M.; Crinier, A.; Vély, F.; Vivier, E. Innate lymphoid cells: Major players in inflammatory diseases. *Nat. Rev. Immunol.* **2017**, *17*, 665–678. [CrossRef] [PubMed]
515. Forkel, M.; Berglin, L.; Kekäläinen, E.; Carlsson, A.; Svedin, E.; Michaëlsson, J.; Nagasawa, M.; Erjefält, J.S.; Mori, M.; Flodström-Tullberg, M.; et al. Composition and functionality of the intrahepatic innate lymphoid cell-compartment in human nonfibrotic and fibrotic livers. *Eur. J. Immunol.* **2017**, *47*, 1280–1294. [CrossRef]
516. Godfrey, D.I.; Koay, H.F.; McCluskey, J.; Gherardin, N.A. The biology and functional importance of MAIT cells. *Nat. Immunol.* **2019**, *20*, 1110–1128. [CrossRef]
517. Hegde, P.; Weiss, E.; Paradis, V.; Wan, J.; Mabire, M.; Sukriti, S.; Rautou, P.E.; Albuquerque, M.; Picq, O.; Gupta, A.C.; et al. Mucosal-associated invariant T cells are a profibrogenic immune cell population in the liver. *Nat. Commun.* **2018**, *9*, 2146. [CrossRef]
518. Li, Y.; Huang, B.; Jiang, X.; Chen, W.; Zhang, J.; Wei, Y.; Chen, Y.; Lian, M.; Bian, Z.; Miao, Q.; et al. Mucosal-Associated Invariant T Cells Improve Nonalcoholic Fatty Liver Disease Through Regulating Macrophage Polarization. *Front. Immunol.* **2018**, *9*, 1994. [CrossRef]
519. Guan, H.; Zhang, X.; Kuang, M.; Yu, J. The gut-liver axis in immune remodeling of hepatic cirrhosis. *Front. Immunol.* **2022**, *13*, 946628. [CrossRef]
520. Tranah, T.H.; Edwards, L.A.; Schnabl, B.; Shawcross, D.L. Targeting the gut-liver-immune axis to treat cirrhosis. *Gut* **2021**, *70*, 982–994. [CrossRef]
521. Koda, Y.; Teratani, T.; Chu, P.S.; Hagihara, Y.; Mikami, Y.; Harada, Y.; Tsujikawa, H.; Miyamoto, K.; Suzuki, T.; Taniki, N.; et al. CD8+ tissue-resident memory T cells promote liver fibrosis resolution by inducing apoptosis of hepatic stellate cells. *Nat. Commun.* **2021**, *12*, 4474. [CrossRef] [PubMed]
522. Vallianou, N.G.; Kounatidis, D.; Psallida, S.; Vythoulkas-Biotis, N.; Adamou, A.; Zachariadou, T.; Kargioti, S.; Karampela, I.; Dalamaga, M. NAFLD/MASLD and the Gut-Liver Axis: From Pathogenesis to Treatment Options. *Metabolites* **2024**, *14*, 366. [CrossRef] [PubMed]
523. Zhang, S.; Lu, S.; Li, Z. Extrahepatic factors in hepatic immune regulation. *Front. Immunol.* **2022**, *13*, 941721. [CrossRef] [PubMed]

524. Bonneville, M.; O'Brien, R.L.; Born, W.K. Gammadelta T cell effector functions: A blend of innate programming and acquired plasticity. *Nat. Rev. Immunol.* **2010**, *10*, 467–478. [CrossRef]
525. Yang, F.; Li, H.; Li, Y.; Hao, Y.; Wang, C.; Jia, P.; Chen, X.; Ma, S.; Xiao, Z. Crosstalk between hepatic stellate cells and surrounding cells in hepatic fibrosis. *Int. Immunopharmacol.* **2021**, *99*, 108051. [CrossRef]
526. Guo, Z.; Zhang, R.; Yang, A.G.; Zheng, G. Diversity of immune checkpoints in cancer immunotherapy. *Front. Immunol.* **2023**, *14*, 1121285. [CrossRef]
527. Qin, W.; Hu, L.; Zhang, X.; Jiang, S.; Li, J.; Zhang, Z.; Wang, X. The Diverse Function of PD-1/PD-L Pathway Beyond Cancer. *Front. Immunol.* **2019**, *10*, 2298. [CrossRef]
528. Sharpe, A.H.; Pauken, K.E. The diverse functions of the PD1 inhibitory pathway. *Nat. Rev. Immunol.* **2018**, *18*, 153–167. [CrossRef]
529. Zhong, Z.; Vong, C.T.; Chen, F.; Tan, H.; Zhang, C.; Wang, N.; Cui, L.; Wang, Y.; Feng, Y. Immunomodulatory potential of natural products from herbal medicines as immune checkpoints inhibitors: Helping to fight against cancer via multiple targets. *Med. Res. Rev.* **2022**, *42*, 1246–1279. [CrossRef]
530. Chow, A.; Perica, K.; Klebanoff, C.A.; Wolchok, J.D. Clinical implications of T cell exhaustion for cancer immunotherapy. *Nat. Rev. Clin. Oncol.* **2022**, *19*, 775–790. [CrossRef]
531. Zhao, Y.; Shao, Q.; Peng, G. Exhaustion and senescence: Two crucial dysfunctional states of T cells in the tumor microenvironment. *Cell Mol. Immunol.* **2020**, *17*, 27–35. [CrossRef] [PubMed]
532. Schwartz, J.C.; Zhang, X.; Fedorov, A.A.; Nathenson, S.G.; Almo, S.C. Structural basis for co-stimulation by the human CTLA-4/B7-2 complex. *Nature* **2001**, *410*, 604–608. [CrossRef] [PubMed]
533. Linsley, P.S.; Bradshaw, J.; Greene, J.; Peach, R.; Bennett, K.L.; Mittler, R.S. Intracellular trafficking of CTLA-4 and focal localization towards sites of TCR engagement. *Immunity* **1996**, *4*, 535–543. [CrossRef] [PubMed]
534. Marin-Acevedo, J.A.; Kimbrough, E.O.; Lou, Y. Next generation of immune checkpoint inhibitors and beyond. *J. Hematol. Oncol.* **2021**, *14*, 45. [CrossRef]
535. Seidel, J.A.; Otsuka, A.; Kabashima, K. Anti-PD-1 and Anti-CTLA-4 Therapies in Cancer: Mechanisms of Action, Efficacy, and Limitations. *Front. Oncol.* **2018**, *8*, 86. [CrossRef]
536. Ruff, S.M.; Pawlik, T.M. Emerging data on immune checkpoint inhibitors in the neoadjuvant and adjuvant setting for patients with hepatocellular carcinoma. *Hepatoma Res.* **2024**, *10*, 22. [CrossRef]
537. Baldanzi, G. Immune Checkpoint Receptors Signaling in T Cells. *Int. J. Mol. Sci.* **2022**, *23*, 3529. [CrossRef]
538. Cai, J.; Qi, Q.; Qian, X.; Han, J.; Zhu, X.; Zhang, Q.; Xia, R. The role of PD-1/PD-L1 axis and macrophage in the progression and treatment of cancer. *J. Cancer Res. Clin. Oncol.* **2019**, *145*, 1377–1385. [CrossRef]
539. Gianchecchi, E.; Delfino, D.V.; Fierabracci, A. Recent insights into the role of the PD-1/PD-L1 pathway in immunological tolerance and autoimmunity. *Autoimmun. Rev.* **2013**, *12*, 1091–1100. [CrossRef]
540. Keir, M.E.; Butte, M.J.; Freeman, G.J.; Sharpe, A.H. PD-1 and its ligands in tolerance and immunity. *Annu. Rev. Immunol.* **2008**, *26*, 677–704. [CrossRef]
541. Agata, Y.; Kawasaki, A.; Nishimura, H.; Ishida, Y.; Tsubata, T.; Yagita, H.; Honjo, T. Expression of the PD-1 antigen on the surface of stimulated mouse T and B lymphocytes. *Int. Immunol.* **1996**, *8*, 765–772. [CrossRef] [PubMed]
542. Barber, D.L.; Wherry, E.J.; Masopust, D.; Zhu, B.; Allison, J.P.; Sharpe, A.H.; Freeman, G.J.; Ahmed, R. Restoring function in exhausted CD8 T cells during chronic viral infection. *Nature* **2006**, *439*, 682–687. [CrossRef] [PubMed]
543. Park, B.V.; Freeman, Z.T.; Ghasemzadeh, A.; Chattergoon, M.A.; Rutebemberwa, A.; Steigner, J.; Winter, M.E.; Huynh, T.V.; Sebald, S.M.; Lee, S.J.; et al. TGFβ1-Mediated SMAD3 Enhances PD-1 Expression on Antigen-Specific T Cells in Cancer. *Cancer Discov.* **2016**, *6*, 1366–1381. [CrossRef] [PubMed]
544. Sun, Z.; Fourcade, J.; Pagliano, O.; Chauvin, J.M.; Sander, C.; Kirkwood, J.M.; Zarour, H.M. IL10 and PD-1 Cooperate to Limit the Activity of Tumor-Specific CD8+ T Cells. *Cancer Res.* **2015**, *75*, 1635–1644. [CrossRef]
545. Sun, C.; Mezzadra, R.; Schumacher, T.N. Regulation and Function of the PD-L1 Checkpoint. *Immunity* **2018**, *48*, 434–452. [CrossRef]
546. Yamazaki, T.; Akiba, H.; Iwai, H.; Matsuda, H.; Aoki, M.; Tanno, Y.; Shin, T.; Tsuchiya, H.; Pardoll, D.M.; Okumura, K.; et al. Expression of programmed death 1 ligands by murine T cells and APC. *J. Immunol.* **2002**, *169*, 5538–5545. [CrossRef]
547. Li, K.; Yuan, Z.; Lyu, J.; Ahn, E.; Davis, S.J.; Ahmed, R.; Zhu, C. PD-1 suppresses TCR-CD8 cooperativity during T-cell antigen recognition. *Nat. Commun.* **2021**, *12*, 2746. [CrossRef]
548. Apol, Á.D.; Winckelmann, A.A.; Duus, R.B.; Bukh, J.; Weis, N. The Role of CTLA-4 in T Cell Exhaustion in Chronic Hepatitis B Virus Infection. *Viruses* **2023**, *15*, 1141. [CrossRef]
549. Gordon, S.R.; Maute, R.L.; Dulken, B.W.; Hutter, G.; George, B.M.; McCracken, M.N.; Gupta, R.; Tsai, J.M.; Sinha, R.; Corey, D.; et al. PD-1 expression by tumour-associated macrophages inhibits phagocytosis and tumour immunity. *Nature* **2017**, *545*, 495–499. [CrossRef]

550. Qorraj, M.; Bruns, H.; Böttcher, M.; Weigand, L.; Saul, D.; Mackensen, A.; Jitschin, R.; Mougiakakos, D. The PD-1/PD-L1 axis contributes to immune metabolic dysfunctions of monocytes in chronic lymphocytic leukemia. *Leukemia* **2017**, *31*, 470–478. [CrossRef]
551. Liu, J.; Xu, X.; Zhong, H.; Yu, M.; Abuduaini, N.; Zhang, S.; Yang, X.; Feng, B. Glycosylation and Its Role in Immune Checkpoint Proteins: From Molecular Mechanisms to Clinical Implications. *Biomedicines* **2024**, *12*, 1446. [CrossRef] [PubMed]
552. Hsu, J.M.; Xia, W.; Hsu, Y.H.; Chan, L.C.; Yu, W.H.; Cha, J.H.; Chen, C.T.; Liao, H.W.; Kuo, C.W.; Khoo, K.H.; et al. STT3-dependent PD-L1 accumulation on cancer stem cells promotes immune evasion. *Nat. Commun.* **2018**, *9*, 1908. [CrossRef] [PubMed]
553. Zhao, Y.; Qu, Y.; Hao, C.; Yao, W. PD-1/PD-L1 axis in organ fibrosis. *Front. Immunol.* **2023**, *14*, 1145682. [CrossRef]
554. Aoki, T.; Nishida, N.; Kudo, M. Current Perspectives on the Immunosuppressive Niche and Role of Fibrosis in Hepatocellular Carcinoma and the Development of Antitumor Immunity. *J. Histochem. Cytochem.* **2022**, *70*, 53–81. [CrossRef]
555. Zhang, Y.C.; Zhang, Y.T.; Wang, Y.; Zhao, Y.; He, L.J. What role does PDL1 play in EMT changes in tumors and fibrosis? *Front Immunol.* **2023**, *14*, 1226038. [CrossRef]
556. Ke, M.Y.; Xu, T.; Fang, Y.; Ye, Y.P.; Li, Z.J.; Ren, F.G.; Lu, S.Y.; Zhang, X.F.; Wu, R.Q.; Lv, Y.; et al. Liver fibrosis promotes immune escape in hepatocellular carcinoma via GOLM1-mediated PD-L1 upregulation. *Cancer Lett.* **2021**, *513*, 14–25. [CrossRef]
557. Xiang, M.; Liu, T.; Tian, C.; Ma, K.; Gou, J.; Huang, R.; Li, S.; Li, Q.; Xu, C.; Li, L.; et al. Kinsenoside attenuates liver fibro-inflammation by suppressing dendritic cells via the PI3K-AKT-FoxO1 pathway. *Pharmacol. Res.* **2022**, *177*, 106092. [CrossRef]
558. Dong, Y.; Li, X.; Zhang, L.; Zhu, Q.; Chen, C.; Bao, J.; Chen, Y. CD4+ T cell exhaustion revealed by high PD-1 and LAG-3 expression and the loss of helper T cell function in chronic hepatitis B. *BMC Immunol.* **2019**, *20*, 27. [CrossRef]
559. Ye, B.; Liu, X.; Li, X.; Kong, H.; Tian, L.; Chen, Y. T-cell exhaustion in chronic hepatitis B infection: Current knowledge and clinical significance. *Cell Death Dis.* **2015**, *6*, e1694. [CrossRef]
560. Cho, H.; Kang, H.; Lee, H.H.; Kim, C.W. Programmed Cell Death 1 (PD-1) and Cytotoxic T Lymphocyte-Associated Antigen 4 (CTLA-4) in Viral Hepatitis. *Int. J. Mol. Sci.* **2017**, *18*, 1517. [CrossRef]
561. Huang, D.; Yan, W.; Han, M.; Yuan, W.; Wang, P.; Chen, Y.; Wan, X.; Luo, X.; Wu, D.; Ning, Q. Insufficient immunity led to virologic breakthrough in NAs-treated chronic hepatitis B patients switching to Peg-IFN-α. *Antiviral Res.* **2022**, *197*, 105220. [CrossRef] [PubMed]
562. Ferrando-Martinez, S.; Huang, K.; Bennett, A.S.; Sterba, P.; Yu, L.; Suzich, J.A.; Janssen, H.L.A.; Robbins, S.H. HBeAg seroconversion is associated with a more effective PD-L1 blockade during chronic hepatitis B infection. *JHEP Rep.* **2019**, *1*, 170–178. [CrossRef] [PubMed]
563. Cui, D.; Jiang, D.; Yan, C.; Liu, X.; Lv, Y.; Xie, J.; Chen, Y. Immune Checkpoint Molecules Expressed on CD4+ T Cell Subsets in Chronic Asymptomatic Hepatitis B Virus Carriers With Hepatitis B e Antigen-Negative. *Front. Microbiol.* **2022**, *13*, 887408. [CrossRef] [PubMed]
564. Salem, M.L.; El-Badawy, A. Programmed death-1/programmed death-L1 signaling pathway and its blockade in hepatitis C virus immunotherapy. *World J. Hepatol.* **2015**, *7*, 2449–2458. [CrossRef]
565. Park, S.J.; Hahn, Y.S. Hepatocytes infected with hepatitis C virus change immunological features in the liver microenvironment. *Clin. Mol. Hepatol.* **2023**, *29*, 65–76. [CrossRef]
566. Liu, X.; Zhou, J.; Wu, H.; Chen, S.; Zhang, L.; Tang, W.; Duan, L.; Wang, Y.; McCabe, E.; Hu, M.; et al. Fibrotic immune microenvironment remodeling mediates superior anti-tumor efficacy of a nano-PD-L1 trap in hepatocellular carcinoma. *Mol. Ther.* **2023**, *31*, 119–133. [CrossRef]
567. Zhou, L.; Li, X.; Huang, X.; Chen, L.; Gu, L.; Huang, Y. Soluble programmed death-1 is a useful indicator for inflammatory and fibrosis severity in chronic hepatitis B. *J. Viral Hepat.* **2019**, *26*, 795–802. [CrossRef]
568. Huang, N.; Zhou, R.; Chen, H.; Zhang, S.; Li, J.; Wei, W.; Sun, J.; Ren, S.; Li, B.; Deng, H.; et al. Splenic CD4+ and CD8+ T-cells highly expressed PD-1 and Tim-3 in cirrhotic patients with HCV infection and portal hypertension. *Int. J. Immunopathol. Pharmacol.* **2021**, *35*, 20587384211061051. [CrossRef]
569. Jiang, A.; Liu, N.; Wang, J.; Zheng, X.; Ren, M.; Zhang, W.; Yao, Y. The role of PD-1/PD-L1 axis in idiopathic pulmonary fibrosis: Friend or foe? *Front. Immunol.* **2022**, *13*, 1022228. [CrossRef]
570. Lu, Y.; Zhong, W.; Liu, Y.; Chen, W.; Zhang, J.; Zeng, Z.; Huang, H.; Qiao, Y.; Wan, X.; Meng, X.; et al. Anti-PD-L1 antibody alleviates pulmonary fibrosis by inducing autophagy via inhibition of the PI3K/Akt/mTOR pathway. *Int. Immunopharmacol.* **2022**, *104*, 108504. [CrossRef]
571. Paskeh, M.D.A.; Ghadyani, F.; Hashemi, M.; Abbaspour, A.; Zabolian, A.; Javanshir, S.; Razzazan, M.; Mirzaei, S.; Entezari, M.; Goharrizi, M.A.S.B.; et al. Biological impact and therapeutic perspective of targeting PI3K/Akt signaling in hepatocellular carcinoma: Promises and Challenges. *Pharmacol. Res.* **2023**, *187*, 106553. [CrossRef] [PubMed]
572. Song, L.; Chen, T.Y.; Zhao, X.J.; Xu, Q.; Jiao, R.Q.; Li, J.M.; Kong, L.D. Pterostilbene prevents hepatocyte epithelial-mesenchymal transition in fructose-induced liver fibrosis through suppressing miR-34a/Sirt1/p53 and TGF-β1/Smads signalling. *Br. J. Pharmacol.* **2019**, *176*, 1619–1634. [CrossRef] [PubMed]

573. Yang, Y.Z.; Zhao, X.J.; Xu, H.J.; Wang, S.C.; Pan, Y.; Wang, S.J.; Xu, Q.; Jiao, R.Q.; Gu, H.M.; Kong, L.D. Magnesium isoglycyrrhizinate ameliorates high fructose-induced liver fibrosis in rat by increasing miR-375-3p to suppress JAK2/STAT3 pathway and TGF-β1/Smad signaling. *Acta Pharmacol. Sin.* **2019**, *40*, 879–894. [CrossRef]
574. Zhou, W.C.; Zhang, Q.B.; Qiao, L. Pathogenesis of liver cirrhosis. *World J. Gastroenterol.* **2014**, *20*, 7312–7324. [CrossRef]
575. Ye, Y.; Xu, Y.; Lai, Y.; He, W.; Li, Y.; Wang, R.; Luo, X.; Chen, R.; Chen, T. Long non-coding RNA cox-2 prevents immune evasion and metastasis of hepatocellular carcinoma by altering M1/M2 macrophage polarization. *J. Cell Biochem.* **2018**, *119*, 2951–2963. [CrossRef]
576. Li, Q.; Deng, M.S.; Wang, R.T.; Luo, H.; Luo, Y.Y.; Zhang, D.D.; Chen, K.J.; Cao, X.F.; Yang, G.M.; Zhao, T.M.; et al. PD-L1 upregulation promotes drug-induced pulmonary fibrosis by inhibiting vimentin degradation. *Pharmacol. Res.* **2023**, *187*, 106636. [CrossRef]
577. Kong, X.; Peng, H.; Liu, P.; Fu, X.; Wang, N.; Zhang, D. Programmed death ligand 1 regulates epithelial-mesenchymal transition and cancer stem cell phenotypes in hepatocellular carcinoma through the serum and glucocorticoid kinase 2/β-catenin signaling pathway. *Cancer Sci.* **2023**, *114*, 2265–2276. [CrossRef]
578. Nakamoto, N.; Cho, H.; Shaked, A.; Olthoff, K.; Valiga, M.E.; Kaminski, M.; Gostick, E.; Price, D.A.; Freeman, G.J.; Wherry, E.J.; et al. Synergistic reversal of intrahepatic HCV-specific CD8 T cell exhaustion by combined PD-1/CTLA-4 blockade. *PLoS Pathog.* **2009**, *5*, 1000313. [CrossRef]
579. Hazrati, A.; Malekpour, K.; Khorramdelazad, H.; Rajaei, S.; Hashemi, S.M. Therapeutic and immunomodulatory potentials of mesenchymal stromal/stem cells and immune checkpoints related molecules. *Biomark. Res.* **2024**, *12*, 35. [CrossRef]
580. Bally, A.P.; Lu, P.; Tang, Y.; Austin, J.W.; Scharer, C.D.; Ahmed, R.; Boss, J.M. NF-κB regulates PD-1 expression in macrophages. *J. Immunol.* **2015**, *194*, 4545–4554. [CrossRef]
581. Said, E.A.; Dupuy, F.P.; Trautmann, L.; Zhang, Y.; Shi, Y.; El-Far, M.; Hill, B.J.; Noto, A.; Ancuta, P.; Peretz, Y.; et al. Programmed death-1-induced interleukin-10 production by monocytes impairs CD4+ T cell activation during HIV infection. *Nat. Med.* **2010**, *16*, 452–459. [CrossRef]
582. Huang, X.; Venet, F.; Wang, Y.L.; Lepape, A.; Yuan, Z.; Chen, Y.; Swan, R.; Kherouf, H.; Monneret, G.; Chung, C.S.; et al. PD-1 expression by macrophages plays a pathologic role in altering microbial clearance and the innate inflammatory response to sepsis. *Proc. Natl. Acad. Sci. USA* **2009**, *106*, 6303–6308. [CrossRef] [PubMed]
583. Shen, L.; Gao, Y.; Liu, Y.; Zhang, B.; Liu, Q.; Wu, J.; Fan, L.; Ou, Q.; Zhang, W.; Shao, L. PD-1/PD-L pathway inhibits M.tb-specific CD4+ T-cell functions and phagocytosis of macrophages in active tuberculosis. *Sci. Rep.* **2016**, *6*, 38362. [CrossRef] [PubMed]
584. Hartley, G.P.; Chow, L.; Ammons, D.T.; Wheat, W.H.; Dow, S.W. Programmed Cell Death Ligand 1 (PD-L1) Signaling Regulates Macrophage Proliferation and Activation. *Cancer Immunol. Res.* **2018**, *6*, 1260–1273. [CrossRef] [PubMed]
585. Kassel, R.; Cruise, M.W.; Iezzoni, J.C.; Taylor, N.A.; Pruett, T.L.; Hahn, Y.S. Chronically inflamed livers up-regulate expression of inhibitory B7 family members. *Hepatology* **2009**, *50*, 1625–1637. [CrossRef]
586. Triantafyllou, E.; Gudd, C.L.; Mawhin, M.A.; Husbyn, H.C.; Trovato, F.M.; Siggins, M.K.; O'Connor, T.; Kudo, H.; Mukherjee, S.K.; Wendon, J.A.; et al. PD-1 blockade improves Kupffer cell bacterial clearance in acute liver injury. *J. Clin. Investig.* **2021**, *131*, 140196. [CrossRef]
587. Triantafyllou, E.; Woollard, K.J.; McPhail, M.J.W.; Antoniades, C.G.; Possamai, L.A. The Role of Monocytes and Macrophages in Acute and Acute-on-Chronic Liver Failure. *Front. Immunol.* **2018**, *9*, 2948. [CrossRef]
588. Charles, R.; Chou, H.S.; Wang, L.; Fung, J.J.; Lu, L.; Qian, S. Human hepatic stellate cells inhibit T-cell response through B7-H1 pathway. *Transplantation* **2013**, *96*, 17–24. [CrossRef]
589. Onorati, A.; Havas, A.P.; Lin, B.; Rajagopal, J.; Sen, P.; Adams, P.D.; Dou, Z. Upregulation of PD-L1 in Senescence and Aging. *Mol. Cell Biol.* **2022**, *42*, 0017122. [CrossRef] [PubMed]
590. Salminen, A. Inhibitory immune checkpoints suppress the surveillance of senescent cells promoting their accumulation with aging and in age-related diseases. *Biogerontology* **2024**, *25*, 749–773. [CrossRef]
591. Salminen, A. The role of the immunosuppressive PD-1/PD-L1 checkpoint pathway in the aging process and age-related diseases. *J. Mol. Med.* **2024**, *102*, 733–750. [CrossRef] [PubMed]
592. Wang, T.W.; Johmura, Y.; Suzuki, N.; Omori, S.; Migita, T.; Yamaguchi, K.; Hatakeyama, S.; Yamazaki, S.; Shimizu, E.; Imoto, S.; et al. Blocking PD-L1-PD-1 improves senescence surveillance and ageing phenotypes. *Nature* **2022**, *611*, 358–364. [CrossRef] [PubMed]
593. Sun, L.; Wang, Y.; Wang, X.; Navarro-Corcuera, A.; Ilyas, S.; Jalan-Sakrikar, N.; Gan, C.; Tu, X.; Shi, Y.; Tu, K.; et al. PD-L1 promotes myofibroblastic activation of hepatic stellate cells by distinct mechanisms selective for TGF-β receptor I versus II. *Cell Rep.* **2022**, *38*, 110349. [CrossRef] [PubMed]
594. Kontos, F.; Michelakos, T.; Kurokawa, T.; Sadagopan, A.; Schwab, J.H.; Ferrone, C.R.; Ferrone, S. B7-H3: An Attractive Target for Antibody-based Immunotherapy. *Clin. Cancer Res.* **2021**, *27*, 1227–1235. [CrossRef]
595. Picarda, E.; Ohaegbulam, K.C.; Zang, X. Molecular Pathways: Targeting B7-H3 (CD276) for Human Cancer Immunotherapy. *Clin. Cancer Res.* **2016**, *22*, 3425–3431. [CrossRef]

596. Podojil, J.R.; Miller, S.D. Potential targeting of B7-H4 for the treatment of cancer. *Immunol. Rev.* **2017**, *276*, 40–51. [CrossRef]
597. Sica, G.L.; Choi, I.H.; Zhu, G.; Tamada, K.; Wang, S.D.; Tamura, H.; Chapoval, A.I.; Flies, D.B.; Bajorath, J.; Chen, L. B7-H4, a molecule of the B7 family, negatively regulates T cell immunity. *Immunity.* **2003**, *18*, 849–861. [CrossRef]
598. Jiang, D.; Chen, C.; Yan, D.; Zhang, X.; Liu, X.; Yan, D.; Cui, D.; Yang, S. Exhausted phenotype of circulating CD8+ T cell subsets in hepatitis B virus carriers. *BMC Immunol.* **2022**, *23*, 18. [CrossRef]
599. Mohammadizad, H.; Shahbazi, M.; Hasanjani Roushan, M.R.; Soltanzadeh-Yamchi, M.; Mohammadnia-Afrouzi, M. TIM-3 as a marker of exhaustion in CD8+ T cells of active chronic hepatitis B patients. *Microb. Pathog.* **2019**, *128*, 323–328. [CrossRef]
600. Arvanitakis, K.; Papadakos, S.P.; Vakadaris, G.; Chatzikalil, E.; Stergiou, I.E.; Kalopitas, G.; Theocharis, S.; Germanidis, G. Shedding light on the role of LAG-3 in hepatocellular carcinoma: Unraveling immunomodulatory pathways. *Hepatoma Res.* **2024**, *10*, 21. [CrossRef]
601. Heim, K.; Neumann-Haefelin, C.; Thimme, R.; Hofmann, M. Heterogeneity of HBV-Specific CD8+ T-Cell Failure: Implications for Immunotherapy. *Front. Immunol.* **2019**, *10*, 2240. [CrossRef] [PubMed]
602. Ogiso, H.; Ito, H.; Ando, T.; Arioka, Y.; Kanbe, A.; Ando, K.; Ishikawa, T.; Saito, K.; Hara, A.; Moriwaki, H.; et al. The Deficiency of Indoleamine 2,3-Dioxygenase Aggravates the CCl4-Induced Liver Fibrosis in Mice. *PLoS ONE* **2016**, *11*, 0162183. [CrossRef] [PubMed]
603. Hoshi, M.; Osawa, Y.; Nakamoto, K.; Morita, N.; Yamamoto, Y.; Ando, T.; Tashita, C.; Nabeshima, T.; Saito, K. Kynurenine produced by indoleamine 2,3-dioxygenase 2 exacerbates acute liver injury by carbon tetrachloride in mice. *Toxicology* **2020**, *438*, 152458. [CrossRef]
604. Nebbia, G.; Peppa, D.; Schurich, A.; Khanna, P.; Singh, H.D.; Cheng, Y.; Rosenberg, W.; Dusheiko, G.; Gilson, R.; ChinAleong, J.; et al. Upregulation of the Tim-3/galectin-9 pathway of T cell exhaustion in chronic hepatitis B virus infection. *PLoS ONE* **2012**, *7*, e47648. [CrossRef]
605. Fisicaro, P.; Valdatta, C.; Massari, M.; Loggi, E.; Biasini, E.; Sacchelli, L.; Cavallo, M.C.; Silini, E.M.; Andreone, P.; Missale, G.; et al. Antiviral intrahepatic T-cell responses can be restored by blocking programmed death-1 pathway in chronic hepatitis B. *Gastroenterology* **2010**, *138*, 682–693. [CrossRef]
606. Wu, W.; Shi, Y.; Li, S.; Zhang, Y.; Liu, Y.; Wu, Y.; Chen, Z. Blockade of Tim-3 signaling restores the virus-specific $CD8^+$ T-cell response in patients with chronic hepatitis B. *Eur. J. Immunol.* **2012**, *42*, 1180–1191. [CrossRef]
607. Zong, L.; Peng, H.; Sun, C.; Li, F.; Zheng, M.; Chen, Y.; Wei, H.; Sun, R.; Tian, Z. Breakdown of adaptive immunotolerance induces hepatocellular carcinoma in HBsAg-tg mice. *Nat. Commun.* **2019**, *10*, 221. [CrossRef]
608. Li, Q.; Han, J.; Yang, Y.; Chen, Y. PD-1/PD-L1 checkpoint inhibitors in advanced hepatocellular carcinoma immunotherapy. *Front. Immunol.* **2022**, *13*, 1070961. [CrossRef]
609. Abou-Alfa, G.K.; Chan, S.L.; Kudo, M.; Lau, G.; Kelley, R.K.; Furuse, J.; Sukeepaisarnjaroen, W.; Kang, Y.K.; Dao, T.V.; De Toni, E.N.; et al. Phase 3 randomized, open-label, multicenter study of tremelimumab (T) and durvalumab (D) as first-line therapy in patients (pts) with unresectable hepatocellular carcinoma (uHCC): HIMALAYA. *J. Clin. Oncol.* **2022**, *40*, 379. [CrossRef]
610. Gupta, T.; Jarpula, N.S. Hepatocellular carcinoma immune microenvironment and check point inhibitors-current status. *World J. Hepatol.* **2024**, *16*, 353–365. [CrossRef]
611. Haber, P.K.; Puigvehí, M.; Castet, F.; Lourdusamy, V.; Montal, R.; Tabrizian, P.; Buckstein, M.; Kim, E.; Villanueva, A.; Schwartz, M.; et al. Evidence-Based Management of Hepatocellular Carcinoma: Systematic Review and Meta-analysis of Randomized Controlled Trials (2002–2020). *Gastroenterology* **2021**, *161*, 879–898. [CrossRef]
612. Li, X.; Gao, L.; Wang, B.; Hu, J.; Yu, Y.; Gu, B.; Xiang, L.; Li, X.; Li, H.; Zhang, T.; et al. FXa-mediated PAR-2 promotes the efficacy of immunotherapy for hepatocellular carcinoma through immune escape and anoikis resistance by inducing PD-L1 transcription. *J. Immunother. Cancer* **2024**, *12*, e009565. [CrossRef] [PubMed]
613. Oliveira, C.; Mainoli, B.; Duarte, G.S.; Machado, T.; Tinoco, R.G.; Esperança-Martins, M.; Ferreira, J.J.; Costa, J. Immune-related serious adverse events with immune checkpoint inhibitors: Systematic review and network meta-analysis. *Eur. J. Clin. Pharmacol.* **2024**, *80*, 677–684. [CrossRef] [PubMed]
614. Liang, X.; Xiao, H.; Li, H.; Chen, X.; Li, Y. Adverse events associated with immune checkpoint inhibitors in non-small cell lung cancer: A safety analysis of clinical trials and FDA pharmacovigilance system. *Front. Immunol.* **2024**, *15*, 1396752. [CrossRef] [PubMed]
615. Godbert, B.; Petitpain, N.; Lopez, A.; Nisse, Y.E.; Gillet, P. Hepatitis B reactivation and immune check point inhibitors. *Dig. Liver Dis.* **2021**, *53*, 452–455. [CrossRef] [PubMed]
616. Ren, X.; Wang, H.; Deng, L.; Wang, W.; Wang, Y. Immune-related adverse events of immune checkpoint inhibitors combined with angiogenesis inhibitors: A real-world pharmacovigilance analysis of the FDA Adverse Event Reporting System (FAERS) database (2014–2022). *Int. Immunopharmacol.* **2024**, *136*, 112301. [CrossRef]

livers

MDPI

Article

Advancing Chronic Liver Disease Diagnoses: Targeted Proteomics for the Non-Invasive Detection of Fibrosis

Andrea Villanueva Raisman [1,2], David Kotol [3], Ozlem Altay [1,2], Adil Mardinoglu [1,2], Dila Atak [4], Cihan Yurdaydin [5], Murat Akyildiz [5], Murat Dayangac [6], Hale Kirimlioglu [7], Müjdat Zeybel [5,6] and Fredrik Edfors [1,2,*]

1 SciLifeLab, KTH Royal Institute of Technology, 114 28 Stockholm, Sweden; andrea.villanueva@scilifelab.se (A.V.R.); havva.altay@scilifelab.se (O.A.); adilm@scilifelab.se (A.M.)
2 Department of Protein Science, Division of Systems Biology, School of Chemistry, Biotechnology and Health, KTH Royal Institute of Technology, 114 28 Stockholm, Sweden
3 ProteomEdge AB, 106 91 Stockholm, Sweden
4 Translational Medicine Research Center, Koç University, Istanbul 34010, Turkey; dilatak@ku.edu.tr
5 Department of Gastroenterology and Hepatology, School of Medicine, Koç University, Istanbul 34450, Turkey; cyurdaydin@ku.edu.tr (C.Y.); makyildiz@kuh.ku.edu.tr (M.A.); mzeybel@ku.edu.tr (M.Z.)
6 Department of General Surgery, Faculty of Medicine, Medipol University, Istanbul 34010, Turkey; mdayangac@medipol.edu.tr
7 Department of Pathology, School of Medicine, Acibadem Mehmet Ali Aydinlar University, Istanbul 34752, Turkey
* Correspondence: edfors@kth.se

Abstract: Chronic liver disease poses significant challenges to healthcare systems, which frequently struggle to meet the needs of end-stage liver disease patients. Early detection and management are essential because liver damage and fibrosis are potentially reversible. However, the implementation of population-wide screenings is hindered by the asymptomatic nature of early chronic liver disease, along with the risks and costs associated with traditional diagnostics, such as liver biopsies. This study pioneers the development of innovative, minimally invasive methods capable of improving the outcomes of liver disease patients by identifying liver disease biomarkers using quantification methods with translational potential. A targeted mass spectrometry assay based on stable isotope standard protein epitope signature tags (SIS-PrESTs) was employed for the absolute quantification of 108 proteins in just two microliters of plasma. The plasma profiles were derived from patients of various liver disease stages and etiologies, including healthy controls. A set of potential biomarkers for stratifying liver fibrosis was identified through differential expression analysis and supervised machine learning. These findings offer promising alternatives for improved diagnostics and personalized treatment strategies in liver disease management. Moreover, our approach is fully compatible with existing technologies that facilitate the robust quantification of clinically relevant protein targets via minimally disruptive sampling methods.

Keywords: chronic liver disease (CLD); fibrosis biomarkers; targeted proteomics; plasma proteome profiling; mass spectrometry

1. Introduction

Liver diseases claim approximately 2 million lives globally every year [1], representing a significant clinical and economic challenge to healthcare systems worldwide [2,3]. Most of the cases are attributed to cirrhosis and hepatocellular carcinoma (HCC), followed by a smaller fraction from acute liver failure [4–7]. Chronic liver disease (CLD) is a broad term, which includes many disease etiologies, such as alcohol-related liver disease (ARLD), metabolic dysfunction-associated steatotic liver disease (MASLD), and chronic viral hepatitis (VHB). The common ground among these disease etiologies is that they tend to progress in sequential stages, which do not necessarily have distinct bounds, making the classification challenging [1,4]. CLD progresses from hepatic steatosis (steatotic liver), through hepatitis (which can also start without steatosis), to fibrosis (excessive buildup of extracellular matrix), and finally to cirrhosis (severe liver scarring) [4]. Normally, fibrogenesis is meant to maintain the integrity of tissue during the wound-healing response [8]. However, when it is progressive or chronic, it may lead to the disruption of the liver parenchymal architecture. This progression is often slow and asymptomatic, delaying the diagnosis until advanced stages, like cirrhosis or HCC, are reached [8–10], which together account for about 3.5% of all global deaths [6].

The liver, the largest internal organ in the body, has a complex functionality [11], including nutrient metabolism, the synthesis of diverse biomolecules (e.g., proteins, hormones), detoxification, fat digestion, red blood cell breakdown and removal, and the immune system front line [2,11,12]. This functional intricacy is achieved by a composite, multicellular tissue, which has not yet been replicated by any artificial systems [13]. Liver transplantation is the only solution for long-term survival.

Despite the high mortality rate of CLD, early and correct management of the disease cannot only stop or decelerate fibrosis progression, but even reverse it, reducing the possibility of decompensated cirrhosis, HCC, and liver failure [4]. With a timely diagnosis, appropriate measures can be taken to hinder disease progression and increase survival chances. These measures can go from lifestyle changes (e.g., alcohol abstinence, increased physical activity) to antiviral therapy for hepatitis B or C, diabetes treatment, and surveillance for HCC [9]. An early diagnosis enables effective interventions that slow liver disease progression and enhance survival.

However, the often slow and symptom-free progression of these diseases makes early detection challenging [14]. Liver fibrosis, a critical structural and functional change in CLD, helps predict the progression from a healthy liver to cirrhosis. While non-invasive methods are helpful, the histological analysis of liver biopsies has traditionally been considered the gold standard for evaluating necro-inflammation and hepatic fibrosis [4,15]. These analyses rely on systematic, semi-quantitative measurements to grade and stage the histologic progression of the disease [16]. Notably, liver biopsies have significant limitations. Besides technical difficulties, it is an expensive and invasive procedure, which poses the risk of life-threatening complications [8,14,15]. Other limitations include that (i) it does not provide insight into the dynamic changes of fibrogenesis, (ii) it only provides information for a comparatively small part of the liver, risking not being representative of the real level of fibrosis, which has a heterogeneous distribution, and (iii) there is inherent variability in the interpretation between pathologists. Not being apt for population-wide screenings, only a small number of patients are identified as being at risk [8]. Furthermore, other clinical complications can emerge as fibrosis progresses, and fibrosis staging does not necessarily reflect these outcomes [16]. This presents a strong case to move to less invasive and more informative tests to improve individual patient outcomes and make population-wide screening more feasible and reduce the clinical and economic burden for healthcare systems [9].

This has led to the move towards minimally invasive procedures, such as blood analysis and imaging [8]. Blood is a key source for molecular analyses in both clinical and research settings [17]. It holds immense potential for biomarker discovery and therapeutic targeting. Currently, some non-invasive methods for the assessment of liver fibrosis are used in patients for first-line assessments [15]. However, biomarker-discovery efforts have centered on single molecules [14]. This has been an obstacle to their success since the multiplicity of the liver's biochemical, synthetic, and excretory functions cannot be captured by a single biomarker [18].

Mass spectrometry enhances biomarker discovery by allowing for the simultaneous quantitative analysis of multiple targets with high specificity. It is particularly effective in proteomic research, where it is used to gather comprehensive data across different biological systems. Mass spectrometry-based proteomics are suitable to obtain system-wide information, which can be used in hypothesis testing and for differential expression analysis, as well as supervised machine learning. These algorithms can leverage comprehensive data to generate disease-classification models and extract features suitable for a patient's health assessment. This makes mass spectrometry a fitting strategy to be used in healthcare and biomarker discovery. In this context, the integration of targeted proteomics and specifically selected reaction monitoring (SRM) with stable isotope standard protein epitope signature tags (SIS-PrESTs) presents a relevant solution for the highly specific and reproducible quantification of proteins [19]. This high-throughput method consists of using a predefined multiplex panel of SIS-PrESTs, targeting a set of medium-to-high-abundant blood plasma proteins. SIS-PrESTs are recombinant internal protein standards that are spiked in known quantities into patients' blood plasma samples and digested altogether to peptides prior to MS analysis. From the extracted chromatograms, the ratio of areas under the curves from endogenous peptides to SIS-PrEST signals are calculated and converted to absolute protein quantities. The integration of this technology into clinical practice could provide clinicians with a more precise and comprehensive liver health assessment, allowing for early fibrosis and CLD treatment while being minimally invasive and affordable.

2. Materials and Methods

This study is part of the Human Disease Blood Atlas (HDBA), received approval from the Swedish Ethical Review Authority (EPM dnr 2019-00222), and adheres to relevant ethical regulations. Collection procedures align with participants having provided their informed written consent. The Swedish Ethical Review Board granted ethical approval, authorizing a proteomics analysis on previously collected samples.

The study protocol adheres to the ethical guidelines of the 1975 Declaration of Helsinki. For the liver disease sample cohort, collected at Koç University and Medipol University, the study received approval from the Ethics Committees of Koç University in Istanbul. Prior to clinical sample and data collection, patients were informed, and their written consent was taken, ensuring that ethical guidelines were followed across all participating centers (2015.053.IRB1.014, 2016.024.IRB2.005, 2017.139.IRB2.048, 2018.351.IRB1.043, 2022.246.IRB2.040).

2.1. Sample Collection

A total of 277 EDTA plasma aliquots were sourced, and a patient subset was randomly selected from larger cohorts from within the HDBA program. The samples were categorized according to international medical classification standards. After collection and centrifugation, they were stored at −80 °C.

2.2. Cohort Composition and Disease Groups

The obesity cohort (OBES) included patients with a BMI > 35 kg/m^2, with or without type 2 diabetes, not diagnosed with liver disease. Individuals from the liver disease (LIVD) cohort were patients with chronic liver disease chosen based on disease etiology. The cohort is composed of (i) steatotic liver disease (SLD), (ii) other-etiology chronic liver disease (OLD), (iii) VHB, (iv) HCC, and (v) healthy-liver patients. The SLD group includes patients with ARLD or MASLD, which involve the accumulation of excess fat in liver cells. The OLD group includes other, less common, chronic liver disease etiologies, such as primary biliary cholangitis, drug-induced liver injury, and hepatic venous outflow tract obstruction (Budd–Chiari Syndrome).

Fibrosis stratification data, based on liver histopathological assessments, were available for most individuals (n = 199) from the LIVD cohort, though no biopsies were performed on the healthy-liver or obese patients. The healthy-liver group consisted of individuals between 21 and 54 years of age with a BMI between 19 and 27.5 who did not have any indications of liver disease and who had a normal liver biochemistry, while individuals with abnormal biochemistry or FIB-4 levels higher than 1.33, as well as diabetic and obese individuals, were excluded from this group. On the other hand, the obese patients chosen for the study had no diagnoses of liver disease. For the rest of the LIVD cohort, fibrosis levels ranged from F0 to F4 in the meta-analysis of histological data in viral hepatitis (METAVIR) score and 0 to 6 in the Ishak score. Following the clinicians' stratification indications, Ishak 0 was taken as the equivalent of F0, Ishak 1 and 2 as F1; Ishak 3 as F2, Ishak 4 and 5 as F3, and Ishak 6 as F4. According to the NCI's SEER Registrar Staging Assistant, F0 to 3 indicate no-to-moderate fibrosis, while F4 indicates severe fibrosis and the transition to cirrhosis. Based on this, samples were classified into four fibrosis groups, where F0 was taken as no fibrosis, F1 and F2 as mild fibrosis, F3 as moderate fibrosis, and F4 as severe fibrosis. For the analyses, the healthy-liver and obesity patients were taken as having F0. Most patients from the OLD, VHB, and HCC groups presented severe fibrosis (F4), while the SLD group was more mixed.

2.3. Sample Preparation

A plasma digestion protocol with spiked-in SIS-PrESTs was adopted by the HDBA from Geyer et al. (2016) [20]. Proteins were quantified using SIS-PrESTs mixed in near-healthy levels [19], forming a synthetic heavy-labeled plasma. This mixture was aliquoted into 96-well plates, vacuum dried at 35 °C for 16 h, and stored at −20 °C [21].

For the analysis, patient plasma samples were thawed on ice for an hour and randomized into 96-well plates. Additionally, de-identified in-house plasma was added to empty wells on all plates to serve as biological replicates for intra- and inter-plate quality control. Plasma samples were diluted 10-fold in 1× phosphate-buffered saline (PBS) (Sigma Aldrich, St. Louis, MI, USA). Diluted plasma was mixed for 1:1 volume units with re-suspended SIS-PrESTs, and sodium deoxycholate (SDC) (Sigma Aldrich, St. Louis, MI, USA) and dithiothreitol (DTT) (Sigma Aldrich, St. Louis, MI, USA) were added for a final concentration of 0.66% (w/v) SDC and 10 mM DTT. This mixture was incubated at 37 °C, undergoing a reduction process for an hour, and alkylated with 50 mM chloroacetamide (CAA) (Sigma Aldrich, St. Louis, MI, USA) in the dark for 30 min. Digestion occurred overnight using Trypsin (Thermo Fisher Scientific, Santa Clara, CA, USA) at a 1:50 enzyme-to-substrate ratio and quenched by adding trifluoroacetic acid (TFA) (Sigma Aldrich, St. Louis, MI, USA) to 0.5% (v/v). Half of the sample volume was solid-phase extracted using C18 StageTips packed in-house [22]. Solid phase extraction involved the activation of the C18 matrix (Supelco, Sigma Aldrich, St. Louis, MI, USA) with 100% acetonitrile (ACN), equilibration with 0.1% TFA, sample loading, and subsequently washing and eluting the digested peptides. Eluates were vacuum-dried at 45 °C for 30 min and stored at −20 °C upon analysis. Each plate was reconstituted in Solvent A (3% ACN, 0.1% formic acid (FA)) prior to the analysis.

2.4. LC-SRM/MS

Quantitative analysis and assay development were conducted using an UltiMate 3000 nano-LC system (Thermo Fisher Scientific, Santa Clara, CA, USA) equipped with an EASY-Spray ion source and coupled to a TSQ Altis mass spectrometer (Thermo Fisher Scientific, Santa Clara, CA, USA). The samples were loaded onto an Acclaim PepMap 100 trap column (75 μm × 2 cm, C18, 3 μm, 100 Å, Thermo Fisher Scientific, Santa Clara, CA, USA) and washed for 0.75 min at a flow rate of 15 μL/min with 1% Solvent B (95% ACN, 0.1% FA, water). Peptides were separated using an analytical PepMap RSLC C18 column (150 μm × 15 cm, 2 μm, 100 Å, Thermo Fisher Scientific, Santa Clara, CA, USA) and a gradient from 1% to 30% Solvent B over 29.25 min at 3 μL/min. The columns were subjected to three 30 s washes with 95% Solvent B, followed by a wash with 1% Solvent B. The columns were re-equilibrated for 1.4 min with 1% Solvent B. Total cycle times, including sample loading, analysis, and column re-equilibration, were 15 min for method development and 35 min for plasma quantification. Column oven temperatures were set at 40 °C for the analytical column and 60 °C for the column oven, with the autosampler temperature held at 10 °C.

Totals of 125 proteins and 294 peptides were targeted (Supplementary Table S1) using a peptide assay library provided by ProteomEdge (ProteomEdge AB, Stockholm, Sweden) for peptide identification and quantification. The library was developed towards the SIS-PrESTs sequences using their proprietary qRePS (quantitative recombinant protein standard) technology. The heavy signals from all SIS-PrEST peptides were used as internal standards for the one-point calibration and calculation of the light-to-heavy peptide ratios and subsequent absolute quantification.

2.5. Data Pre-Processing

The raw data from the mass spectrometer were imported into Skyline (beta version 23.1.1.459) [23] for peak integration and initial quality control. During this process, the areas under the curve (AUCs) for both heavy and light peptides were extracted, enabling relative quantification through the calculation of ratios between the heavy and light signal intensities. Using ratios as a measure of the protein concentration—as opposed to using the AUC of the endogenous protein directly—mitigates the variability commonly encountered in mass spectrometry. Annotated reports were exported from Skyline for downstream bioinformatic analyses in R (version 4.3.1) [24]. These reports indicate the sample, peptide being measured, protein it belongs to, and light-to-heavy peptide ratio, which can later be used for a calculation of the absolute concentration. This is achieved through a simple transformation of the endogenous-to-standard protein ratios into blood plasma concentrations by multiplying the ratios by the known spiked-in amounts of each SIS-PrEST. The LC-SRM/MS data were subjected to quality control using the heavy SIS-PrEST signals for filtering out datapoints with a library dot product (dotp) or a peptide peak found ratio (rdotp) below 0.8. Also, peptides identified in fewer than 50% of the samples were excluded, together with samples where fewer than 80% of the targeted standards were detected.

The in-house biological control samples distributed among the four plates were used to perform a batch effect analysis, based on which the harmonizR function from the HarmonizR package (v 1.0.0) [25] was used to correct the detected batch effects, using Combat_mode = 2. After quality control and batch effect correction, the quantitative data used for the analyses were the ratios of the light-to-heavy precursors. The median of the peptide ratios from a single protein was then used as the final representative measurement for that protein in downstream analyses. Missing values were imputed using the hotdeck() function from the VIM package (v 6.2.2) [26].

2.6. Differential Expression Analysis

The differential expression of proteins was estimated with two-sided *t*-tests. Multiple hypothesis correction was performed using a false discovery rate (FDR) adjustment, with a significance cutoff of $q < 0.05$. Volcano plots were used to summarize the q-values and expression fold-changes for each of the disease groups compared to the rest.

2.7. Machine Learning and Classification

There were three approaches to generate the classification models. The binary models included (i) classifying patients with any level of fibrosis against those deemed healthy or with no fibrosis (F0) and (ii) classifying patients with a specific level of fibrosis against those deemed healthy or with no fibrosis (F0), while the multi-classification model consisted of classifying patients with different fibrosis levels simultaneously.

The models were generated using the tidymodels package (v 1.1.1) [27]. In every case, the class sizes were balanced. This was determined based on the group with the fewest samples. For instance, in the mild fibrosis model, the subset of data consisted of all samples belonging to patients from the mild liver fibrosis group ($n = 30$) and a same-sized group of samples, which were a random mix of all the F0, healthy-liver, and obesity cohort patients, obtained with the basic sample() function (v 4.3.1) [26]. Then, 70% of this data was used for training and 30% was used for testing, using the initial_split() function in tidymodels. This data size balance and split were the same for all models. Overall fibrosis and each level of fibrosis were classified against the healthy and obesity controls and the samples marked with no fibrosis, always balancing group sizes. For the multiclassification model, patients were put into four groups, which consisted of no fibrosis (healthy, obese and F0), mild fibrosis (F1 and F2), moderate fibrosis (F3), and severe fibrosis (F4). These were simultaneously classified against each other.

The classification models were generated with the selected training sets using a pipeline of tidymodel functions. First, a recipe was created using recipe(), which specifies the data set that will be used and the column with the true classification information. Here, step_corr() is used to eliminate proteins with a correlation of more than 0.8. Then, a model was specified where rand_forest() (trees = 500) was the chosen classification algorithm, set_engine() was used to determine the system to fit the model, with "ranger" as the engine and "permutation" as the mode to determine feature importance, and set_mode() was used to establish that the model should be a "classification" one. After this, a workflow() container is created that uses add_recipe() and add_model() to include the previously formulated recipe and parsnip model. Finally, the fit() [23] function takes the workflow container with all the specifications and uses the chosen data to train the model. Each protein's contribution was retrieved using the vi_model() function from the vip package (v 0.4.1) [28].

Random forest is an algorithm where multiple decision trees are generated during training, so the result of the classification task is the one reached by most trees [29,30]. When generating classification models, random forest estimates each protein's importance for that model. Permutation-based importance measures the decrease in model performance (e.g., accuracy) when the values of a feature are randomly shuffled. Thus, it quantifies the importance of a feature by assessing how much the model's predictive performance deteriorates when the relationship between that feature and the target is disrupted [31]. For all models, the input data were iteratively restricted to a subset of proteins, where the pipeline was run and the proteins with negative permutation importance were eliminated until the model only contained proteins with positive scores. Then, thresholds were used to keep only the topmost important proteins that could maintain at least the same performance as the model with all the positively scoring proteins. These changes were made on the recipe step, using the functions remove_role() and update_role() to eliminate the previous proteins and add the new subset of proteins.

The predict() function from the stats package (v 4.3.1) [24] was used to estimate each of the test sets samples' probabilities of belonging to a given class. Since these samples were not used for training, they can be used to determine model performance. The sensitivity and specificity of the classifications were evaluated with confusion matrices, performed with the confusionMatrix() function from caret (v 6.0.94) [32], with ROC analyses with AUC scores using the roc() function from pROC (v 1.18.5) [33].

2.8. Data Visualization

Graphs were generated with R (version 4.3.1) [24], using the ggplot2 (v 3.5.0) [34], ggpubr (v 0.6.0) [35], factoextra (v 1.7.0) [36], ggstatsplot (v 0.12.2) [37], UpSetR (v 1.4.0) [38], ggrepel (version 0.9.5) [39], and patchwork (v 1.2.0) [40] packages.

2.9. Data Availability

The data supporting the findings of this study are available upon request, subject to a review for validation purposes. We are committed to facilitating access within the limits established by patient consent agreements.

3. Results

This study analyzed a diverse cohort of 277 plasma samples in which 125 target proteins were absolutely quantified with 294 peptides using SIS-PrESTs internal protein standards. The absolute concentration data were processed to select potential biomarkers and classifiers for liver disease patients' stratification (Figure 1a). After stringent quality control, 243 samples and 212 peptides from 108 proteins were selected for further analysis. Measuring more than one peptide per protein is a way to ensure that the protein has indeed been detected. Visual inspection of the data in Skyline and quality control steps make it possible to determine if the measurements of different peptides support each other. After filtering low-quality samples, the liver disease (LIVD) cohort included patients with HCC (n = 54), chronic VHB (n = 59), OLD (n = 28), and SLD (n = 57) who had been stratified by fibrosis levels (METAVIR F0 to F4, Ishak 0 to 6), and healthy-liver controls (n = 31), while the OBES cohort included individuals with a BMI > 35 (n = 14), with or without diabetes, but no diagnosis of liver damage. The proteomic data further supported this assumption, as the profile of the OBES group was markedly distinct from that of the liver disease patients and aligned more closely with the healthy-liver group. Thus, both the healthy-liver and the obese patients were taken as controls (F0). Figure 1b summarizes the age, BMI, and sex distribution for each fibrosis group (healthy, mild-to-moderate, and severe).

3.1. Identification of Fibrosis-Specific Biomarkers Through Differential Expression Analysis

Fibrosis progression proteome profiling was performed through differential expression analyses. Each fibrosis group (mild, moderate, and severe) was compared to the control group. The summary of the proteins up- or downregulated at each fibrosis stage is represented by volcano plots (Figure 2a). Most of the proteins downregulated with mild or moderate fibrosis continue to be downregulated at the next stage of fibrosis (Figure 2b). This analysis revealed a pattern of increasing dysregulation with more advanced fibrosis, with the fold-changes in protein expression becoming more pronounced as the disease progressed. A clear example of both patterns is apolipoprotein M (APOM), a well-known liver-enriched protein, which is specific to hepatocytes and has been associated with high-density lipoproteins (HDLs) according to the Human Protein Atlas (HPA) (v23, www.proteinatlas.org) [41]. On the other hand, while most of the differentially expressed proteins are downregulated, a handful of them show elevated levels in advanced fibrosis. Such is the case for von Willebrand Factor (VWF), a protein involved in blood coagulation, hemostasis, and cell adhesion, for which upregulation has been associated with an increased risk of arterial thrombosis [42]. Thus, the analysis of protein expression in liver fibrosis reveals key changes in both upregulated and downregulated proteins, shedding light on their diverse roles in disease progression and liver-specific impacts as the fibrosis severity increases. The differentially expressed proteins for the different fibrosis levels are included in the Supplementary Materials (Supplementary Table S2).

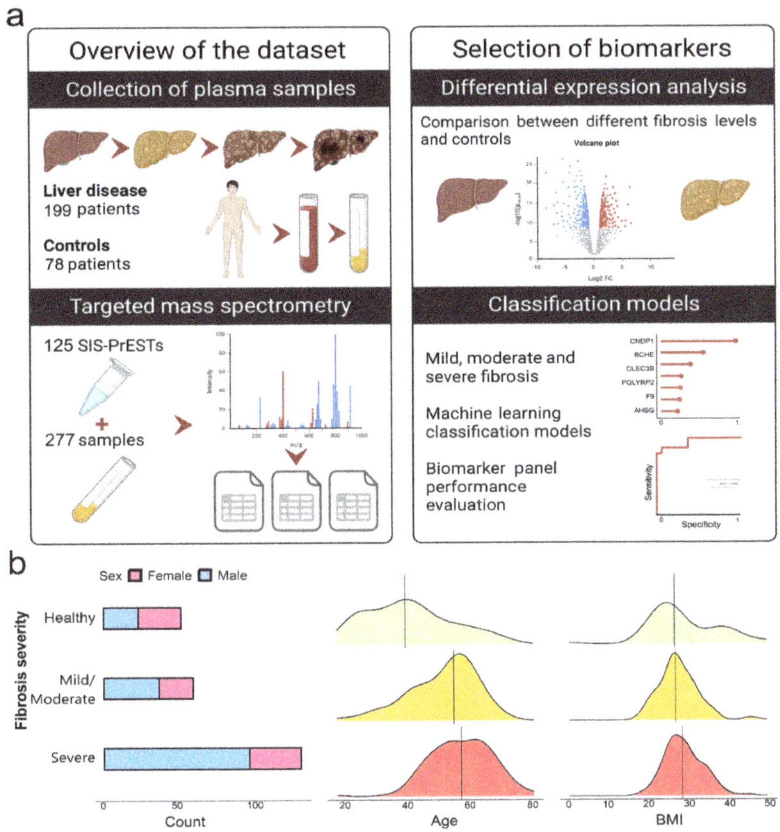

Figure 1. Overview of the study. (**a**) Summarization of the study. Targeted mass spectrometry and SIS-PrESTs were used to profile the plasma proteomes from 277 liver disease and 78 liver-healthy individuals, which were analyzed. Skyline was the first step for data analysis. Peptide intensity spectra were visually inspected, and quantitative reports were exported for downstream bioinformatic analyses. Liver fibrosis samples were compared to the controls using differential expression analysis to find statistical differences, summarized by volcano plots. Important feature selection was performed through classification models, which were generated using a random forest algorithm trained on 70% of the data. Model performance was assessed on the other 30% of the data using confusion matrices and ROC curves (shown). (**b**) Sample distribution of patient samples from Healthy, Mild/Moderate, or Severe Fibrosis.

Figure 2c shows the number of up- and downregulated proteins as the fibrosis severity increases. In total, 84 out of 108 proteins were differentially expressed in at least one level of fibrosis compared to the controls. A functional gene ontology (GO) analysis reveals that the downregulated proteins are involved in wound healing and the wound response, coagulation and fibrinolysis, hemostasis, regulation of body fluid levels, blood pressure homeostasis, immune response, and complement activation, among others (Figure S1a).

This is in line with liver disease symptoms, such as coagulopathies, edema, and an increased risk of sepsis [6,13]. Instead, the upregulated proteins are mainly involved in coagulation, extracellular matrix assembly and organization, and cell–substrate adhesion (Figure S1b). According to the HPA tissue specificity classification, most of the downregulated proteins are enriched or enhanced in the liver. This reflects how CLD progresses regardless of its etiology. The liver fibrosis stratification indicates the level of structural and functional alterations in the liver. Mild fibrosis is essentially asymptomatic, while once fibrosis transitions into cirrhosis and cancer emerges, the liver becomes severely impaired.

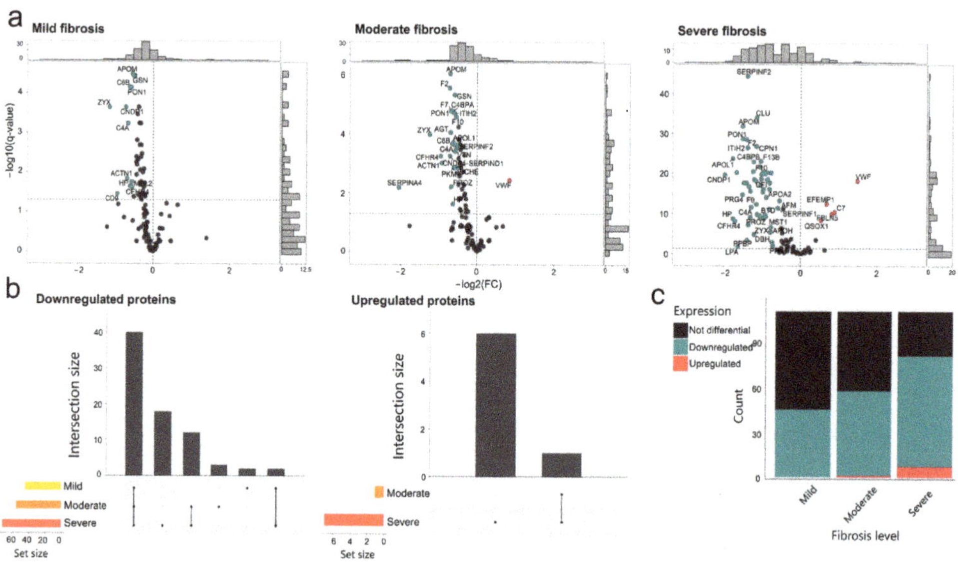

Figure 2. Differential expression analysis. (**a**) Volcano plots summarizing the results for differentially expressed proteins for each fibrosis level against the controls (healthy, obese, and F0), with the fold-change (FC) on the x-axis and the significance (q-value) on the y-axis. Each dot represents a protein. Two-sided t-tests were applied for each protein and a q-value obtained after FDR-correction. The proteins above the established level of significance (q-value > 0.05) and of expression ($\log_2$ (FC) > 0.5) are marked with red (upregulated) or blue (downregulated). (**b**) Upset plots show the number of upregulated and downregulated proteins that overlap between fibrosis levels. The bars on the side show the number of differentially expressed proteins per fibrosis level and, on top, how many of them overlap between fibrosis levels. (**c**) Bar plot with the counts of significantly upregulated (red) and downregulated (blue) proteins for each fibrosis level.

We performed dimensionality reduction using principal component analysis (PCA) to identify proteins driving the protein profile changes. Figure 3a shows the PCA plot (PC1 vs. PC2) for all samples with the distinct clustering of data points, indicating specific proteins that differentiate the samples based on the progression of the disease, particularly in severe cases.

A GO analysis indicated that the most critical proteins in PC1 are mainly involved in the negative regulation of fibrinolysis and positive regulation of wound healing and hemostasis. The four proteins involved in these processes, vitronectin (VTN), coagulation factor II (F2), alpha-2-antiplasmin (SERPINF2), and kininogen 1 (KNG1), are significantly and increasingly downregulated in mild, moderate, and severe fibrosis compared to the controls. Their low levels could lead to increased fibrinolysis and decreased wound healing, which is in line with symptoms, such as excessive bleeding, observed in advanced liver disease patients [43]. The same GO search does not render any significant results for the variables of PC 2. However, the proteins in PC3 are shown to be involved in inflammation processes—such as neutrophil aggregation and the chronic and acute inflammatory response (Figure 3b). In fact, neutrophil aggregation can cause pseudoleukopenia, a condition in which the neutrophils present in the body migrate towards a specific site, making it look like there is a decrease in the circulating leukocytes, despite the bone marrow's later production of more white blood cells. Liver disorders have been observed to be an underlying cause of this condition [44]. Thus, the most important proteins in the PCA seem to have biological relevance.

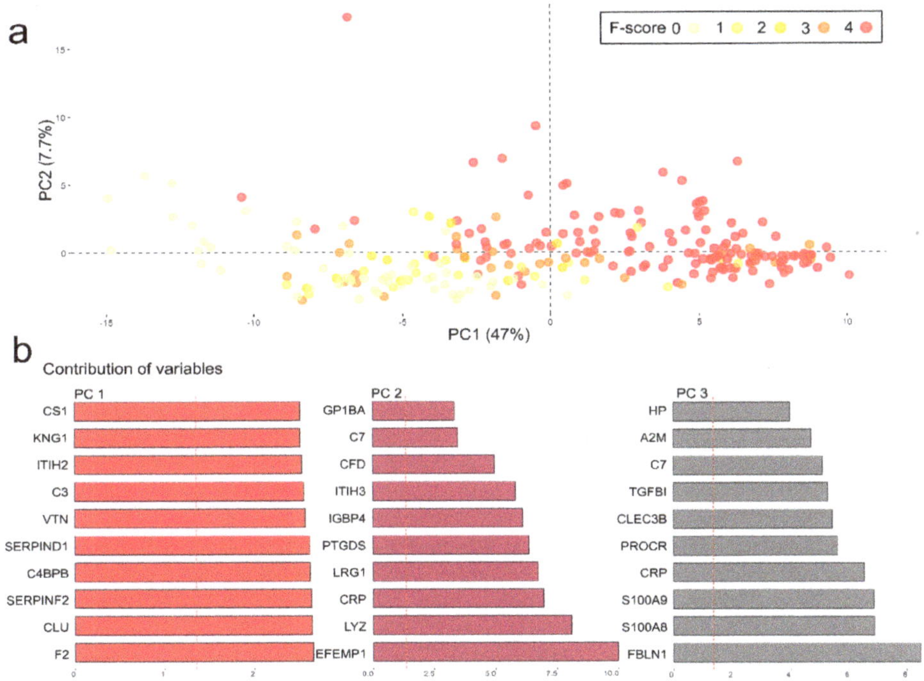

Figure 3. Principal component analysis. (**a**) PCA plot for PC 1 and 2. The data points (n = 243), representing all samples, are colored by fibrosis severity (red = severe fibrosis, orange = moderate fibrosis, yellow = mild fibrosis, green = no fibrosis). (**b**) Top ten contributing proteins for PCs 1, 2, and 3.

3.2. Fibrosis Classification Models

While the PCA provides valuable insights into the overall variance and patterns in the data, it is not specifically tailored to identify biomarkers that are directly associated with fibrosis severity. A supervised machine learning strategy was used to build models to identify the most relevant proteins to classify samples as belonging to the control group or to the mild, moderate, or severe fibrosis patients. All proteins were used as input (n = 108), while a 70:30 split of the samples was used to establish training and testing sets (Figure 4). In each case, the model was trained with a weighted number of samples per group. Thus, the sample size of the smallest group would determine how many samples were to be included from the larger groups to ensure a balanced set. Random forest was used to establish a fibrosis model based on protein levels; a same-sample size mix of all fibrosis levels was classified against the control group of F0, healthy-liver, and obese patients with the goal of separating patients as presenting any level of fibrosis or having a fibrosis-free liver.

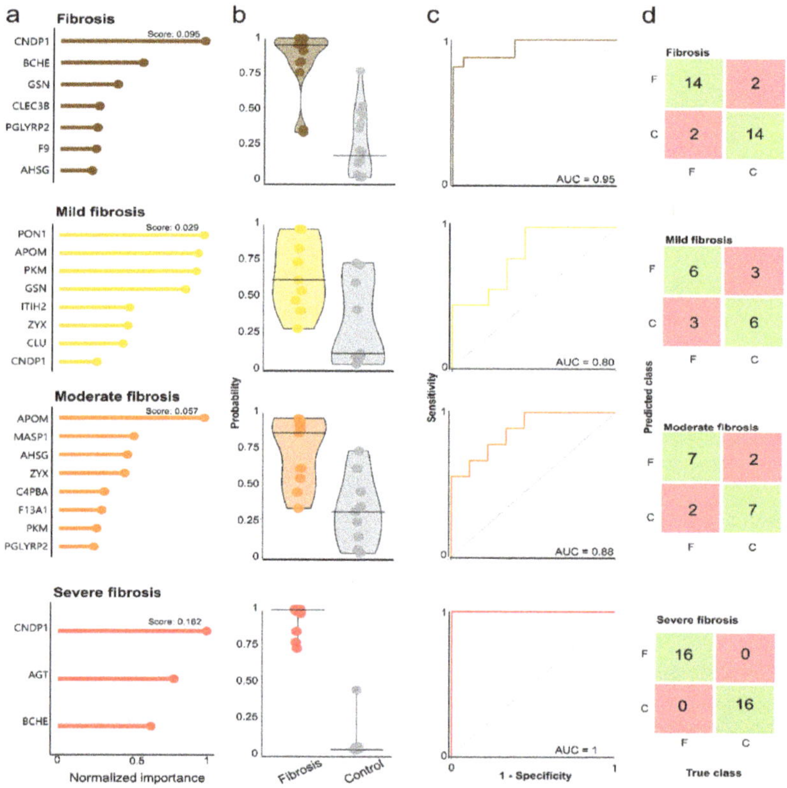

Figure 4. Fibrosis models' selected features and performance. (**a**) Lollipop charts of the selected proteins per model with their normalized importance as a fraction of the top scoring protein, for which the permutation score is shown at the top of each plot. (**b**) Probabilities of general fibrosis or specific fibrosis levels for the samples in the test set. (**c**) ROC curves with AUCs to indicate model performance. (**d**) Confusion matrices with classification results for each model, where F = fibrosis group and C = control group.

The features (i.e., proteins) selected for each classification model are shown in Figure 4a. The objective of these models was to obtain a minimal protein panel that maintained at least the same sensitivity and specificity as previous iterations, which included more proteins. The starting points were models that comprised all the proteins with positive permutation importance, excluding highly correlated proteins (>0.8) for minimally redundant biomarkers (Figure S3 illustrates the protein correlation in this study). The most important proteins for the models include examples, such as (i) carnosine dipeptidase 1 (CNDP1), involved in the metabolism of dipeptides; (ii) paraoxonase 1 (PON1), which hydrolyzes toxic metabolites; (iii) APOM, which is involved in lipid transportation; and (iv) angiotensinogen (AGT), which regulates blood pressure [41]. PON1, APOM, and AGT are enriched in the liver and CNDP1 in the brain. The functions associated with these proteins, with all of their levels seeming to drop as fibrosis progresses, reflect some of the symptoms observed in chronic liver disease patients, such as abnormalities in the regulation of blood pressure and cognitive symptoms related to the accumulation of toxic metabolites (i.e., confusion or drowsiness) [45].

The performance of the classification models was tested on the 30% of the data not used for training. The probabilities of the plasma samples belonging to the disease group for each disease model are shown in Figure 4b. The first model would classify samples as having any level of fibrosis against having no fibrosis with an AUC of 0.95, while the rest could classify specific levels of fibrosis (F1-2, mild; F3, moderate; and F4, severe) against no fibrosis with an AUC between 0.80 and 1 (Figure 4c). For these last three models, the model performance and the distance between the classification probabilities for the disease and the healthy samples increase with the fibrosis severity. The confusion matrices show the number of samples from the test set correctly and incorrectly classified by the model (Figure 4d). The results show high specificity and sensitivity, especially for the general fibrosis and the severe fibrosis models, despite sample size limitations, which should be addressed to further validate the models. On the other hand, the results for the mild fibrosis model were poorer than for the others. This would be in line with the PCA results (Figure 3), where some of the mild fibrosis samples were closer to the controls than to the moderate or severe fibrosis samples.

3.3. *Data-Driven Fibrosis Stratification*

The models generated up to this point have been binary. While they could be used to determine whether a sample belongs to a liver fibrosis patient, they would not be applicable as a stratification strategy. Therefore, a multiclassification model was generated for this purpose, using the same number of samples for all groups. Figure 5a shows the minimal panel of selected features that enabled the model to maintain at least the same specificity and sensitivity as models including larger sets of proteins. The multiclassification model can classify test set samples as having a specific level of fibrosis with an AUC between 0.62 and 0.91 (Figure 5b). While only 18 of the 36 samples were correctly classified (Figure 5c), the model is placing samples next to the true class. Importantly, no healthy samples were classified as having either moderate or severe fibrosis, and no severe samples were classified as healthy. The most problematic group seemed to be the moderate fibrosis group, where only two of the samples were correctly classified, but most were assigned to another fibrosis class. Figure 5d shows the comparison between the probabilities for the different fibrosis groups of being classified as healthy. The severe fibrosis samples show the smallest probabilities of being classified as healthy, while the opposite is the case for some of the moderate samples. A relevant consideration here, beyond the adequacy of the model, is the potential variability in the biopsy-based clinical stratification itself.

The top proteins selected for this model are (i) CNDP1, involved in the metabolism of dipeptides; (ii) butyrylcholinesterase (BCHE), a liver-enriched protein that can degrade neurotoxins; (iii) gelsolin (GSN), a heart-enhanced protein involved in the modulation of actin; (iv) C-type lectin domain family 3 member B (CLEC3B), an adipose-tissue enhanced protein involved in retinal function; (v) peptidoglycan recognition protein 2 (PGLYRP2), a liver-enriched protein involved in the immune response; (vi) coagulation factor 9 (F9), a liver-enriched protein that participates in blood coagulation and hemostasis; and (vii) alpha 2-HS glycoprotein (AHSG), a liver-enriched associated with the mineral balance [41] (Figures 5e and S2). The seven selected proteins had a significant q-value in the non-parametric Kruskal–Wallis test comparing fibrosis levels (Supplementary Table S3).

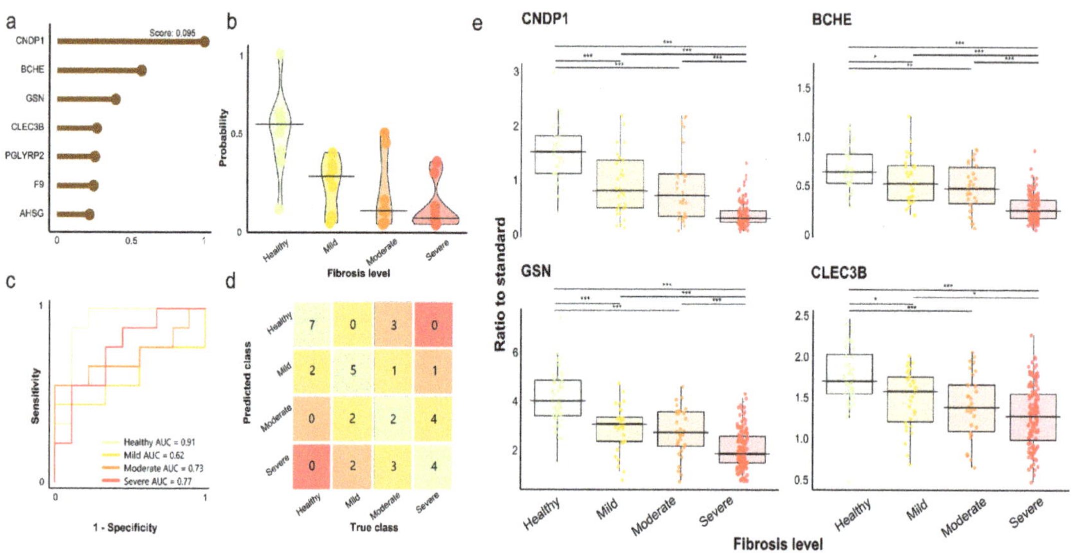

Figure 5. Multiclassification model for fibrosis stratification. (**a**) Lollipop chart of the proteins selected for the model with their normalized importance as a fraction of the top scoring protein for which the permutation importance score is shown at the top of the plot. (**b**) Probabilities for each sample of being classified as healthy by the fibrosis level group. (**c**) ROC curves and AUC show the performance of the model for each fibrosis class. (**d**) Confusion matrix with stratification classification results for the model. (**e**) Boxplots of the topmost important proteins selected for the fibrosis stratification model. The median value and first and third quartiles of the ratio to standard are summarized by the boxplots, and the whiskers mark the minimum and maximum values per group. Samples are grouped by fibrosis level (healthy, n = 52; mild fibrosis, n = 30; moderate fibrosis, n = 30; severe fibrosis, n = 131). The horizontal lines indicate which level pairwise comparisons are significant. p-values were calculated using the post-hoc Wilcox test and FDR-adjusted, and the asterisks indicate the level of significance, where * is significant (q-value < 0.05), ** is very significant (q-value < 0.01), and *** is highly significant (q-value < 0.001).

3.4. Selection of Liver Fibrosis Biomarker Panel

We outline a 20-protein panel (Figure 6) based on the features selected by the random forest models. Most of these proteins show liver specificity, except for (i) CLEC3B, enhanced in the adipose tissue; (ii) GSN, enhanced in the heart muscle; (iii) pyruvate kinase (PKM), enhanced in the skeletal muscle and the tongue; (iv) zyxin (ZYX), with low tissue specificity; (v) coagulation factor XIII A chain (F13A1), enhanced in the adipose tissue and the placenta; and (vi) CNDP1, enriched in the brain, according to the HPA. Following the criteria for the biomarker panel minimization, these proteins all had positive permutation importance and allowed each model to maintain the performance of previous model iterations that included more proteins. Furthermore, the two-sided t-tests, the ANOVA, and the post-hoc tests indicated that these proteins were significantly dysregulated at different levels of fibrosis (Tables S2 and S3). However, it is important to mention that the results of the post-hoc tests performed after the non-parametric Kruskal–Wallis test comparing fibrosis levels were not significant between mild and moderate fibrosis for most proteins, with the exception of MASP1, which was the only protein in the dataset for which this was the case. This lack of significant differences in protein levels could largely explain the problematic classification of patients with mild or moderate liver fibrosis.

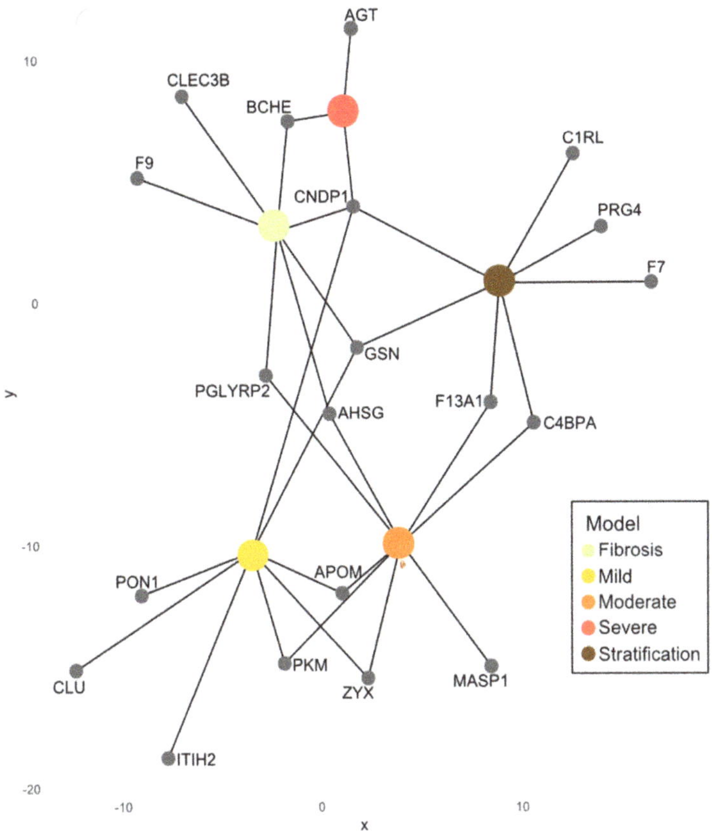

Figure 6. Liver fibrosis protein panel. Network visualization of the proteins selected for each fibrosis model. The distance from the protein to the model node is inversely proportional to the permutation importance score for the model—the longer the distance, the smaller the importance score.

4. Discussion

The high incidence of CLD emphasizes the urgent need for better diagnostic tools to improve patient outcomes, particularly given that many chronic liver diseases can be controlled. The identification and further investigation of the plasma proteins driving the progression of the disease is crucial for developing a less invasive method to assess the presence and severity of liver fibrosis, which could significantly enhance the diagnosis and management of CLD. This study presents an attractive strategy for plasma protein profiling to detect liver fibrosis at an early stage. It advances the search for optimal plasma protein biomarkers by deploying a highly multiplexable targeted mass spectrometry approach that requires small plasma volumes. We analyzed the plasma protein expression of a total of 108 proteins across various liver conditions in 243 samples and obtained reliable quantitative data. This strategy highlights the necessity of the absolute quantification of plasma proteins and facilitates the identification of protein states linked to liver fibrosis progression through differential expression analysis and machine learning techniques.

Our findings demonstrate that targeted mass spectrometry with use of heavy internal protein standards can effectively assess the plasma proteome on a system-wide scale by precisely quantifying medium-to-high-abundance proteins important for liver fibrosis and its progression. This capability is crucial for developing clinical assays that can be used to monitor liver health, marking a significant step towards screening procedures where high-risk patients can be followed up with a confirmatory assay, such as a liver biopsy.

Previous studies from the HDBA [46,47] have shown the potential of using highly multiplexable methods for plasma proteome profiling to generate pan-disease biomarker panels, while other studies have focused on specific liver diseases [14]. This study is a continuation of the above, harnessing the pan-disease approach to study liver diseases with different etiologies and fibrosis progression comprehensively.

The overall liver fibrosis classification model, which separated F0—healthy and obese patients—from F1 to F4 samples, had high performance (AUC = 0.95). Binary classification models were also generated based on the presence of specific levels of fibrosis. The moderate and severe fibrosis models showed good specificity and sensitivity (AUC = 0.80 and AUC = 0.88), while the severe fibrosis model showed the best performance (AUC = 1). The number of selected features was reduced up to the point where a decrease in model performance was observed. This deterioration of the model performance can also be taken as a reminder of the increased reliability that biomarker panels provide against single biomarkers. At the same time, while these results are promising, the search for biomarkers that can better reflect liver disease progression must continue in order to obtain more reliable panels. Currently available commercial options, such as the LiverEdge panel (ProteomEdge AB, Stockholm, Sweden), facilitate this process.

The seven-feature multiclassification model, which was built to stratify samples showing severe, moderate, mild, or no fibrosis, allowed for the correct stratification of the test set plasma samples with a 0.50 accuracy. Being a four-class model, this is better than random classification, which would have a 0.25 accuracy score. Furthermore, the classification errors were between healthy and mild/moderate or between mild/moderate and severe, but there were no misclassifications between healthy and severe. At the same time, supervised machine learning depends completely on the quality of the training data. This means that the results are also impacted by the inherent variability of the clinical assessment of fibrosis in liver biopsies.

Here, we recognize that it is possible that a subset of the OBES patients could have undiagnosed mild fibrosis or early liver damage, particularly given the known risk of metabolic comorbidities, such as MASLD in obesity. However, given the distinct separation of the control group from the liver disease group, this is unlikely to have significantly impacted the conclusions of the study. Most importantly, treating the OBES group as F0 reduced the probabilities of incorrectly identifying biomarkers that may be confounded by an obesity-related pathophysiology rather than liver fibrosis. On the other hand, while the aspect of disease progression that has been explored here is liver fibrosis, it is not possible to conclude from this study that the selected proteins indicate fibrosis, since they could be indicating other aspects of liver disease progression that accompany it instead. To connect the protein expression to its ultimate cause, it would be necessary to include clinical metadata that accounted for other progression metrics of liver disease, such as steatosis and inflammation [14], as well as a higher number of stratified samples. Overall, the sample size is a limitation of this study. This was especially apparent for the test sets used to evaluate model performance. Prior to any contemplation of the applicability of the biomarker panel in a clinical setting, it would be necessary to validate it using larger, independent patient cohorts.

Another aspect to consider in this study is the characteristics of the targeted proteins. Proteins with medium-to-high-abundant concentrations in blood were analyzed, this being the range in which targeted mass spectrometry delivers more reliable measurements [48]. Almost 60% of the targeted proteins are enriched or enhanced in the liver, according to the HDBA. However, this seemingly biased selection has, at least partly, a biological explanation, since genome-scale metabolic models indicate that the liver is the most metabolically active tissue in the body [41]. Here, as liver disease progresses, most of the targeted proteins that show differential expression are downregulated, reflecting the impairment of liver function. This is in line with Niu et al.'s previous 2019 and 2022 [2,14] mass spectrometry-based liver disease studies, which, through data-independent acquisition (DIA), found that most of the liver-specific proteins were downregulated in liver disease and that most of these had metabolic and bloodstream-related functions. This included proteins, such as (i) prothrombin (F2), which converts fibrinogen to fibrin in the coagulation cascade, (ii) protein S (PROS), an anticoagulant protein, or (iii) apolipoprotein M (APOM), involved in lipid transportation [41]. All of these proteins were also found to be increasingly down-regulated as liver fibrosis progressed in this study. On the other hand, proteins involved in cell–extracellular matrix interactions, immunity, and inflammation, which had been found to be upregulated in liver disease [2,14], followed the same tendency in this study. These include examples include (i) quiescin sulfhydryl oxidase 1 (QSOX), which plays a role in cell adhesion and migration, and (ii) complement 7 (C7), which is involved in the innate and adaptive immune response [41]. Both proteins' levels seemed to increase with fibrosis progression in this study.

In summary, targeted proteomics and the use of SIS-PrESTs increase accuracy and reliability in protein identification and quantification. This method addresses issues that could hinder clinical translation, such as the lack of absolute quantification in DIA mass spectrometry. Thus, it presents itself as a more competitive option for proteome profiling in the clinic.

Supplementary Materials: The following supporting information can be downloaded at: https://www.mdpi.com/article/10.3390/livers5010002/s1, Figure S1: Overrepresentation analysis, Figure S2: Multiclassification model for fibrosis stratification, Figure S3: Protein expression correlation, Table S1: List of targets, Table S2: De-identified list of samples with diagnose and fibrosis staging, Table S3: Differentially expressed proteins and regulation type, Table S4: Kruskal-Wallis and Wilcox post-hoc tests *q*-values by protein.

Author Contributions: Conceptualization, A.V.R., D.K., O.A., A.M., D.A., C.Y., M.A., M.D., H.K., M.Z. and F.E.; Methodology, A.V.R., D.K. and F.E.; Formal analysis, A.V.R.; Investigation, A.V.R. and F.E.; Resources, D.K., O.A., A.M., C.Y., M.A., M.D., H.K., M.Z. and F.E.; Data curation, A.V.R. and F.E.; Writing—original draft, A.V.R., D.K. and F.E.; Writing—review & editing, A.V.R., D.K., O.A., A.M., D.A., M.Z. and F.E.; Visualization, A.V.R. and F.E.; Supervision, F.E.; Project administration, A.V.R., A.M. and F.E.; Funding acquisition, F.E. All authors have read and agreed to the published version of the manuscript.

Funding: This research received no external funding.

Institutional Review Board Statement: The study was conducted in accordance with the Declaration of Helsinki, and approved by the Institutional Review Board of Koç University (protocol codes 2015.053.IRB1.014: 30 March 2015), (2016.024.IRB2.005: 4 February 2016), (2017.139.IRB2.048: 5 September 2017), (2018.351.IRB1.043: 15 May 2019), (2022.246.IRB2.040: 28 July 2022).

Informed Consent Statement: Informed consent was obtained from all subjects involved in the study.

Data Availability Statement: The data supporting the findings of this study are not publicly available due to ethical restrictions related to patient confidentiality and data protection policies. However, de-identified data may be made available upon reasonable request to the corresponding author, subject to appropriate ethical approvals and data-sharing agreements.

Acknowledgments: We thank the entire staff of the Human Protein Atlas program (www.proteinatlas.org) and Proteome Edge AB (Stockholm, Sweden) for their valuable contributions. We gratefully acknowledge the scientists, services, and facilities of the Koç University Research Center for Translational Medicine (KUTTAM), funded by the Presidency of Turkey, Head of Strategy and Budget.

Conflicts of Interest: DK is employed by ProteomeEdge AB (Stockholm, Sweden). DK and FE are co-founders of ProteomeEdge AB (Stockholm, Sweden).

References

1. Devarbhavi, H.; Asrani, S.K.; Arab, J.P.; Nartey, Y.A.; Pose, E.; Kamath, P.S. Global burden of liver disease: 2023 update. *J. Hepatol.* **2023**, *79*, 516–537. [CrossRef] [PubMed]
2. Niu, L.; Geyer, P.E.; Wewer Albrechtsen, N.J.; Gluud, L.L.; Santos, A.; Doll, S.; Treit, P.V.; Holst, J.J.; Knop, F.K.; Vilsbøll, T.; et al. Plasma proteome profiling discovers novel proteins associated with non-alcoholic fatty liver disease. *Mol. Syst. Biol.* **2019**, *15*, e8793. [CrossRef] [PubMed]
3. Underhill, G.H.; Khetani, S.R. Emerging trends in modeling human liver disease in vitro. *APL Bioeng.* **2019**, *3*, 040902. [CrossRef] [PubMed]
4. Chowdhury, A.B.; Mehta, K.J. Liver biopsy for assessment of chronic liver diseases: A synopsis. *Clin. Exp. Med.* **2023**, *23*, 273–285. [CrossRef] [PubMed]
5. Cheemerla, S.; Balakrishnan, M. Global epidemiology of chronic liver disease. *Clin. Liver Dis.* **2021**, *17*, 365–370. [CrossRef]
6. Asrani, S.K.; Devarbhavi, H.; Eaton, J.; Kamath, P.S. Burden of liver diseases in the world. *J. Hepatol.* **2019**, *70*, 151–171. [CrossRef]
7. Mokdad, A.A.; Lopez, A.D.; Shahraz, S.; Lozano, R.; Mokdad, A.H.; Stanaway, J.; Murray, C.; Naghavi, M. Liver cirrhosis mortality in 187 countries between 1980 and 2010: A systematic analysis. *BMC Med.* **2014**, *12*, 145. [CrossRef]
8. Heyens, L.J.; Busschots, D.; Koek, G.H.; Robaeys, G.; Francque, S. Liver fibrosis in non-alcoholic fatty liver disease: From liver biopsy to non-invasive biomarkers in diagnosis and treatment. *Front. Med.* **2021**, *8*, 615978. [CrossRef]
9. Ginès, P.; Castera, L.; Lammert, F.; Graupera, I.; Serra-Burriel, M.; Allen, A.M.; Wai-Sun Wong, V.; Hartmann, P.; Thiele, M.; Caballeria, L.; et al. Population screening for liver fibrosis: Toward early diagnosis and intervention for chronic liver diseases. *Hepatology* **2022**, *75*, 219–228. [CrossRef]
10. Huang, D.Q.; Terrault, N.A.; Tacke, F.; Gluud, L.L.; Arrese, M.; Bugianesi, E.; Loomba, R. Global epidemiology of cirrhosis—Aetiology, trends and predictions. *Nat. Rev. Gastroenterol. Hepatol.* **2023**, *20*, 388–398. [CrossRef]
11. Nagy, P.; Thorgeirsson, S.S.; Grisham, J.W. Organizational principles of the liver. In *The Liver: Biology and Pathobiology*; Arias, I.M., Alter, H.J., Boyer, J.L., Cohen, D.E., Shafritz, D.A., Thorgeirsson, S.S., Wolkoff, A.W., Eds.; John Wiley & Sons Ltd.: Hoboken, NJ, USA, 2020; pp. 1–13.
12. Abdel-Misih, S.R.; Bloomston, M. Liver anatomy. *Surg. Clin. N. Am.* **2010**, *90*, 643–653. [CrossRef] [PubMed]
13. Larsen, F.S.; Saliba, F. Liver support systems and liver transplantation in acute liver failure. *Liver Int.* **2023**. [CrossRef] [PubMed]
14. Niu, L.; Thiele, M.; Geyer, P.E.; Rasmussen, D.N.; Webel, H.E.; Santos, A.; Gupta, R.; Meier, F.; Strauss, M.; Kjaergaard, M.; et al. Noninvasive proteomic biomarkers for alcohol-related liver disease. *Nat. Med.* **2022**, *28*, 1277–1287. [CrossRef] [PubMed]
15. European Association for the Study of the Liver. EASL-ALEH Clinical Practice Guidelines: Non-invasive tests for evaluation of liver disease severity and prognosis. *J. Hepatol.* **2015**, *63*, 237–264. [CrossRef]
16. Everhart, J.E.; Wright, E.C.; Goodman, Z.D.; Dienstag, J.L.; Hoefs, J.C.; Kleiner, D.E.; Ghany, M.G.; Mills, A.S.; Nash, S.R.; Govindarajan, S.; et al. Prognostic value of Ishak fibrosis stage: Findings from the hepatitis C antiviral long-term treatment against cirrhosis trial. *Hepatology* **2010**, *51*, 585–594. [CrossRef]
17. Uhlén, M.; Karlsson, M.J.; Zhong, W.; Tebani, A.; Pou, C.; Mikes, J.; Lakshmikanth, T.; Forsström, B.; Edfors, F.; Odeberg, J.; et al. A genome-wide transcriptomic analysis of protein-coding genes in human blood cells. *Science* **2019**, *366*, eaax9198. [CrossRef]
18. Thapa, B.R.; Walia, A. Liver function tests and their interpretation. *Indian J. Pediatr.* **2007**, *74*, 663–671. [CrossRef]
19. Hober, A.; Edfors, F.; Ryaboshapkina, M.; Malmqvist, J.; Rosengren, L.; Percy, A.J.; Lind, L.; Forsström, B.; Uhlén, M.; Oscarsson, J.; et al. Absolute quantification of apolipoproteins following treatment with omega-3 carboxylic acids and fenofibrate using a high precision stable isotope-labeled recombinant protein fragments based SRM assay. *Mol. Cell. Proteom.* **2019**, *18*, 2433–2446. [CrossRef]
20. Geyer, P.E.; Kulak, N.A.; Pichler, G.; Holdt, L.M.; Teupser, D.; Mann, M. Plasma proteome profiling to assess human health and disease. *Cell Syst.* **2016**, *2*, 185–195. [CrossRef]
21. Kotol, D.; Hober, A.; Strandberg, L.; Svensson, A.S.; Uhlén, M.; Edfors, F. Targeted proteomics analysis of plasma proteins using recombinant protein standards for addition only workflows. *Biotechniques* **2021**, *71*, 473–483. [CrossRef]
22. Callesen, A.K.; Mohammed, S.; Bunkenborg, J.; Kruse, T.A.; Cold, S.; Mogensen, O.; dePont Christensen, R.; Vach, W.; Jørgensen, P.E.; Jensen, O.N. Serum protein profiling by miniaturized solid-phase extraction and matrix-assisted laser desorption/ionization mass spectrometry. *Rapid Commun. Mass Spectrom.* **2005**, *19*, 1578–1586. [CrossRef] [PubMed]
23. MacLean, B.; Tomazela, D.M.; Shulman, N.; Chambers, M.; Finney, G.L.; Frewen, B.; Kern, R.; Tabb, D.; Liebler, D.; MacCoss, M.J. Skyline: An open source document editor for creating and analyzing targeted proteomics experiments. *Bioinformatics* **2010**, *26*, 966–968. [CrossRef] [PubMed]
24. R Core Team. *R: A Language and Environment for Statistical Computing*; R Foundation for Statistical Computing: Vienna, Austria, 2023.

25. Voß, H.; Schlumbohm, S.; Barwikowski, P.; Wurlitzer, M.; Dottermusch, M.; Neumann, P.; Krisp, C. HarmonizR enables data harmonization across independent proteomic datasets with appropriate handling of missing values. *Nat. Commun.* **2022**, *13*, 3523. [CrossRef] [PubMed]
26. Kowarik, A.; Templ, M. Imputation with the R Package VIM. *J. Stat. Softw.* **2016**, *74*, 1–16. [CrossRef]
27. Kuhn, M.; Wickham, H. Tidymodels: A Collection of Packages for Modeling and Machine Learning Using Tidyverse Principles. Available online: https://www.tidymodels.org (accessed on 10 January 2025).
28. Greenwell, B.M.; Boehmke, B.C.; Gray, B. Variable Importance Plots-An Introduction to the vip Package. *R J.* **2020**, *12*, 343. [CrossRef]
29. Ho, T.K. Random decision forests. In Proceedings of the 3rd International Conference on Document Analysis and Recognition, Montreal, QC, Canada, 14–16 August 1995; IEEE: Piscataway, NJ, USA, 1995; Volume 1, pp. 278–282.
30. Breiman, L. Random forests. *Mach. Learn.* **2001**, *45*, 5–32. [CrossRef]
31. Zhu, R.; Zeng, D.; Kosorok, M.R. Reinforcement learning trees. *J. Am. Stat. Assoc.* **2015**, *110*, 1770–1784. [CrossRef]
32. Kuhn, M. Building Predictive Models in R Using the caret Package. *J. Stat. Softw.* **2008**, *28*, 1–26. [CrossRef]
33. Robin, X.; Turck, N.; Hainard, A.; Tiberti, N.; Lisacek, F.; Sanchez, J.C.; Müller, M. pROC: An open-source package for R and S+ to analyze and compare ROC curves. *BMC Bioinform.* **2011**, *12*, 77. [CrossRef]
34. Wickham, H. *ggplot2: Elegant Graphics for Data Analysis*; Springer: New York, NY, USA, 2016.
35. Kassambara, A. ggpubr: 'ggplot2' Based Publication Ready Plots. Available online: https://cran.r-project.org/web/packages/ggpubr/index.html (accessed on 10 January 2025).
36. Kassambara, A.; Mundt, F. Factoextra: Extract and Visualize the Results of Multivariate Data Analyses. R Package Version 1.0.7. Available online: https://CRAN.R-project.org/package=factoextra (accessed on 10 January 2025).
37. Patil, I. Visualizations with statistical details: The 'ggstatsplot' approach. *J. Open Source Softw.* **2021**, *6*, 3167. [CrossRef]
38. Conway, J.R.; Lex, A.; Gehlenborg, N. UpSetR: An R package for the visualization of intersecting sets and their properties. *Bioinformatics* **2017**, *33*, 2938–2940. [CrossRef] [PubMed]
39. Slowikowski, K.; Schep, A.; Hughes, S. ggrepel: Automatically Position Non-Overlapping Text Labels with 'ggplot2'. R Package Version 0.9. Available online: https://cran.r-project.org/web/packages/ggrepel/ggrepel.pdf (accessed on 10 January 2025).
40. Pedersen, T. Patchwork: The Composer of Plots. R Package Version 1.3.0.9000. Available online: https://github.com/thomasp85/patchwork (accessed on 10 January 2025).
41. Uhlén, M.; Fagerberg, L.; Hallström, B.; Lindskog, C.; Oksvold, P.; Mardinoglu, A.; Sivertsson, Å.; Kampf, C.; Sjöstedt, E.; Asplund, A.; et al. Proteomics. Tissue-based map of the human proteome. *Science* **2015**, *347*, 1260419. [CrossRef] [PubMed]
42. Shahidi, M. Thrombosis and von Willebrand factor. *Thromb. Embolism Res. Clin. Pract.* **2017**, *1*, 285–306.
43. Rodríguez-Castro, K.I.; Antonello, A.; Ferrarese, A. Spontaneous bleeding or thrombosis in cirrhosis: What should be feared the most? *World J. Hepatol.* **2015**, *7*, 1818. [CrossRef]
44. Claviez, A.; Horst, H.A.; Santer, R.; Suttorp, M. Neutrophil aggregates in a 13-year-old girl: A rare hematological phenomenon. *Ann. Hematol.* **2003**, *82*, 251–253. [CrossRef]
45. Newton, J.L.; Jones, D.E. Managing systemic symptoms in chronic liver disease. *J. Hepatol.* **2012**, *56*, S46–S55. [CrossRef]
46. Álvez, M.B.; Edfors, F.; von Feilitzen, K.; Zwahlen, M.; Mardinoglu, A.; Edqvist, P.H.; Sjöblom, T.; Lundin, E.; Rameika, N.; Enblad, G.; et al. Next generation pan-cancer blood proteome profiling using proximity extension assay. *Nat. Commun.* **2023**, *14*, 4308. [CrossRef]
47. Kotol, D.; Woessmann, J.; Hober, A.; Álvez, M.B.; Tran Minh, K.H.; Pontén, F.; Fagerberg, L.; Edfors, F. Absolute Quantification of Pan-Cancer Plasma Proteomes Reveals Unique Signature in Multiple Myeloma. *Cancers* **2023**, *15*, 4764. [CrossRef]
48. Tu, C.; Rudnick, P.A.; Martinez, M.Y.; Cheek, K.L.; Stein, S.E.; Slebos, R.J.; Liebler, D.C. Depletion of abundant plasma proteins and limitations of plasma proteomics. *J. Proteome Res.* **2010**, *9*, 4982–4991. [CrossRef]

livers

MDPI

Article

Innovative Elastography Measuring Cap for Ex Vivo Liver Condition Assessment: Numerical and Preclinical Studies in a Porcine Model

Dariusz Pyka [1,*], Agnieszka Noszczyk-Nowak [2], Karina Krawiec [1], Tomasz Świetlik [3] and Krzysztof J. Opieliński [3]

[1] Department of Mechanics, Materials and Biomedical Engineering, Wroclaw University of Science and Technology, Smoluchowskiego 25 Str., 50-370 Wroclaw, Poland; karina.krawiec@pwr.edu.pl
[2] Division of Translational Medicine, Department of Internal Medicine and Clinic of Diseases of Horses, Dogs and Cats, Faculty of Veterinary Medicine, Wrocław University of Environmental and Life Sciences, Grunwaldzki sq. 47, 50-366 Wrocław, Poland; agnieszka.noszczyk-nowak@upwr.edu.pl
[3] Department of Acoustics, Multimedia and Signal Processing, Faculty of Electronics, Photonics and Microsystems, Wroclaw University of Science and Technology, Wybrzeze Wyspianskiego 2627, 50-370 Wroclaw, Poland; tomasz.swietlik@pwr.edu.pl (T.Ś.); krzysztof.opielinski@pwr.edu.pl (K.J.O.)
* Correspondence: dariusz.pyka@pwr.edu.pl; Tel.: +48-71-320-27-60

Abstract: The authors of this study focused their research on developing cap geometries for the FibroScan® elastograph (FibroScan, EchoSens, Paris, France) measuring head aimed at a non-invasive assessment of liver condition for transplantation using a pig animal model. Numerical models were created to simulate the propagation of a mechanical wave through a biological medium induced by the FibroScan® elastograph measuring head. The designed caps were intended to replicate the skin–muscle–rib–liver structures to minimize the risk of damage caused by mechanical wave excitation when directly applied to liver tissue. The construction process of numerical models for the liver and surrounding tissues is presented, along with simulations reflecting the mechanical and acoustic properties of the wave propagation process. The results obtained from in vivo measurements on pigs were validated through a numerical analysis, confirming a high level of agreement between the test results and the numerical model.

Keywords: elastography; pig liver; FibroScan®; liver fibrosis; FEM/SPH analysis

1. Introduction

Tools designed for diagnosing the condition of human organs can also be utilized to evaluate the health of livers intended for transplantation. One such device is the FibroScan® elastograph, which allows for the non-invasive evaluation of the liver by generating mechanical waves and measuring their propagation speed and attenuation using ultrasound. There are two types of ultrasound probes: the M for general applications and the XL which was specifically designed for obese individuals. The test performed with this device is characterized by a high reproducibility of the results, the speed of the process, and a high diagnostic value [1,2].

Liver transplantation studies require non-invasive evaluation methods as existing tests fail to fully meet this need. Liver biopsy currently remains the best method, but it is invasive, and the time needed to analyze the results is lengthy. The FibroScan® device can be a valuable tool for assessing the condition of the organ before transplantation, particularly due to the limited time available for evaluation [3].

Currently, there is limited studies on the application of transient elastography, including the FibroScan® device, for assessing liver fibrosis [4]. Studies indicate that the device demonstrates potential effectiveness; however, its performance is significantly limited in patients with obesity. Animal studies, including pig livers, may provide valuable data on the effectiveness of the device and its potential limitations. Attention is drawn to the need for further research to improve the device to allow for a more accurate assessment of the organ's condition before transplantation.

The anatomy of the porcine digestive system shows significant differences from that of humans; nevertheless, the physiology of digestion and, more specifically, the course of digestive processes in both species are similar. Despite the presence of anatomical discrepancies, pigs are a frequently used gastrointestinal model for clinical studies. Figure 1 shows an overview of the distribution of organs in the thorax of the domestic pig. Depending on the age and species, the geometric dimensions of organs such as the liver vary.

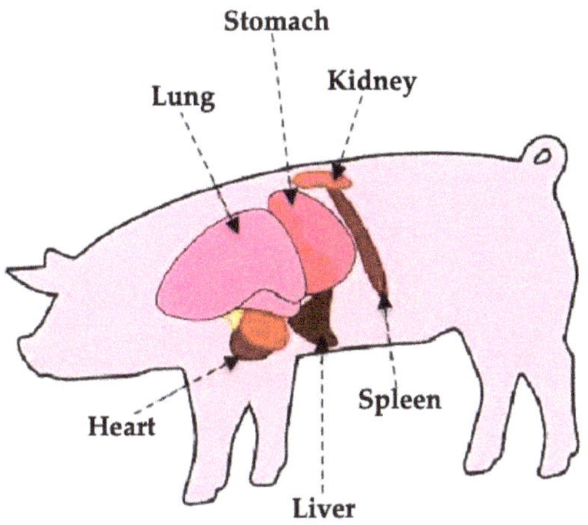

Figure 1. Distribution of organs in the thorax of the pig [5].

A French–German research group conducted a study on "Non-Invasive Assessment of Liver Fibrosis by Vibration-Controlled Transient Elastography (Fibroscan®)" using fresh pig livers [6]. It has been observed that liver stiffness increases with the rise in shear wave frequency. Consequently, higher frequencies result in greater measured stiffness values. Key findings from the use of the FibroScan® device include its capability to differentiate between early and advanced cirrhosis, its strong prognostic value for predicting patient survival, and its utility in monitoring patients undergoing treatment. However, the presence of ascites has been identified as a significant physical limitation to elastography, as fluid accumulation obstructs the propagation of shear waves, preventing them from reaching the liver.

A team representing the University of Heidelberg presented a study in the *Journal of Hepatology* indicating that liver stiffness is directly influenced by central venous pressure [7]. They conducted elastography studies using the Fibroscan® device for 10 landrace pigs. In their study, liver stiffness was evaluated as a function of venous pressure in an isolated pig liver by clamping the superior and inferior vena cava, the reflux vein, and the hepatic artery. Their findings demonstrated that central venous pressure directly and reversibly regulates liver stiffness. Over a wide range, liver stiffness exhibited a linear relationship with intravenous pressure, reaching an upper detection limit of 75 kPa at an intravenous pressure of 36 cm in a water column. This pronounced dependence of stiffness on venous pressure highlights the necessity of excluding hepatic congestion before assessing fibrosis.

Given the research problem outlined above, the aim of this article is to perform preliminary analyses of mechanical wave propagation within the studied system, specifically the porcine skin–liver system. The primary objective is to achieve satisfactory outcomes through a proposed modification to the measurement head overlay of the FibroScan® device. This modification is designed to ensure that its application does not cause structural damage to the organ as a result of mechanical wave excitation.

Therefore, it is necessary to develop numerical models that will allow for a rapid preliminary assessment of the propagation of mechanical waves in liver tissue and other relevant parameters. This requires constructing accurate geometric representations of the liver system and incorporating materials that mimic the properties of the skin and adjacent tissues. These models will then be enhanced by applying suitable initial and boundary conditions to replicate the environment observed during in vivo animal experiments.

2. Research Material

2.1. Liver

The liver of the pig is located in the abdominal cavity, on the right side of the body. It occupies most of the abdominal space and is surrounded by other organs. The average weight of the liver in pigs is approximately 1 kg, with its volume ranging between 640 and 910 mL in pigs aged 9 to 12 weeks and weighing between 25 and 35 kg [8].

In the structure of the pig liver, 5–6 lobes are distinguished. Their number depends on the breed under consideration. Regardless of the species, their minimum number is always 5, and they are defined as the left lateral, left medial, right lateral, right medial, and caudal lobes. From a ventral perspective, four lobes can be observed in the following order from left to right: left lateral, left medial, right medial, and right lateral. When these are elevated, it is possible to observe the caudal lobe surrounding the vena cava [9]. The sections are separated by deep interlobular fissures and can be further subdivided into eight segments, which are determined by the patterns of blood supply and bile duct drainage. The different parts of the liver are numbered in a counterclockwise direction. Segment I corresponds to the caudate lobe. The left lateral lobe comprises segments II and III, while segment IV represents the left medial lobe. The right medial lobe is associated with segments V and VIII, and the right lateral lobe consists of segments VI and VII [10,11]. Figure 2 shows the anatomy of the liver divided into segments observed from the diaphragmatic (A) and abdominal (B) surfaces.

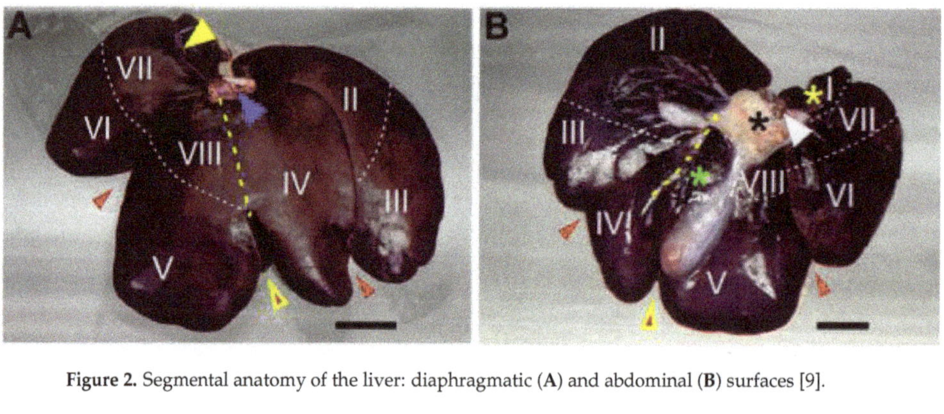

Figure 2. Segmental anatomy of the liver: diaphragmatic (**A**) and abdominal (**B**) surfaces [9].

The pig liver has a specific system of reflux veins that differs from that of humans. In the case of the porcine liver, the arterial blood supplying oxygen and nutrients to the organ combines with the blood of the reflux vein, and then the two bloods mix in vessels called hepatic glomeruli. This process allows the porcine liver to access nutrients and oxygen and allows for the removal of metabolic products [12].

2.2. Bone System

Ribs are long, arched bones that form a ring around the rib cage (Figure 3). Depending on the species, a pig's rib cage consists of 13–17 pairs of ribs (Figure 4). The last two pairs are known as free ribs, which are not connected to the sternum. In the structure of a single rib, the shaft and the two tips—anterior and posterior—are distinguished. The diameter of the bone changes with length, where the anterior end is much thicker. This phenomenon is the result of more bone tissue, which provides a stronger connection between the ribs and the rest of the rib cage [13].

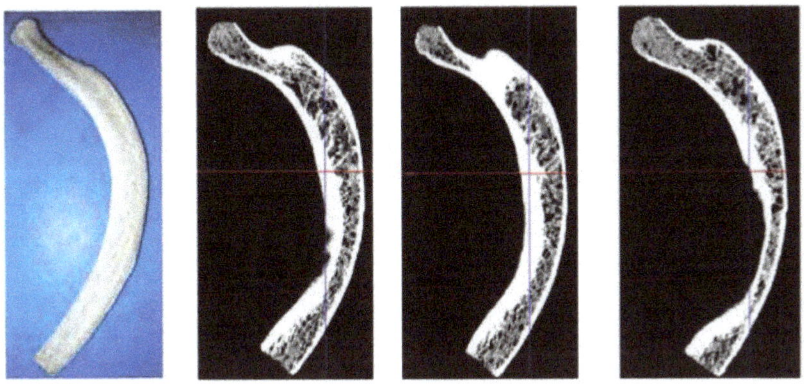

Figure 3. Pig's rib and CT images [14].

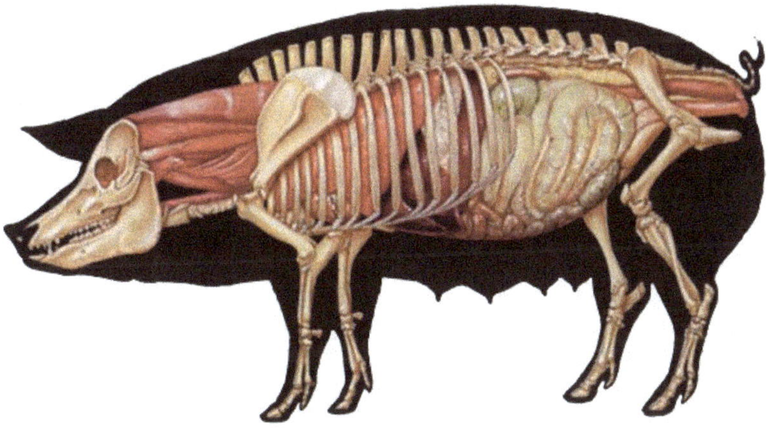

Figure 4. The bone system of a pig [15].

The rib shaft is the main part of the bone, which is a long and curved structure. It consists of a dense bone tissue, which provides it with strength and protection for the organs in the rib cage. It has two rib processes on the sides facing backward. The rib processes are shaped like hooks that connect to the spinous processes of the spinal vertebrae, which hold the ribs in place. The back of the rib connects to the spine through the rib–vertebral joint, which allows for a mobile connection to the corresponding vertebra of the spine. This connection provides flexibility and allows the chest to move during breathing. The front ends of the ribs connect to the sternum, which is a flat, horizontal bone located at the front of the rib cage, using rib cartilage. This is a flexible connection that allows some degree of rib movement and cushions forces during breathing. Encasing the ribs are the rib muscles, which are crucial for facilitating the movement of the rib cage during breathing. These muscles help raise and lower the ribs, allowing the space inside the rib cage to expand and contract [13].

The structure of a single rib consists of two primary layers: an outer compact layer and an inner spongy layer. The compact part, also called the cortical substance of the bone, accounts for most of the mass and volume of the bone. It mainly consists of compact bone tissue, which is a densely packed, hard, and durable form of bone tissue. It surrounds the inner spongy substance of the bone and is mainly found in the middle part of the bone. It is a porous, plexiform structure, which makes bones lighter but maintains their strength. This structure allows the body to maintain mobility while reducing stress on the body. Tables 1 and 2 show the selected mechanical properties of a cortical and spongy bone structure.

Table 1. Mechanical parameters of the pig's cortical bone material [14].

Parameter	Value	Unit
Density ρ	1691.0	kg/m^3
Young's modulus E	9.38	GPa
Poisson's ratio ν	0.3	-
Yield strength R_E	70.88	MPa
Exponent of consolidation n	1.2	-

Table 2. Mechanical parameters of the pig's spongy bone material [14].

Parameter	Value	Unit
Density ρ	773.0	kg/m^3
Young's modulus E	1.8	GPa
Poisson's ratio ν	0.45	-
Yield strength R_E	20.48	MPa
Exponent of consolidation n	2.0	-

2.3. *Pig's Skin*

The pig's skin is an external, durable, and flexible organ that covers almost its entire body. It is a heterogeneous material composed of three primary layers: the epidermis, dermis, and subcutaneous tissue (Figure 5). The epidermis, the outermost layer, is primarily composed of dead cells, with a thickness ranging from 30 to 140 μm [16]. The dermis lies directly beneath the epidermis and contains collagen fibers, elastin fibers, blood vessels, sebaceous glands, and sweat glands. The innermost layer, known as subcutaneous tissue, is a fatty layer situated beneath the dermis. The average thickness of the skin in the thoracic region is 2.3 mm, and its density is 1000–1300 kg/m^3, depending on the species studied [17].

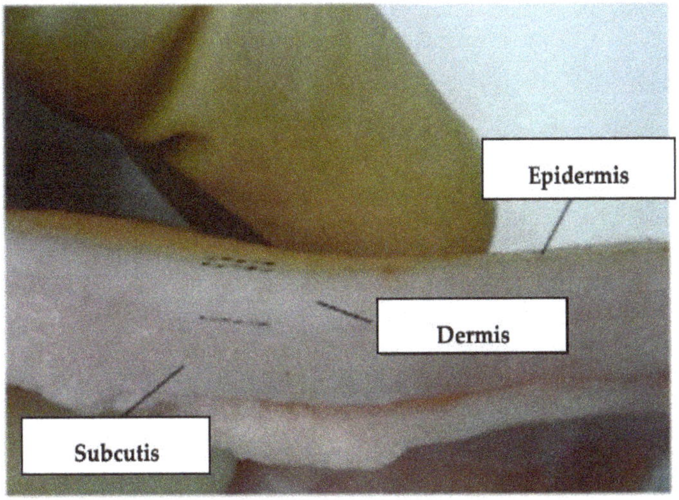

Figure 5. Pig's skin divided into layers [18].

From a mechanical perspective, leather is regarded as a composite material characterized by a highly hierarchical structure. Its multilayered nature also makes it a highly anisotropic material. Skin tissues exhibit viscoelastic mechanical properties, and under the action of pre-stress, it shows an uneven distribution of changes on its surface [19]. Collagen fibers play a significant role in determining the mechanical properties of the skin, particularly in their structural arrangement and orientation. The orientation of collagen fibers is not indifferent. There is a preferred orientation described as Langer lines, where there is optimal tension in the skin.

The viscoelastic properties of skin tissue are demonstrated by the hysteresis observed in the stress–strain relationship as depicted in Figure 6. The graph illustrates the energy lost within the tissue during the loading and unloading process. This phenomenon occurs as a result of internal friction, where the energy of mechanical deformation is converted to heat [20]. Skin tissue hardening under uniaxial tension begins at lower stress levels when aligned parallel to the preload direction compared to stresses transverse to the preload direction. This behavior is explained by defining skin as an orthropic material.

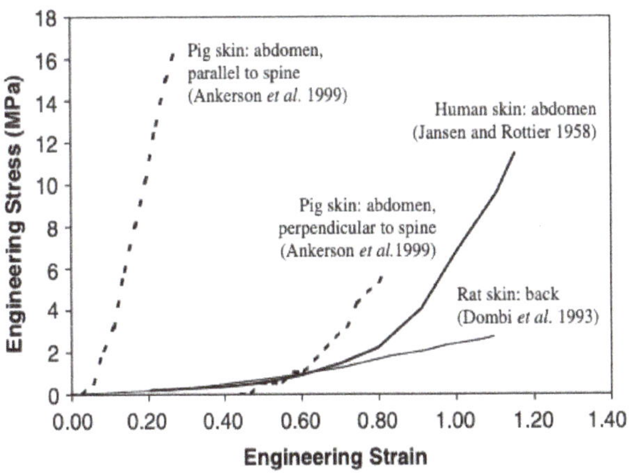

Figure 6. Uniaxial tension for stretching human, pig, and rat skin [21–23].

Determining the values of the mechanical parameters of skin tissue is challenging. Young's modulus is estimated to range between 7.6 and 62.6 MPa, where tensile strength for samples taken parallel to the spine is 2.5–15.7 MPa [17].

3. Assumptions for Numerical Modeling

A hybrid numerical approach was used in the modeling, combining features of the finite element method (FEM) and smoothed particle hydrodynamics (SPHs). The FEM was used to simulate bodies with a homogeneous and continuous structure, characterized by a compact material structure. In contrast, the SPH method was used for materials with a discontinuous structure, such as porous materials. The porosity of these materials was only a small fraction of the total volume of the component under study, which made it impossible to accurately model the pores using the conventional FEM due to the need for a very fine discretization mesh. As a result, the two methods were combined to effectively represent the various structural properties of the materials under analysis.

Rheological models are mathematical or physical models that describe the behavior of materials under stress and strain. Nonlinear rheological models are a type of these models that account for nonlinear stress–strain relationships in a material. In studies of the properties of soft tissues such as the liver, simplified models such as the linear-elastic model are often used to describe their behavior. The linear-elastic model is versatile and allows for the analysis of a material's behavior under different types of loading. However, this general idea has some limitations due to the assumption of a linear rheological response of the material, which can lead to errors.

In contrast, another approach describes hyper-stress models as dominant when related to viscosity. Basic diagrams of the most commonly used viscoelastic models in the mathematical description of liver tissue and the strain energy density functions of hyperelastic models are presented in Table 3.

Table 3. Deformation energy density functions of models.

Model	Equation
Neo-Hooke	$W = C_1(I_1 - 3)$
Mooney-Rivlin	$W = \sum C_{ij}(I_1 - 3)^i (I_2 - 3)^j$
Ogden	$W = \sum\left(\frac{\mu_k}{\alpha_k}\right)\left(\lambda_1^{\alpha k} + \lambda_2^{\alpha k} + \lambda_3^{\alpha k} - 3\right)$
Yeoh	$W = \sum C_k(I_1 - 3)^k$
Arruda-Boyce	$W = nkB\theta\left[\frac{1}{2}(I_1 - 3) + \left(\frac{1}{20N}\right)(I_1^2 - 9) + \left(\frac{11}{1050N^2}\right)(I_1^3 - 27) + \ldots\right]$
Veronda-Westmann	$W = C_1\left(e^{C_3(I_1-3)} - 1\right) + C_2(I_2 - 3)$

Among the hyperelastic models presented in Table 3, except for the last one, all models represent polynomial functions, describing rubber-like materials subjected to large deformations. The Veronda–Westmann model, on the other hand, is an exponential model.

In order to reduce the likelihood of erroneous analysis results, a different approach is used to study the structure of the tissues. It involves describing their properties using hyperelastic and hyperelastic models [24]. These models enable more precise predictions of the mechanical behavior of various elastomers or soft tissues. Given the complexity of rheological models and the extensive input data required, the focus was narrowed to two hyperelastic rheological models: the Yeoh model and the Ogden model. Both models are widely referenced in the literature for accurately characterizing the mechanical response of the liver. A mathematical approach was selected to compare these models, emphasizing simplicity in calculations while still providing valuable data for simulations.

Yeoh's hyperelastic material model provides a phenomenological representation of the deformation behavior of nearly incompressible and nonlinear elastic materials, such as rubber. This model builds on Ronald Rivlin's observation that the elastic properties of rubber can be characterized using the strain energy density function, which is expressed as a power series of strain invariants.

Yeoh's model, often referred to as the reduced polynomial model due to its polynomial format of the strain energy density function, was originally proposed in a cubic form. This formulation considers only the first strain invariant I_1 and is specifically designed for completely incompressible materials. The strain energy density function for Yeoh's model is expressed as follows:

$$W = \sum C_k \left(I_1 - 3 \right)^k \tag{1}$$

where C_k is the material's constants (Table 4). The quantity $2C_1$ can be interpreted as the initial shear modulus.

Table 4. Yeoh model's material constants.

Sample	Material Constants		
	C_{10}	C_{20}	C_{30}
1	1.414	51.352	189.630
2	1.571	36.782	452.368
3	0.418	89.325	−8.329
4	0.952	25.984	5.219

The Yeoh mathematical model is presented below.

$$U = C_{10}(I_1 - 3) + C_{20}(I_1 - 3)^2 + C_{30}(I_1 - 3)^3 + \frac{1}{D_1}(J^{el} - 1)^2 + \frac{1}{D_2}(J^{el} - 1)^4 + \frac{1}{D_3}(J^{el} - 1)^6 \tag{2}$$

$$I_1 = \lambda_1^2 + \lambda_2^2 + \lambda_3^2,\ \mu_0 = 2C_{10},\ K_0 = \frac{2}{D_1} \tag{3}$$

The Ogden material model is a hyperelastic framework designed to characterize the nonlinear stress–strain behavior of complex materials, including polymers and biological tissues. This model was developed by Raymond Ogden in 1972 and has since become a widely used approach for modeling the mechanical properties of such materials. The model plays a key role in determining stress–strain relationships in hyperelastic materials. It characterizes materials as isotropic, incompressible, and hyperelastic.

Similar to other hyperelastic models, Ogden's model assumes that a material's behavior can be characterized by a strain energy density function, which forms the basis for deriving stress–strain relationships. In Ogden's model, the strain energy density W is expressed in terms of the principal stretches $\lambda_{i,j} = 1,\ 2,\ 3$.

$$W = \sum \left(\frac{\mu_k}{\alpha_k} \right) \left(\lambda_1^{\alpha k} + \lambda_2^{\alpha k} + \lambda_3^{\alpha k} - 3 \right) \tag{4}$$

Analyzing a material that is not in compression during uniaxial stretching uses a stretching factor, defined as $\lambda = l/l_0$. Here, l represents the length after stretching, and l_0 is the original, unstretched length of the material.

$$U = \sum_{i=1}^{N} \frac{2\mu_i}{\alpha_i^2} (\lambda_1^{\alpha_i} + \lambda_2^{\alpha_i} + \lambda_3^{\alpha_i} - 3) + \sum_{i=1}^{N} \frac{1}{D_i} (J^{el} - 1)^{2i} \tag{5}$$

$$\mu_0 = \sum_{i=1}^{N} \mu_i \tag{6}$$

$$K_0 = \frac{2}{D_1} \tag{7}$$

For incompressible materials, the principal stresses satisfy the following condition [25]:

$$\lambda_1 \lambda_2 \lambda_3 = 1 \tag{8}$$

The two constants used in the Ogden model are determined through experimental data. Figure 7 shows the stress–strain curve in pig skin tension fitted to Ogden's one-particle model in quasi-static tension. The experimentally determined Ogden constants are shown in Table 5. Having knowledge of one of the two constants in the Ogden model enables a reasonably accurate approximation of the experimental data.

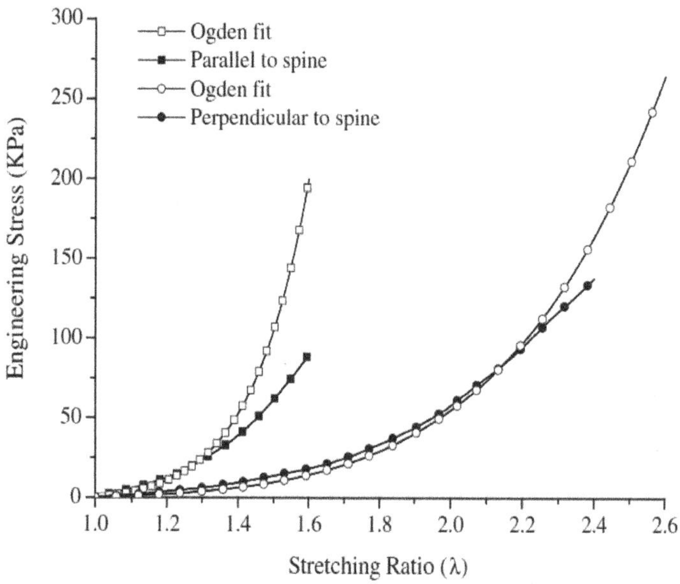

Figure 7. Tensile stress response of pig skin at 0.005 m/s strain rate [25].

Table 5. Material constants of Ogden's model.

Sample	Material Constants					
	μ_1	α_1	μ_2	α_2	μ_3	α_3
1	0.752	53.713	127.595	1.284	41.126	5.055
2	0.242	15.052	5.452	−0.099	42.042	−0.022
3	2.220	8.878	32.485	−0.471	23.779	0.189
4	2.428	10.507	6.411	2.110	16.033	−0.782

Regarding the strength study of the problem under consideration, a numerical analysis was carried out using the Abaqus program. The process began with the creation of geometric models in Inventor, and then these models are exported to a computational environment in .step format. In order to describe the mechanical properties of biological materials, the Johnson–Cook rheological model was used. This is a rheological model used to characterize materials with an elastic–plastic behavior with nonlinear amplification. The initial part of the model describes the linear response of the material under a given load and is characterized by Young's modulus and Poisson's ratio. However, beyond this limit, the material exhibits nonlinear strengthening, which is captured by the Johnson–Cook mathematical model in a numerical analysis. The Johnson-Cook model is based on the von

Mises flow stress and incorporates nonlinear strain-dependent strengthening, strain rate effects, and thermal fatigue. The Johnson–Cook model is typically expressed as follows:

$$\sigma_y = \left(A + B\varepsilon^{p^n}\right)\left(1 + cln\dot{\varepsilon}^*\right)(1 - T^{*m}) \tag{9}$$

where

$$\dot{\varepsilon}^* = \frac{\dot{\underline{\varepsilon}}^p}{\dot{\varepsilon}_0} \tag{10}$$

$$T^* = \frac{T - T_{room}}{T_{melt} - T_{room}} \tag{11}$$

where A is the yield strength of the material; B is the yield strength constant; c is the dynamic strengthening factor; n is the strengthening exponent; m is the thermal weakening factor; $\underline{\varepsilon}^p$ is the effective plastic strain; $\dot{\underline{\varepsilon}}^p$ is the strain rate; $\dot{\varepsilon}^*$ is the dimensionless effective strain rate; $\dot{\varepsilon}_0$ is the reference value for the strain rate; T^* is the dimensionless (homologous) temperature; T_{room} is the reference temperature; T_{melt} is the melting temperature, and T is the base (current) temperature.

4. Numerical Simulations and Results

Given the complexity of the rheological model and the large number of input parameters, the remainder of the paper focuses on the analysis of two specific rheological models: the Yeoh model and the Ogden model. For this purpose, preliminary numerical analyses were carried out by stimulating the process of pressing the penetrator into the liver sample. Due to the lack of available experimental results, we relied on publicly available literature data. This chapter aims to verify the numerical methods used. In order to simplify the calculations, two mathematical models that are effective for simulation applications were selected. The Ogden and Yeoh hyperelastic models, widely referenced in the literature for modeling the mechanical response of the liver, were chosen for our analysis.

The study began by modeling the geometry of the intender and the structure of the liver. The proposed intender was cuboidal in shape with dimensions of 8 × 10 × 30 mm. In order to simplify the simulation, a cuboid of 8 × 32 × 90 mm was assumed as the liver, for which parameters were set corresponding to the mechanical properties given in the table below (Table 6).

Table 6. Mechanical parameters of the pig's liver.

Parameter	Value	Unit
Density ρ	1.075	g/cm^3
Young's modulus E	1.1	kPa
Compressive stress R_C	123.0	kPa
Yield strength R_E	205.0	kPa
Strain energy density	18.19	kJ/m^3

Figure 8 shows the obtained stress results for the simulation of the intender cavity in the liver structure for four time steps. A comparison of the results obtained for the von Mises and Tresca stress results is shown.

Subsequently, a numerical model of the liver structure as an organ with complex structure and geometry was developed. Then, a system was created to simulate the examination of the liver percutaneously. The process was carried out in three stages: the first focused on modeling the soft tissues, such as the skin; the second addressed the modeling of hard tissues, such as the ribs; and the third stage involved integrating the collected data with the liver model and scaling it appropriately.

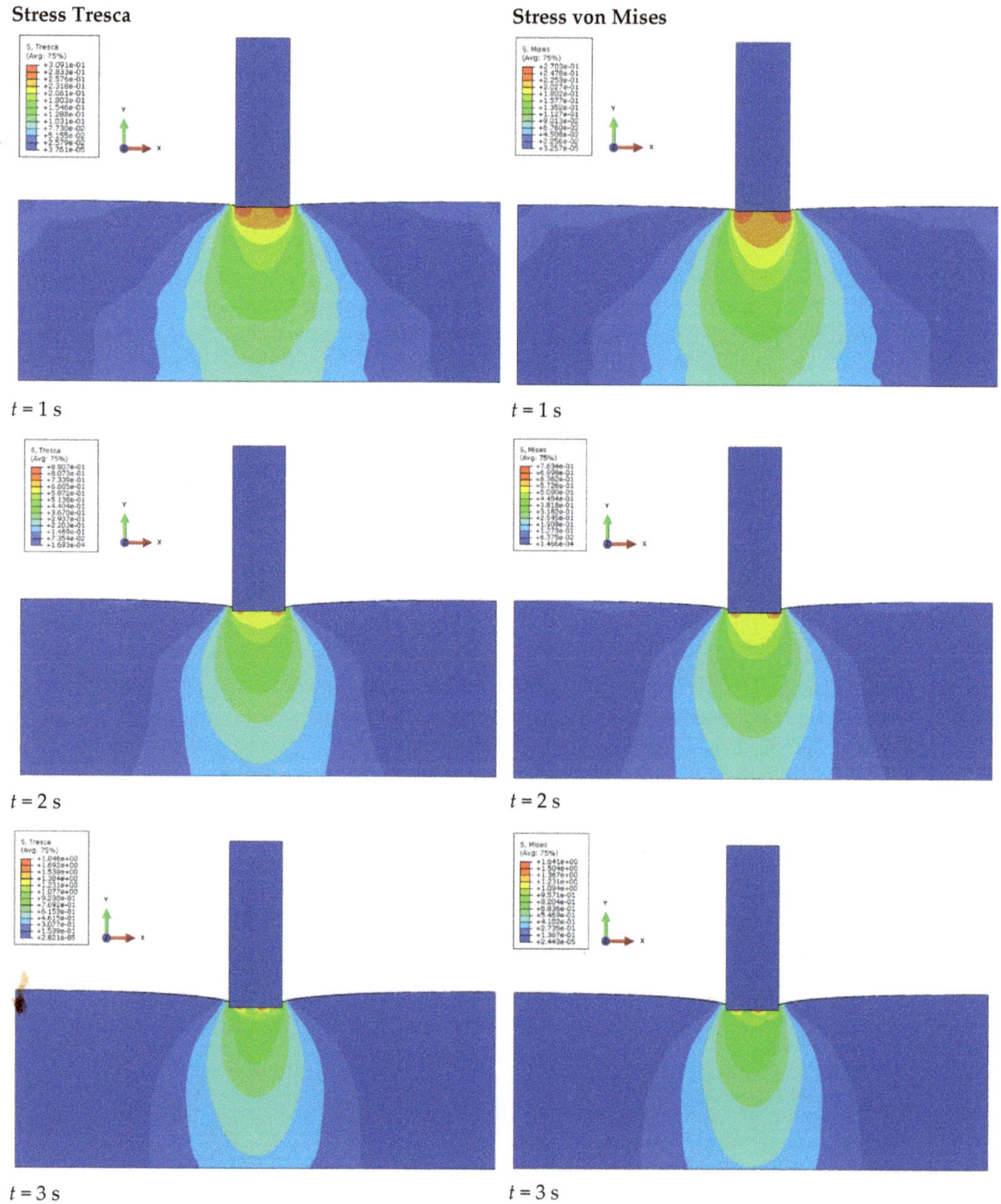

Figure 8. *Cont.*

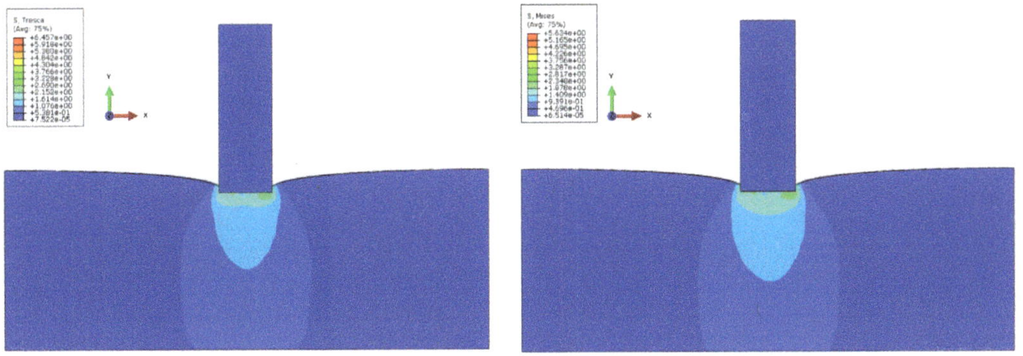

$t = 4$ s $t = 4$ s

Figure 8. Comparison of von Mises and Tresca stress results for a non-deformable penetrator.

In this stage, the rib component was modeled, distinguishing between the external compact layer and the internal spongy layer. The mechanical parameters required for developing the numerical models of these components are provided in Tables 7 and 8. Due to its porous structure, the spongy part of the bone was modeled using smoothed particle hydrodynamic (SPH) elements, while the remaining parts were modeled using the finite element method (FEM).

Table 7. Mechanical parameters of the cortical bone substance.

Parameter	Value	Unit
Density (ρ)	1850.0	kg/m^3
Young's modulus (E)	1.80	GPa
Poisson's ratio (ν)	0.35	-
	Johnson–Cook Model	
Yield strength (A)	160.0	MPa
Fixed fortification (B)	165.0	MPa
Exponent of consolidation (n)	0.1	-

Table 8. Mechanical parameters of the spongy bone substance.

Parameter	Value	Unit
Density (ρ)	900.0	kg/m^3
Young's modulus (E)	18.0	MPa
Poisson's ratio (ν)	0.4	-
	Johnson–Cook Model	
Yield strength (A)	42.0	MPa
Fixed fortification (B)	55.0	MPa
Exponent of consolidation (n)	0.9	-

A series of numerical simulations were performed on the developed geometric models, incorporating initial and boundary conditions, as well as parameters for simulating the liver's loading within the elastic range. The first numerical analysis focused on a single rib. The rib's average length ranged between 30 and 40 cm, with a typical width and depth between 5.5 and 7.5 cm, which was measured along its curved length [13]. For this study, these values were averaged across the majority of the population. The model was discretized with a resolution of 0.5 mm, employing Tetra-type elements for the simulation. The goal was to represent the wave motion that occurs when performing elastography. A rectangular-shaped inductor was used in the analysis.

In addition, numerical simulations were carried out at various signal frequencies, from 1.0 to 5.0 MHz. Based on the results, hard tissues were analyzed to evaluate the accuracy of the modeling for both cortical and spongy structures, as well as the bone's capacity to absorb sound waves. Finally, a comprehensive model combining soft tissues, hard tissues, and liver elements was validated to ensure its accuracy and reliability.

The simulation results of mechanical wave propagation through tissues, ribs, and the liver without an additional cap revealed the occurrence of interference phenomena at the level of the rib bones (Figures 9 and 10). Subsequent stages of the simulation were excluded due to wave reflection at the liver's edge, as the model did not include adjacent organs. The wave's effects were meticulously analyzed within a frequency range of 1.0 to 5.0 MHz, liver tissue stiffness between 2.7 and 16.5 kPa, and a liver steatosis level below 270 dB/m. From this analysis, the speed of sound propagation in the studied environment was determined. Specifically, for an excitation frequency of 3.5 MHz, the simulation yielded a propagation velocity of 1420 m/s.

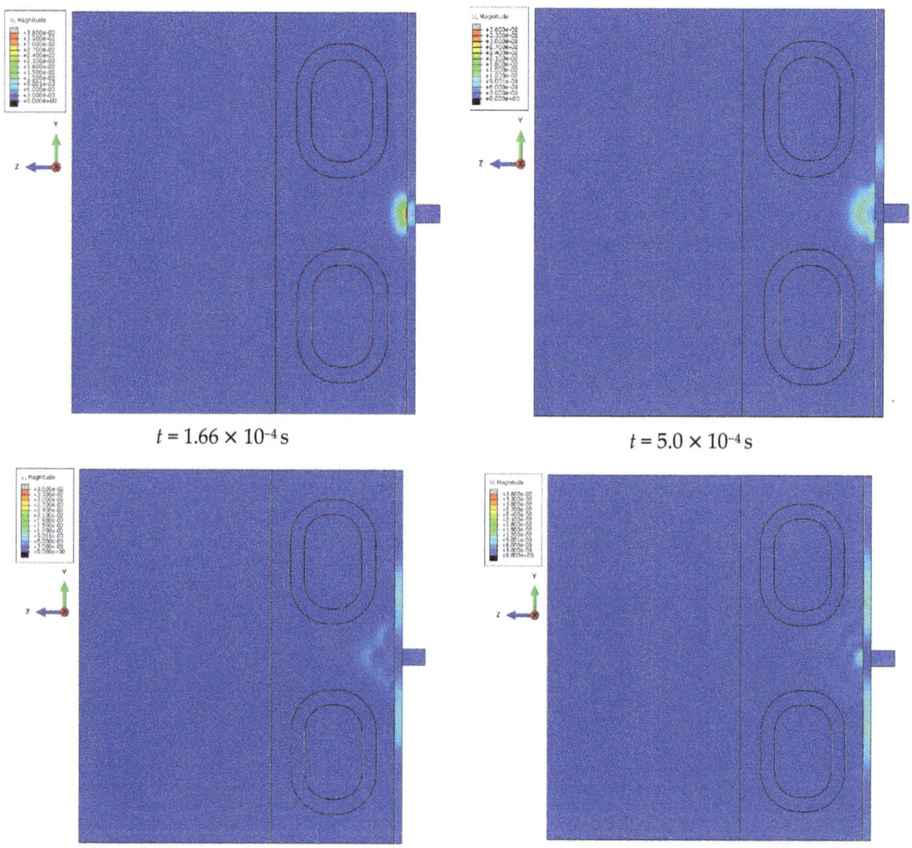

$t = 1.66 \times 10^{-4}$ s

$t = 5.0 \times 10^{-4}$ s

$t = 8.33 \times 10^{-4}$ s

$t = 1.16 \times 10^{-3}$ s

Figure 9. *Cont.*

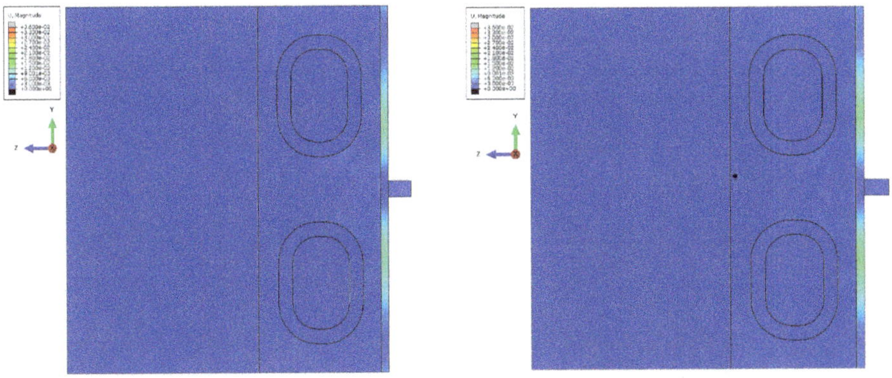

$t = 1.50 \times 10^{-3}$ s $t = 1.83 \times 10^{-3}$ s

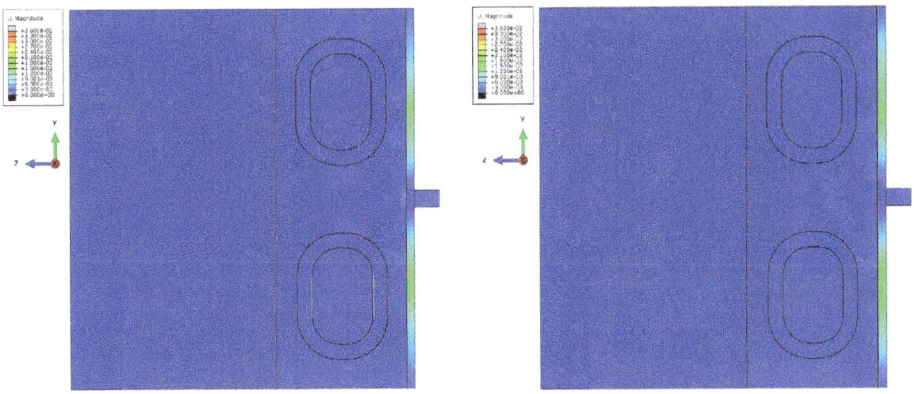

$t = 2.16 \times 10^{-3}$ s $t = 2.50 \times 10^{-3}$ s

Figure 9. Wavefront displacements for the system at individual time steps: $t = 1.66 \times 10^{-4}$ s, $t = 5.0 \times 10^{-4}$ s, $t = 8.33 \times 10^{-4}$ s, $t = 1.16 \times 10^{-3}$ s, $t = 1.50 \times 10^{-3}$ s, $t = 1.83 \times 10^{-3}$ s, $t = 2.16 \times 10^{-3}$ s, and $t = 2.50 \times 10^{-3}$ s.

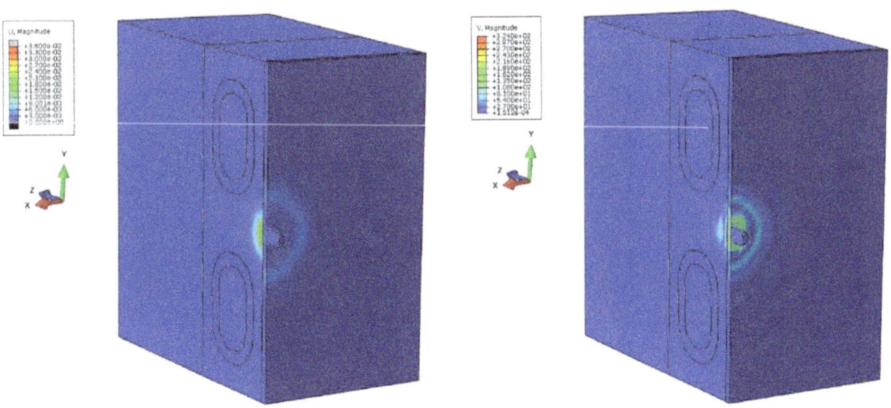

$t = 1.66 \times 10^{-4}$ s

Figure 10. *Cont.*

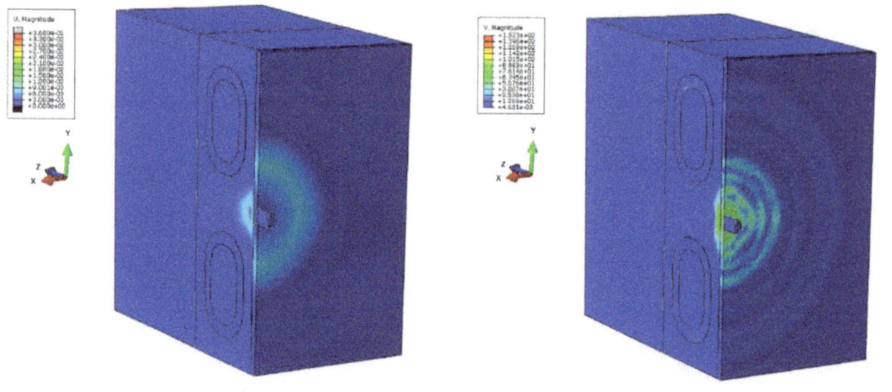

$t = 5.0 \times 10^{-4}$ s

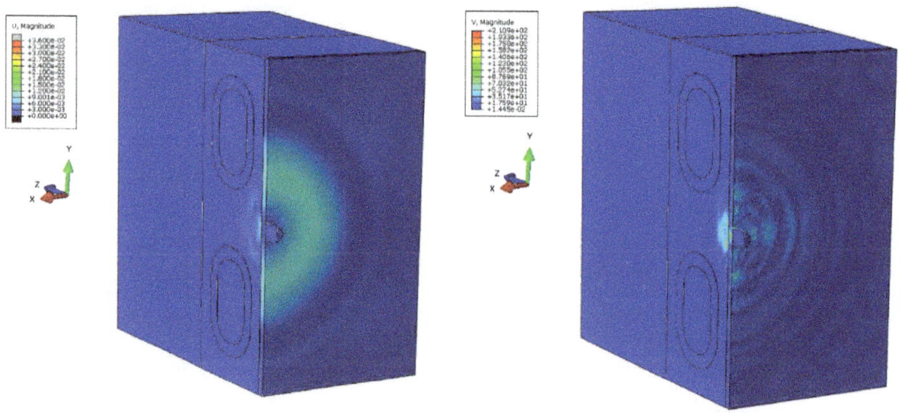

$t = 8.33 \times 10^{-4}$ s

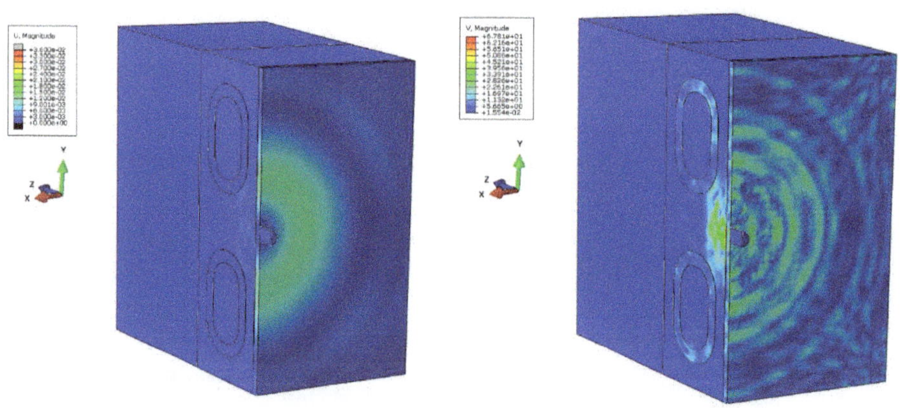

$t = 1.16 \times 10^{-3}$ s

Figure 10. Summary of the propagation of the mechanical wave in each time step: $t = 1.66 \times 10^{-4}$ s, $t = 5.0 \times 10^{-4}$ s, $t = 8.33 \times 10^{-4}$ s, and $t = 1.16 \times 10^{-3}$ s.

Tests were carried out for the use of the FibroScan® device together with the six types of caps designed. Two geometric designs for the caps were selected for analysis: a cylindrical one using the designation E15 and a conical one referred to as D0. Tetra-type elements with an additional node inside were adopted for discretization. Geometric models were made based on technical documentation. Figure 11 shows the adopted layout with the overlays undergoing discretization.

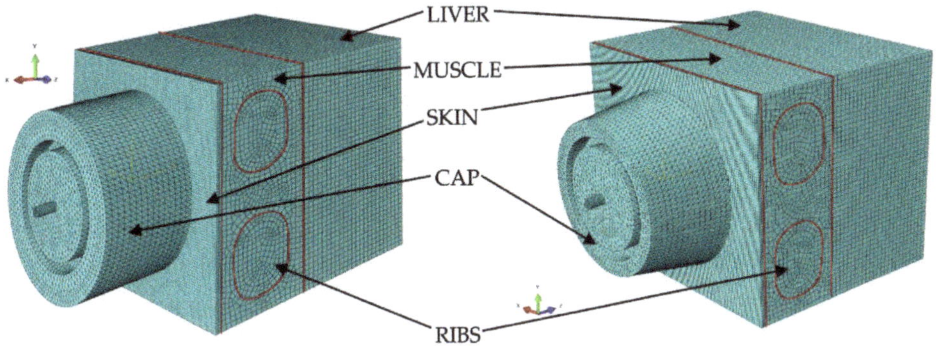

Figure 11. Discretization of caps: (**a**) cylindrical and (**b**) conical [26].

From conducting preliminary simulations, it was noted that the size of the discretization component of the model does not affect the results obtained (Table 9). The individual variables in each frequency occur due to the way the computer software represents the results and does not affect the result (rounding of numbers).

Table 9. Summary of the results for a cylindrical head with different discretization sizes.

Cap	Frequency of the Inductor [MHz]	Wave Velocity [m/s]	0.5 mm	1.0 mm	1.5 mm	2.0 mm
	1.0	843	843	842	842	842
	1.5	906	906	905	905	906
	2.0	969	969	969	969	969
	2.5	992	991	992	991	992
cylindrical	3.0	1050	1050	1051	1050	1050
	3.5	1083	1082	1082	1083	1082
	4.0	1132	1132	1132	1132	1132
	4.5	1183	1182	1182	1183	1184
	5.0	1243	1245	1244	1243	1244
Cap	**Frequency of the inductor [MHz]**	**Wave velocity [m/s]**	**2.5 mm**	**3.0 mm**	**4.0 mm**	**5.0 mm**
	1.0	843	841	843	843	843
	1.5	906	906	905	905	906
	2.0	968	969	968	968	969
	2.5	992	991	992	991	992
cylindrical	3.0	1050	1051	1050	1051	1050
	3.5	1083	1082	1083	1082	1082
	4.0	1132	1132	1132	1132	1132
	4.5	1183	1182	1182	1182	1182
	5.0	1245	1243	1244	1243	1245

In the first stage of wavefront propagation studies, a numerical analysis was conducted on two types of cap geometries: conical and cylindrical, with an assumed wave excitation frequency of 3 MHz. Figure 12 presents a summary of wave propagation for the conical cap at successive time moments: 3.3×10^{-4} s, 6.6×10^{-4} s, and 1.0×10^{-3} s. The observations show how the size and intensity of the wave change as the propagation process continues through the medium.

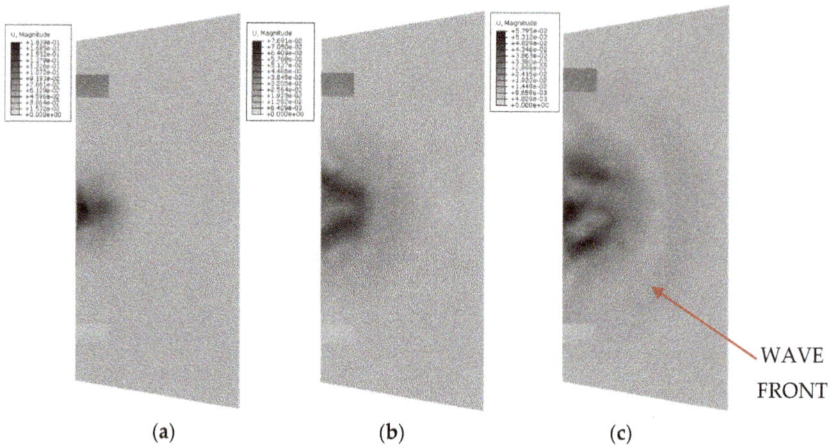

Figure 12. Summary of wave propagation for the conical cap with frequency 3 MHz in time (**a**) 3.3×10^{-4} s, (**b**) 6.6×10^{-4} s, and (**c**) 1.0×10^{-3} s.

In comparison, Figure 13 illustrates the wave propagation for the cylindrical cap at the same time moments: 3.3×10^{-4} s, 6.6×10^{-4} s, and 1.0×10^{-3} s. This comparison allows for an assessment of how the cap geometry influences the shape and scattering of the mechanical wave. The differences in propagation are evident in the way the wave spreads and in the efficiency of energy dispersion within the medium, which is crucial for further analysis of the models' effectiveness.

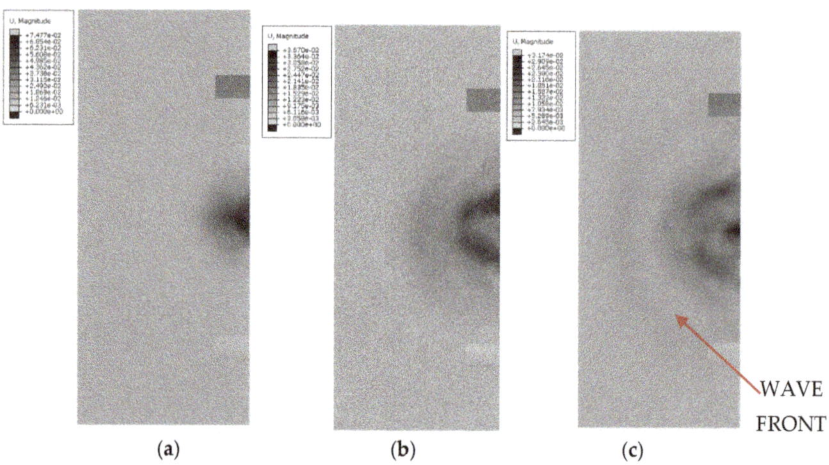

Figure 13. Summary of wave propagation for the cylindrical cap with frequency 3 MHz in time (**a**) 3.3×10^{-4} s, (**b**) 6.6×10^{-4} s, and (**c**) 1.0×10^{-3} s.

This approach enables the evaluation of which geometry better reduces wave intensity, which is significant for applications in non-invasive medical examinations, such as liver assessment using a cap model.

Initially, the caps were made by using three different materials: Agar, Ecoflex 00-20, and Medical Gel. Based on the results obtained on experimental animals and post-mortem organs, the best-fitting material in relation to the tissue under study was selected, which turned out to be Ecoflex 00-20.

A numerical analysis was carried out while maintaining the set frequency for the inductor at 1.0–5.0 MHz. The following is an example of the results obtained for caps made of the Ecoflex 00-20 material using an exciter frequency of 2.0 MHz. The change in displacement during the phenomenon and the value of attenuation (CAP) in relation to the obtained stiffness were analyzed depending on the mathematical model used. The juxtaposition of damping results for different numerical models using a conical cap and a cylindrical cap made of the Ecoflex 00-20 material (Figures 14 and 15) is important in the context of comparing their effectiveness in reducing the intensity of the mechanical wave (Tables 10 and 11).

At specific time steps, i.e., $t = 5.0 \times 10^{-4}$ s, $t = 1.0 \times 10^{-3}$ s, $t = 2.0 \times 10^{-3}$ s, and $t = 3.0 \times 10^{-3}$ s, changes in the displacements of the wavefront within the simulated liver tissue can be observed. These displacement values indicate the evolution of the mechanical wave within the tissue under study. At the initial time step, $t = 5.0 \times 10^{-4}$ s, the wave is in its early propagation phase, traveling along the cylindrical applicator and progressing through the tissue as a longitudinal wave. As time progresses, i.e., at subsequent time steps, the wave gradually spreads through the simulated tissue, moving further from the generating source. By the final time step, in the description of the mechanical wave, the wavefront extends to a greater distance from the cylindrical applicator. A portion of the wave is absorbed by the bony structures present in the system, such as the ribs.

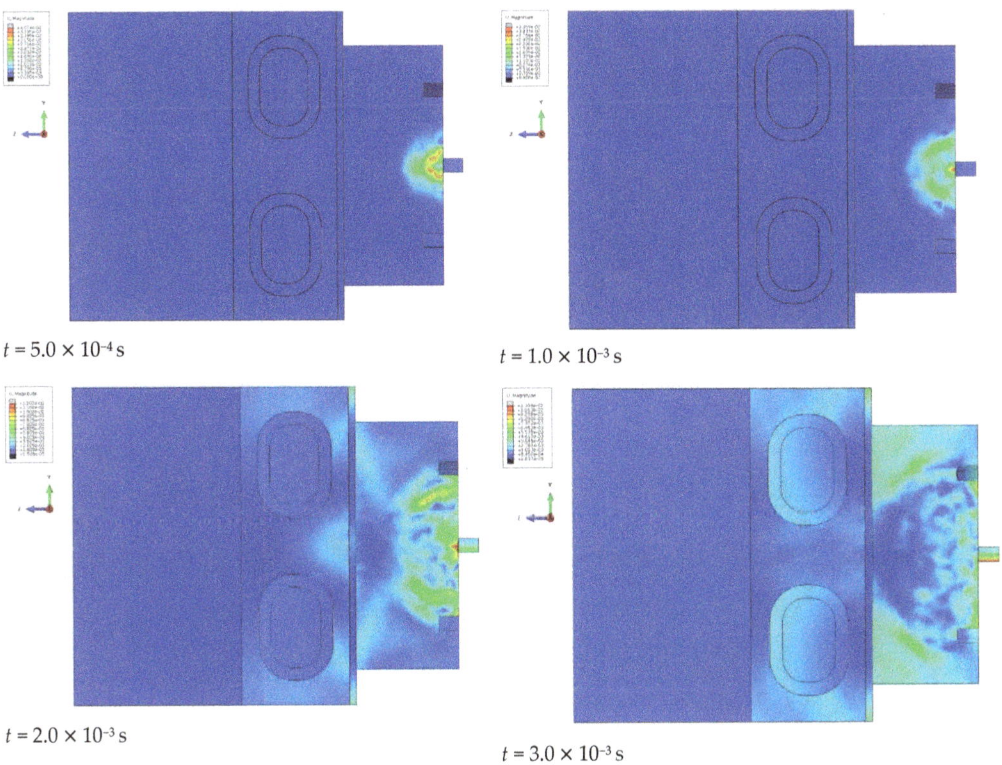

Figure 14. Displacements of the wavefront for the cylindrical cap made of Ecoflex 00-20 material at the following individual time steps: $t = 5.0 \times 10^{-4}$ s, $t = 1.0 \times 10^{-3}$ s, $t = 2.0 \times 10^{-3}$ s, and $t = 3.0 \times 10^{-3}$ s.

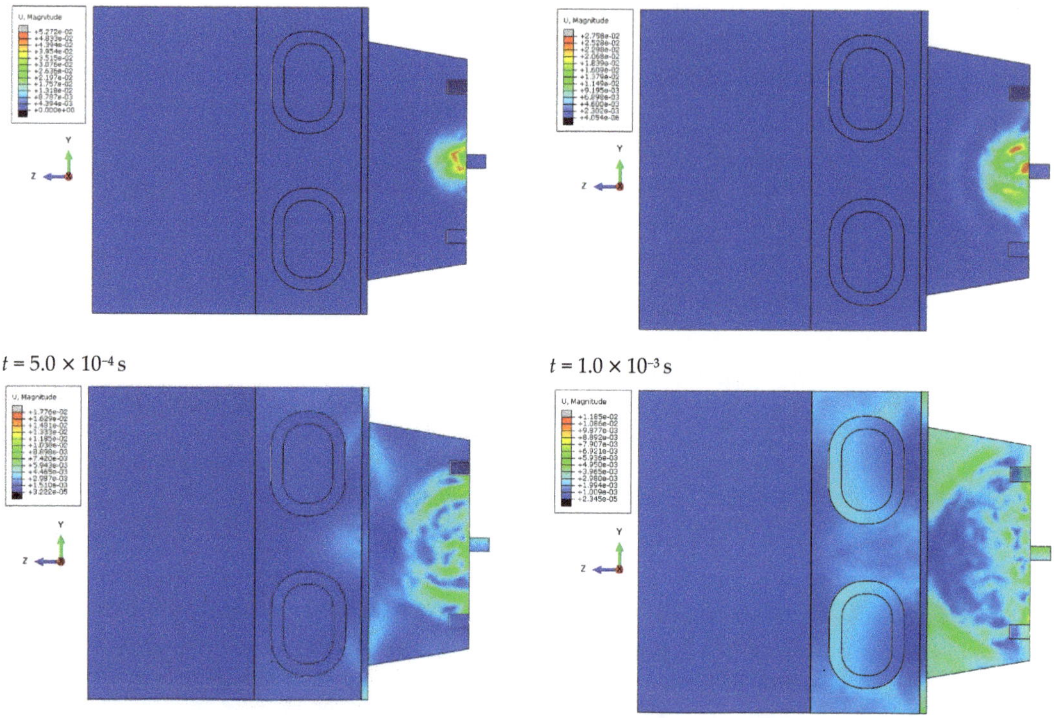

$t = 5.0 \times 10^{-4}$ s $t = 1.0 \times 10^{-3}$ s

$t = 2.0 \times 10^{-3}$ s $t = 3.0 \times 10^{-3}$ s

Figure 15. Wavefront displacements for a conical cap made of the Ecoflex 00-20 material at the following individual time steps: $t = 5.0 \times 10^{-4}$ s, $t = 1.0 \times 10^{-3}$ s, $t = 2.0 \times 10^{-3}$ s, and $t = 3.0 \times 10^{-3}$ s.

The cylindrical design of the applicator directly impacts the mechanics of wave propagation within the tissue. The shape of the tool affects the wave properties, including its amplitude, and plays a significant role in its interaction with the examined tissue during the simulation of a percutaneous liver assessment.

Table 10. Summary of the damping results for the applied numerical models using a cylindrical cap made of the Ecoflex 00-20 material.

Mathematical Model	Name	CAP (dB/m)	*E* (kPA) Median
Yeoh	flank	240	4.7
J-C	breastbone	172	11.2
J-C	back	213	9.7
Yeoh	flank	242	8.2
J-C	breastbone	253	7.5
J-C	back	214	4.3
Odgen	flank	241	6.5
J-C	breastbone	223	8.9
J-C	back	165	7.1
Odgen	flank	264	13.4
J-C	breastbone	241	3.6
J-C	back	157	3.8

Table 11. Summary of the damping results for the numerical models using a conical cap made of the Ecoflex 00-20 material.

Mathematical Model	Name	CAP (dB/m)	*E* (kPA) Median
Yeoh	flank	245	5.1
J-C	breastbone	184	10.2
J-C	back	201	9.3
Yeoh	flank	256	8.5
J-C	breastbone	248	5.9
J-C	back	211	5.1
Odgen	flank	236	6.9
J-C	breastbone	213	7.8
J-C	back	185	8.3
Odgen	flank	281	15.4
J-C	breastbone	223	4.3
J-C	back	157	4.9

The conical applicator represents a geometric form that influences the focusing or scattering of the wave within the examined tissue. At the first time step, $t = 5.0 \times 10^{-4}$ s, an early stage of wave propagation from the conical applicator is observed. The area where the wave is noticeable is limited and does not extend to greater distances, similar to the early stage described in the previous phenomenon. As time advances, at subsequent time steps, the conical shape of the applicator enables the observation of wave dispersion within the studied medium. By the final time step, $t = 3.0 \times 10^{-3}$ s, the area in which the wave is observed reaches its maximum size, but the intensity is significantly diminished. The wavefront displacement values also change over time. At the first time step, the displacement reaches a maximum value of 0.05 mm, while at the final time step, it decreases to 0.01 mm, corresponding to the described decrease in wave intensity as it propagates through the simulated medium.

In conclusion, the shape of the conical applicator has a crucial impact on wave propagation in the tissue during the simulation of a percutaneous liver assessment. This tool shape determines the area and intensity of the wave as well as its behavior in the examined tissue at the different time stages of the simulation.

5. Validation Research

FibroScan® technology represents a leading technique for assessing liver stiffness. This technique utilizes a low-frequency acoustic wave to non-invasively measure the stiffness of liver tissue. One of the key parameters characterizing this technology is tissue elasticity, denoted by the elasticity parameter E. In this study, applicators with two geometric shapes were considered: a cylindrical shape, designated as E15, and a conical shape, referred to as D0, both constructed from the Ecoflex 00-20 material.

Validation studies of liver stiffness measurements were conducted using the FibroScan® device in percutaneous assessments (Figure 16), taking into account the elasticity parameter E, which was expressed in kPa [27]. Advanced numerical models of liver tissues were developed and utilized to perform numerical simulations in the Abaqus software, allowing for the evaluation of the accuracy and effectiveness of this technology under various clinical conditions.

To conduct a comparative analysis of the results obtained from numerical simulations against reference data derived from histological studies and in vivo measurements on pigs using the FibroScan® (Figure 17), the outcomes for the Ecoflex material are presented in Table 12.

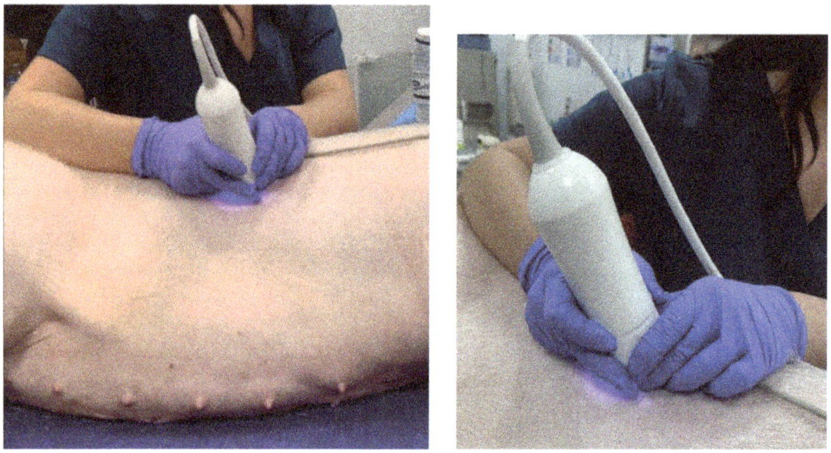

Figure 16. The procedure of liver elastography in pigs using the FibroScan® device.

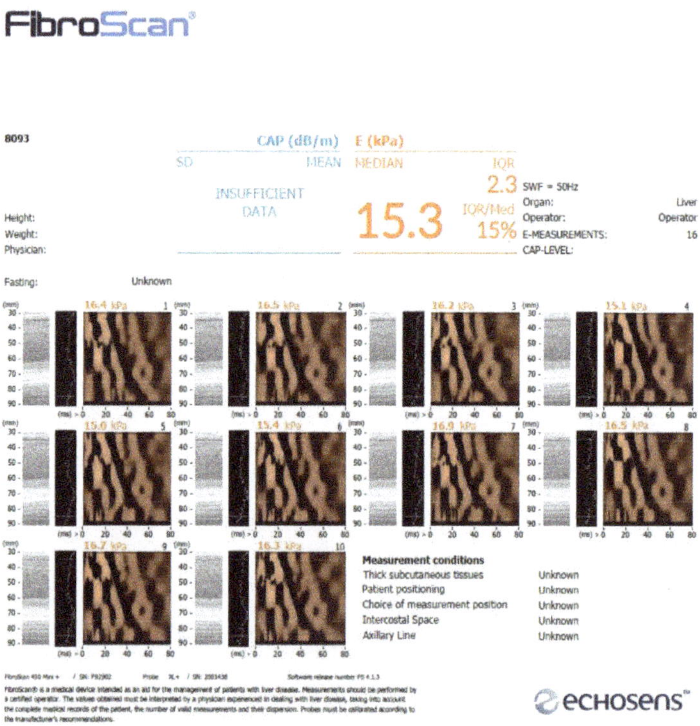

Figure 17. Example results obtained using the FibroScan® device.

The study involved eight Polish landrace pigs sourced from the same breeding facility. Female pigs aged 16–20 weeks with an initial weight of 40–45 kg were selected for the experiments. Elastographic measurements were conducted four times at weekly intervals. Prior to the study, all animals were acclimatized to the handling and grooming procedures. The pigs were fed an identical full-portion feed mixture in accordance with nutritional standards and kept under uniform husbandry conditions. Animal care was conducted in compliance with the National Institutes of Health guidelines for the care and use of laboratory animals. The experiments were approved and carried out in accordance with the regulations set forth by the Local Ethics Committee in Wrocław (Approval No. 46/2022/P1 dated 16 November 2022).

Table 12. Summary of the results for validation.

	Research on Organs			Numerical Simulations	
Pig no.	**Date**	**Cap**	***E* (kPA) Median**	**Cap**	***E* (kPA) Median**
W8 8236	9 March 2023	Ecoflex D0 Ecoflex E15	17.4 19.0	Ecoflex D0	11.1
W7 8337	9 March 2023	Ecoflex D0 Ecoflex E15	11.4 7.7	Ecoflex D0	6.5
W6 8252	9 March 2023	Ecoflex D0 Ecoflex E15	24.7 23.5	Ecoflex D0	17.6
W5 8093	9 March 2023	Ecoflex D0 Ecoflex E15	15.2 15.3	Ecoflex D0	18.2
W2 0590	22 December 2022	Ecoflex D0 Ecoflex E15	14.2 -	Ecoflex E15	7.5
W1 0586	22 December 2022	Ecoflex D0 Ecoflex E15	12.7 -	Ecoflex E15	16.6
W3 0630	22 December 2022	Ecoflex D0 Ecoflex E15	16.5 -	Ecoflex E15	10.2
W4 0661	22 December 2022	Ecoflex D0 Ecoflex E15	19.5 -	Ecoflex E15	13.4

Elastographic examinations were conducted under general anesthesia using propofol (2 mg/kg) and isoflurane (1.5 vol%), following premedication with ketamine (10 mg/kg), midazolam (0.3 mg/kg), and medetomidine (0.03 mg/kg), with the animal positioned on its left side. An example result of liver elasticity measurement in a pig was obtained using the FibroScan® Mini + 430 device equipped with an XL probe (5 MHz) and a stabilization-enhanced applicator, and the liver was placed in a specialized container.

No significant correlation was demonstrated between liver elasticity, measured directly in liver samples (Elasto direct; *E* kPa), and the results were related to non-invasive liver steatosis and liver elasticity obtained from in vivo animal studies (Table 13). The liver elasticity results (direct) were analyzed using a one-way analysis of variance (ANOVA). The application of the FibroScan® device probe in liver stiffness measurement was considered, with the elasticity parameter E expressed in kPa.

Table 13. Pearson correlation coefficients calculated for 8 animals.

			Correlation Coefficient				
Variable	**Mean**	**Std. Deviation**	**Elasto Direct *E* (kPa)**	**CAP (dB/m)**	**SD**	***E* (kPA) Median**	**IQR/Med.**
Elasto direct *E* (kPa)	16.7	5.6	1.000	−0.283	−0.061	−0.258	−0.267
CAP (dB/m)	52.8	11.9	−0.283	1.000	0.174	0.214	0.288
SD	17.9	1.2	−0.061	0.174	1.000	0.407	0.689
E (kPA) median	10.0	3.8	−0.258	0.214	0.407	1.000	0.032
IQR/Med.	0.4	0.2	−0.267	0.288	0.689	0.032	1.000

Figures 18 and 19 show the results of the analysis of the agreement of elasticity measurements in kPa, obtained using the FibroScan® applicator with a conical overlay (D0) and a cylindrical overlay (E15) made of the Ecoflex 00-20 material. The horizontal axis of the graph (x) shows the average elasticity values determined using the direct and simulation methods, while the vertical axis (y) represents the differences between these values for each measurement.

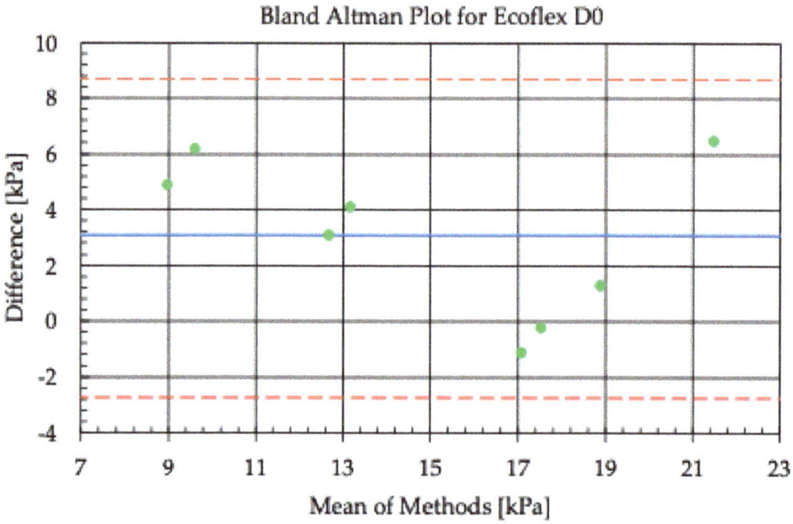

Figure 18. Bland–Altman Plot for Ecoflex D0.

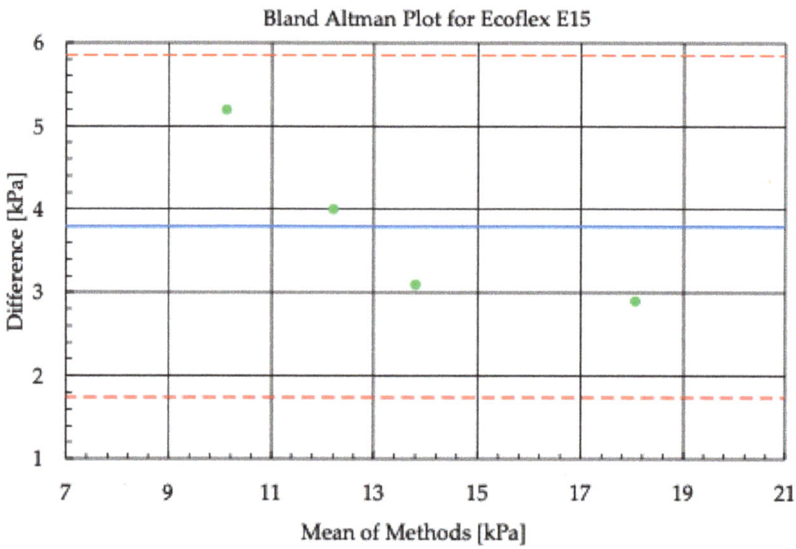

Figure 19. Bland–Altman Plot for Ecoflex E15.

The graph shows the middle line (blue), which represents the average difference (bias) between the results of the two methods, as well as the dashed lines (red) marking the limits of agreement (limits of agreement), calculated as ±1.96 standard deviations from the average difference. Most of the points on the graph are within the limits of agreement, indicating good agreement between the direct and simulation methods.

The variation in results may be due to differences in the geometry of the applicator, the properties of the Ecoflex 00-20 material, and local differences in the mechanical properties of the tissue being tested. The limits of agreement show the range within which the differences between the methods are statistically acceptable, confirming that the measurement and simulation method used is consistent in analyzing the elasticity of the tissue under the specified conditions.

6. Results and Discussion

Numerical analysis results indicate that no significant differences were observed in the outcomes associated with the applied mathematical model. Both the Yeoh and Ogden rheological models produced comparable results, with the differences being negligible. The variance in the results, approximately 8%, represents a very good fit. Greater discrepancies were noted in the constant parameters used in the calculations—the obtained results upon altering these parameters showed larger variations within ±27%. Nevertheless, these results were deemed satisfactory, likely due to significant variability in the initial data of the rheological models. These results were used in further numerical simulations.

In the frequency range of 1.0–5.0 MHz, ultrasound attenuation in the skin increases with frequency, averaging from several to over ten dB/cm. Excessive attenuation within the scanning device's applicator could weaken the ultrasonic wave entering the liver tissue, leading to measurement errors or making measurements impossible. The analysis employed durable gel-like or rubber-like materials with attenuation in the range of several to over ten dB/cm, which enabled accurate results.

The results of the conducted studies indicate that the shear wave velocity increases with increasing tissue stiffness, which is confirmed in the literature [6]. However, it should be noted that higher stiffness does not necessarily mean higher wave frequency, which may be a limitation due to the characteristics of the device and its configuration according to the manufacturer's recommendations. This limitation may affect the interpretation of results under other test conditions. Future studies should consider the possibility of using other device configurations or alternative measurement techniques to compare results.

All elastography studies conducted on experimental animals using the percutaneous technique yielded valid results. In experiments performed on livers collected immediately post-euthanasia, measurements were successfully obtained using all applicator types on four livers placed in a specially prepared container that simulated the shape of a human liver. In the first four cases, where the livers were placed in a standard organ retrieval dish, measurements could not be obtained. Additionally, the first batch of agar-based applicators was prone to damage, preventing measurements, but this issue did not occur with applicators made of Ecoflex 00-20.

Using the Johnson–Cook rheological model resulted in an excellent fit for both the compact and spongy bone structures, such as the ribs. Moreover, applying the hybrid FEM/SPH method in this case yielded very satisfactory results. The spongy bone structure proved to be an excellent model for SPH applications.

The presented numerical analysis results for the preliminary assessment of the effectiveness of mechanical wave propagation, following the application of the scanning device to the examined organ, confirm the correctness of the adopted methodology. The wave velocity result (1420 m/s) correlates well with the healthy liver value (1480 m/s), indicating a very good match.

A comparative analysis between Tables 10 and 11 highlights the differences in attenuation results for various numerical models using two types of Ecoflex 00-20 applicators. For the Yeoh model, in the case of the cylindrical applicator, the attenuation values (CAP) for the side are 240 and 242 dB/m, while for the conical applicator, they are 245 and 256 dB/m. It is noted that the attenuation values are similar for both applicators, but slightly higher for the conical one. For the Johnson–Cook model in different configurations (bridge, back) for cylindrical and conical applicators, the attenuation differences are more varied. Generally, the attenuation results for the cylindrical and conical applicators in this model do not show a consistent pattern—some cases yield similar values, while others differ more. For the Ogden model, side attenuation results for the cylindrical applicator are 241 and 264 dB/m, and for the conical applicator, the values are 236 and 281 dB/m. Attenuation values for this model show some differences between applicators, with the conical applicator sometimes reaching higher values. In summary, the attenuation analysis results for the different numerical models using cylindrical and conical Ecoflex 00-20 applicators show no clear rule for which applicator yields better attenuation results across all models. Attenuation values differ between applicators for different models, indicating the complexity of the applicator geometry's impact on attenuation properties in numerical studies.

Chapter 5 validates the numerical simulation results by comparing them with data from report number N0CBR000.7117.SS.30/Wet/2022 [27]. Liver elasticity measurements with the E15 applicator hover around similar values, regardless of the measurement method (porcine liver measurements or numerical simulations). The average liver elasticity with the E15 applicator (numerical simulations) was 11.6 kPa. Conversely, liver elasticity measurements with the D0 applicator showed variability, both in porcine liver measurements and numerical simulations. The average liver elasticity with the D0 applicator (numerical simulations) was 15.2 kPa. It is noted that the applicator shape significantly affects liver elasticity measurement results. The conical applicator (D0) tends to yield higher liver elasticity values compared to the cylindrical applicator (E15), both for direct organ measurements and numerical simulations. These differences may be due to varying mechanical properties and the interaction of the applicator shapes with liver tissue, as well as their influence on sound wave transmission during measurements.

This study verified applicator geometries using numerical models on animals within the measurement frequency range of 1.0–5.0 MHz, covering the following parameters: liver fibrosis between 1.5 and 12.5 kPa and steatosis < 5%, 5–33%, 33–66%, and above 66%. The numerical simulation results were referenced against a healthy liver baseline value, with liver stiffness at 4.5 kPa and steatosis below 300 dB/m. Experimental and simulation results correlate, confirming the validity of the study.

7. Patents

Elastograph head cap insert, elastography measurement kit, and kit application. PCT application number: PCT/PL2023/050100 from 30 November 2023. Tiba Sp. z o.o., Wroclaw, Poland.

Author Contributions: Conceptualization, D.P. and K.J.O.; Data curation, K.K. and T.Ś.; Formal analysis, D.P. and K.K.; Investigation, A.N.-N. and K.J.O.; Methodology, K.K. and T.Ś.; Project administration, K.J.O.; Resources, D.P.; Supervision, D.P.; Validation, D.P. and A.N.-N.; Writing—original draft, K.K.; Writing—review and editing D.P. and K.J.O. All authors have read and agreed to the published version of the manuscript.

Funding: The work was carried out as part of the project POIR.01.01. 01-00-0462/21 and was co-financed by the European Regional Development Fund under the Smart Growth Operational Program 2014-2020.

Institutional Review Board Statement: The animal study protocol was approved by the Local Ethics Committee for animal experiments in Wroclaw (Resolution No. 046/2022/P1 dated 16 November 2022).

Informed Consent Statement: Not applicable.

Data Availability Statement: Data are contained within the article.

Acknowledgments: Calculations were carried out in Wroclaw Centre for Networking and Supercomputing (http://www.wcss.pl (accessed on 1 April 2023)), grant No. 452.

Conflicts of Interest: There is no conflict of interest declared by the authors.

References

1. De Lédinghen, V.; Wong, V.W.S.; Vergniol, J.; Wong, G.L.H.; Foucher, J.; Chu, S.H.T.; Le Bail, B.; Choi, P.C.L.; Chermak, F.; Yiu, K.K.L.; et al. Diagnosis of Liver Fibrosis and Cirrhosis Using Liver Stiffness Measurement: Comparison between M and XL Probe of FibroScan®. *J. Hepatol.* **2012**, *56*, 833–839. [CrossRef] [PubMed]
2. Barsamian, C.; Carette, C.; Sasso, M.; Poghosyan, T.; Bedossa, P.; Emile, J.F.; Parlier, D.; Miette, V.; Bouillot, J.L.; Czernichow, S.; et al. Diagnostic of Hepatic Fibrosis with the XL Probe of the Fibroscan versus Biopsies in Patients Candidates to Bariatric Surgery. *Clin. Nutr. ESPEN* **2020**, *37*, 226–232. [CrossRef]
3. Romanowska, K.; Pyka, D.; Opieliński, K.; Krawiec, K.; Śliwiński, R.; Jamroziak, K. Preliminary Numerical Analysis of Mechanical Wave Propagation Due to Elastograph Measuring Head Application in Non-Invasive Liver Condition Assessment. *Appl. Sci.* **2023**, *13*, 11843. [CrossRef]
4. Wang, T.; Jirapinyo, P.; Shah, R.; Schuster, K.; Thompson, C.; Lautz, D.; Doyon, L.; Ryou, M. Endoscopic ultrasound shear wave elastography is superior to fibroscan and non-invasive scores for fibrosis staging in patients with obesity and non-alcoholic fatty liver disease: A true virtual biopsy. *Gastrointest. Endosc.* **2023**, *97*, AB872–AB873. [CrossRef]
5. Li, X.; Wu, J.; Zhuang, Z.; Ye, Y.; Zhou, S.; Qiu, Y.; Ruan, D.; Wang, S.; Yang, J.; Wu, Z.; et al. Integrated Single-Trait and Multi-Trait GWASs Reveal the Genetic Architecture of Internal Organ Weight in Pigs. *Animals* **2023**, *13*, 808. [CrossRef]
6. Laurent, S.; Jennifer, O.; Cecile, B.; Celine, F.; Veronique, M.; Sebasti, M. Non-Invasive Assessment of Liver Fibrosis by Vibration-Controlled Transient Elastography (Fibroscan®) . In *Liver Biopsy*; Books on Demand: Norderstedt, Germany, 2011. [CrossRef]
7. Millonig, G.; Friedrich, S.; Adolf, S.; Fonouni, H.; Golriz, M.; Mehrabi, A.; Stiefel, P.; Pöschl, G.; Büchler, M.W.; Seitz, H.K.; et al. Liver Stiffness Is Directly Influenced by Central Venous Pressure. *J. Hepatol.* **2010**, *52*, 206–210. [CrossRef] [PubMed]
8. Junatas, K.L.; Tonar, Z.; Kubíková, T.; Liška, V.; Pálek, R.; Mik, P.; Králíčková, M.; Witter, K. Stereological Analysis of Size and Density of Hepatocytes in the Porcine Liver. *J. Anat.* **2017**, *230*, 575–588. [CrossRef] [PubMed]
9. Lada, E.; Anna, M.; Patrik, M.; Zbynek, T.; Miroslav, J.; Hynek, M.; Richard, P.; Sarah, L.; Vaclav, L. Porcine Liver Anatomy Applied to Biomedicine. *J. Surg. Res.* **2020**, *250*, 70–79. [CrossRef] [PubMed]
10. Skjennald, A. Anatomy of the Liver and Pancreas in the Domestic Swine, with Special Reference to Vascular Structures. *Scand. J. Gastroenterol.* **1982**, *17*, 16–313.
11. Zanchet, D.J.; De Montero, E.F.S. Pig Liver Sectorization and Segmentation and Virtual Reality Depiction. *Acta Cir. Bras.* **2002**, *17*, 381–387. [CrossRef]
12. Swindle, M.M. Comparative Anatomy and Physiology of the Pig. *Scand. J. Lab. Anim. Sci.* **1998**, *25*, 11–21.
13. Nickel, R.; Schummer, A.; Seijerle, E. *Lehrbuch der Anatomie der Haus-Tiere*; Paul Parey: Berlin & Hamburg, Germany, 1968.
14. Ayagara, A.R.; Langlet, A.; Hambli, R. On Dynamic Behavior of Bone: Experimental and Numerical Study of Porcine Ribs Subjected to Impact Loads in Dynamic Three-Point Bending Tests. *J. Mech. Behav. Biomed. Mater.* **2019**, *98*, 336–347. [CrossRef] [PubMed]
15. Mini Pig Health: The Basics—Mini Pig Info. Available online: https://www.minipiginfo.com/mini-pig-health.html (accessed on 13 July 2023).
16. Hamilton, D.W.; Walker, J.T.; Tinney, D.; Grynyshyn, M.; El-Warrak, A.; Truscott, E.; Flynn, L.E. The Pig as a Model System for Investigating the Recruitment and Contribution of Myofibroblasts in Skin Healing. *Wound Repair. Regen.* **2022**, *30*, 45–63. [CrossRef] [PubMed]
17. Wiśniewska, A.; Liber-Kneć, A. Influence of a Skin Tissue Anisotropy on Mechanical Hysteresis/Wpływ Anizotropii Tkanki Skórnej Na Histerezę Mechaniczną. *Czas. Tech. Mech.* **2016**, 125–136. [CrossRef]
18. Rodriguez, N.; Mangiagalli, P.; Persson, B.N.J. Viscoelastic Crack Propagation: Review of Theories and Applications. *Adv. Polym. Sci.* **2021**, *286*, 377–420. [CrossRef]
19. Shergold, O.A.; Fleck, N.A.; Radford, D. The Uniaxial Stress versus Strain Response of Pig Skin and Silicone Rubber at Low and High Strain Rates. *Int. J. Impact Eng.* **2006**, *32*, 1384–1402. [CrossRef]
20. Annaidh, A.N.; Bruyère, K.; Destrade, M.; Gilchrist, M.D.; Maurini, C.; Otténio, M.; Saccomandi, G. Automated Estimation of Collagen Fibre Dispersion in the Dermis and Its Contribution to the Anisotropic Behaviour of Skin. *Ann. Biomed. Eng.* **2012**, *40*, 1666–1678. [CrossRef]
21. Ankersen, J.; Birkbeck, A.E.; Thomson, R.D.; Vanezis, P. Puncture resistance and tensile strength of skin simulants. Proceedings of the Institution of Mechanical Engineers, Part H: Journal of Engineering in Medicine. *Proc. Inst. Mech. Eng. Part H J. Eng. Med.* **1999**, *213*, 493–501. [CrossRef]
22. Dombi, G.W.; Haut, R.C.; Sullivan, W.G. Correlation of high-speed tensile strength with collagen content in control and lathyritic rat skin. *J. Surg. Res.* **1993**, *54*, 21–28. [CrossRef]
23. Jansen, L.H.; Rottier, P.B. Some mechanical properties of human abdominal skin measured on excised strips: A study of their dependence on age and how they are influenced by the presence of striae. *Dermatologica.* **1958**, *117*, 65–83. [CrossRef] [PubMed]

24. Holzapfel, G. Biomechanics of Soft Tissue. In *Handbook of Material Behavior Nonlinear Models and Properties*; LMT-Cachan, Ed.; Academic Press: Paris, France, 2000.
25. Lim, J.; Hong, J.; Chen, W.W.; Weerasooriya, T. Mechanical Response of Pig Skin under Dynamic Tensile Loading. *Int. J. Impact Eng.* **2011**, *38*, 130–135. [CrossRef]
26. Tiba Sp. z o.o. Elastograph Head Cap Insert, Elastography Measurement Kit and Kit Application. PCT/PL2023/050100, 30 November 2023.
27. Tiba Sp. z o.o. Pomiary Realizowane z Zastosowaniem Nasadek Na Głowicę Aparatu FibroScan Na Zwierzętach Doświadczalnych Oraz Pobranych Pośmiertnie Narządach. N0CBR000.7117.SS.30/Wet/2022, 15 May 2023.

livers

MDPI

Article

Comparative Analysis of the Human Proteome Profile in Visceral Adipose and Liver Tissue in Individuals with Obesity with and Without MASLD and MASH

Julie S. Pedersen [1,*], Lili Niu [2], Nicolai J. Wewer Albrechtsen [2,3,4], Viggo B. Kristiansen [5], Inge Marie Poulsen [5], Reza R. Serizawa [6], Torben Hansen [7], Lise Lotte Gluud [1], Sten Madsbad [3,8] and Flemming Bendtsen [1,3]

1 Gastrounit, Medical Division, Copenhagen University Hospital Hvidovre, Kettegaard Allé 30, 2650 Hvidovre, Denmark; lise.lotte.gluud.01@regionh.dk (L.L.G.); flemming.bendtsen@regionh.dk (F.B.)
2 NNF Center for Protein Research, Faculty of Health and Medical Sciences, University of Copenhagen, Blegdamsvej 3B, 2200 Copenhagen, Denmark; lloi@novonordisk.com (L.N.); nicolai.albrechtsen@regionh.dk (N.J.W.A.)
3 Department of Clinical Medicine, Faculty of Health and Medical Sciences, University of Copenhagen, Blegdamsvej 3B, 2200 Copenhagen, Denmark
4 Department of Clinical Biochemistry, Copenhagen University Hospital–Bispebjerg and Frederiksberg, Blegdamsvej 9, 2200 Copenhagen, Denmark
5 Gastrounit, Surgical Division, Copenhagen University Hospital Hvidovre, Kettegaard Allé 30, 2650 Hvidovre, Denmark; viggo.bjerregaard.kristiansen@regionh.dk (V.B.K.); inge.marie.poulsen@regionh.dk (I.M.P.)
6 Department of Pathology, Copenhagen University Hospital Hvidovre, Kettegaard Allé 30, 2650 Hvidovre, Denmark; reza.serizawa@regionh.dk
7 NNF Center for Basic Metabolic Research, Faculty of Health and Medical Sciences, University of Copenhagen, Blegdamsvej 3B, 2200 Copenhagen, Denmark; torben.hansen@sund.ku.dk
8 Department of Endocrinology, Copenhagen University Hospital Hvidovre, Kettegaard Allé 30, 2650 Hvidovre, Denmark; sten.madsbad@regionh.dk
* Correspondence: julie.steen.pedersen@regionh.dk

Abstract: Background/Objectives: Visceral adipose tissue (VAT) may play a direct role in the development of metabolic dysfunction-associated steatotic liver disease (MASLD) and its progression to metabolic dysfunction-associated steatohepatitis (MASH). In this study, we employed untargeted proteomics analyses on paired biopsies from VAT and liver tissues of patients with obesity, MASLD, and MASH. Our objective was to investigate tissue-specific protein expression patterns in search of a potential proteomic signature associated with MASH in both VAT and liver tissue. Methods: VAT and liver tissue were collected from 70 subjects with severe obesity (SWOs) and nine control study subjects without obesity (CON). SWOs were stratified on the basis of liver histology into LS− (no liver steatosis), LS+ (liver steatosis), and MASH. Peptides were extracted from frozen tissue and were analyzed by liquid chromatography coupled to tandem mass spectrometry (LC-MS/MS). Raw files were analyzed with Spectronaut, proteins were searched against the human FASTA Uniprot database, and the significantly expressed proteins in the two tissues were analyzed. The *p*-values were false discovery rate (FDR) corrected. Results: A total of 59 VAT and 42 liver proteins were significantly differentially expressed between the four groups: LS−, LS+, MASH, and CON. The majority were upregulated, and many were related to lipid metabolism. In VAT, only one protein, the mitochondrial sulfide:quinone oxidoreductase (SQOR), was significantly downregulated in the MASH group only. In liver tissue from patients with MASH, six proteins were significantly altered compared with the three other groups. Correlation analyses between the top 10 positive VAT and liver proteins were dominated by inflammatory and detoxification proteins. Conclusions: The presence of MASH was not reflected in the VAT proteome, and both the VAT and the liver proteome were generally affected more by the presence of obesity than by MASLD severity. Several immunomodulating proteins correlated significantly between VAT and liver tissue and could reflect common pathophysiological characteristics.

Keywords: MASLD; MASH; untargeted proteomics; liver tissue; visceral adipose tissue; obesity

1. Introduction

The harmful impact of the excessive deposition of visceral adipose tissue (VAT) on the risk of metabolic disease, type 2 diabetes (T2DM), and cardiovascular disease has been recognized for decades [1,2]. Adipose tissue has major metabolic as well as endocrine functions. Adipose tissue-derived adipocytokines and fat-derived metabolites such as free fatty acids affect the physiology of other organs [3–5], but VAT in particular is associated with metabolic disease risk. In clinical practice, waist circumference, which correlates with truncal VAT mass, is central to identifying patients at increased risk of metabolic comorbidities including metabolic dysfunction-associated steatotic liver disease (MASLD) and metabolic dysfunction-associated steatohepatitis (MASH) [6–8]. An expansion of visceral fat mass negatively impacts adipose tissue physiology and function as the resulting rise in metabolic and oxidative stress contributes to peripheral insulin resistance and disrupts the overall homeostasis of VAT [1]. These alterations are exerted, in part, through changes in the secretion of adipokines and proinflammatory cytokines with the subsequent creation of an inflammatory and metabolic dysfunctional milieu with resultant adipocyte death and fibrosis deposition within the adipose tissue with infiltration and proliferation of macrophages contributing to obesity-associated adipose tissue inflammation [9–13].

In MASLD, triglycerides accumulate within the hepatocytes and cause liver steatosis; the condition may progress to MASH, which is characterized by necroinflammation of the liver tissue and formation of liver fibrosis [14]. In MASLD, the changes that occur in VAT and liver tissue seem to share some pathophysiological characteristics. In addition, mesenteric and omental VAT are venously drained to the liver via the portal vein. According to the portal vein theory, free fatty acid adipocytokines and inflammatory cytokines derived from the VAT access the liver and could contribute to the development of liver steatosis and perhaps impact the progression of MASLD to MASH and liver fibrosis [15].

Mass spectrometry (MS)-based proteomic analyses offer fast and large-scale analyses of the proteomes and can identify alterations in protein abundance in relation to disease. MS-based proteomics could serve as a tool for the identification of proteins that are upregulated or downregulated in patients with MASLD and MASH. However, untargeted proteomics has been applied to adipose tissue in other metabolic diseases, particularly T2DM [16,17].

MASLD remains more unexplored in this context, and most studies have focused on the plasma proteome in relation to MASLD and MASH [18–22], in search of diagnostic markers of MASLD severity. Liver tissue proteomics has previously been applied in human MASLD [23,24], but to a much lesser extent, some studies with focus on MASH associated hepatocarcinogenesis [25,26] and MASH fibrosis [27]. Very limited data exist on the proteomic pattern in adipose tissue in the context of MASLD.

Consequently, the concomitant assessment of VAT and liver tissue allows for a detailed evaluation of the changes that occur in patients with obesity, MASLD, and MASH, and tissue proteomics analyses could provide important information about the underlying pathophysiology of MASLD.

In this cross-sectional study, we conducted tissue proteomics analysis on paired biopsies from omental visceral adipose tissue (VAT) and liver tissues in 70 patients with severe obesity. These patients were categorized based on the presence or absence of varying stages of MASLD and MASH. Additionally, we included nine control subjects without obesity.

Our primary aims were to describe the protein patterns in liver and visceral adipose tissue with increasing severity of MASLD and to explore the potential overlap of proteins that are significantly upregulated or downregulated in both liver tissue and VAT. By identifying potential shared protein changes, we sought to uncover a distinct proteome signature specific to MASH in both tissue types.

2. Materials and Methods

2.1. Cohort and Study Investigations

We collected omental VAT and liver tissue from 70 SWOs undergoing laparoscopic bariatric surgery and control study subjects without obesity (CON) undergoing planned laparoscopic cholecystectomy at Copenhagen University Hospital Hvidovre between December 2016 and October 2019. Tissue samples were collected immediately after induction of anesthesia and trocar placement, before the actual surgical procedure.

After sampling, the VAT was trimmed and cut into smaller pieces of 50–100 mg and immediately snap frozen in liquid nitrogen before storage in a −80-degree freezer until analysis. The liver tissue was similarly trimmed; the capsule was removed; and it was cut into pieces of 50 mg, snap frozen, and stored as described above. In addition, part of the liver biopsy underwent fixation in paraformaldehyde for later paraffin embedment and histological analysis.

The study was conducted according to the Declaration of Helsinki and was approved by the Regional Ethics Committee of Capital Region, Denmark (H-16030784 and H-16020782). All study subjects gave oral and written consent.

2.2. Liver Histology and Grouping of Study Subjects

Liver histology was assessed by three pathologists. The MASLD activity score the (referred to as the NAFLD activity score, NAS) was used to group patients with obesity as follows:

(1) No liver steatosis (LS−): no liver steatosis present in liver biopsies;
(2) Liver steatosis present (LS+): liver steatosis present but without MASH (NAS score < 5);
(3) MASH: NAS $\geq$ 5 with points from all subcategories (steatosis, inflammation, and ballooning).

2.3. Sample Preparation for MS Analysis

Frozen liver and VAT biopsies were homogenized on a Precellys24 homogenizer (Bertin Technologies, Montigny-le-Bretonneux, France) in 300 µL SDC reduction and alkylation buffer (PreOmics GmbH, Martinsried, Germany) containing 1× Roche phosphatase inhibitor with ceramic beads (2.8 and 1.4 mm zirconium oxide beads, Precellys). Approximately 15 mg of liver and 50 mg of VAT were processed as the starting material. The homogenates were incubated at 95 °C for 10 min (1200 rpm) and subsequently transferred to a new 1.5 mL Eppendorf tube, from which 45 µL of homogenate was further transferred to a 96-well plate and sonicated for 5 min using the Covaris Adaptive Focused Acoustics (AFA) sonication system (Covaris, Woburn, MA, USA). The protein content was determined by Tryptophan assay, and an aliquot of 50 µg was digested overnight with LysC and trypsin at a 1:50 ratio (µg of enzyme to µg of protein) at 37 °C (1700 rpm). Peptides were acidified to a final concentration of 0.1% trifluoroacetic acid (TFA). Approximately 20 µg of peptides were loaded on Stage-Tips and washed with isopropanol/1% TFA (200 µL) and then 0.2% TFA (200 µL). Peptides were eluted with 60 µL of elution buffer (80% acetonitrile/1% ammonia) and dried at 60 °C using a SpeedVac centrifuge Concentrator plus) (Eppendorf, Hamborg, Germany) Dried peptides were dissolved and sonicated in 5% acetonitrile/0.1%

TFA, and the concentration was measured using Nanodrop. Peptide mixtures were stored at −80 °C until further analysis. Quality control samples of pooled tissue homogenate were included for measuring the workflow variation.

2.4. LC-MS/MS Analysis (Liquid Chromatography-Mass Spectroscopy/Mass Spectrometry Analysis)

Samples were measured using LC-MS instrumentation consisting of an EASY-nLC 1200 system (Thermo Fisher Scientific, San Jose, CA, USA) interfaced online with a Q Exactive HF-X Orbitrap (Thermo Fisher Scientific, Bremen, Germany). Purified peptides were separated on 42.5 cm HPLC columns (ID: 75 μm; in-house packed into the tip with ReproSil-Pur C18-AQ 1.9 μm resin (Dr. Maisch GmbH)). Approximately 500 ng of peptides were injected for each LC-MS/MS analysis. Peptides were loaded in buffer A (0.1% formic acid) and eluted with a linear 82 min gradient of 3–23% of buffer B (0.1% formic acid, 80% (v/v) acetonitrile), followed by an 8 min increase to 40% of buffer B. The gradients then increased to 98% of buffer B within 6 min, which was maintained for 4 min. Flow rates were maintained at 350 nL/min. Re-equilibration was performed for 4 μL of 0.1% buffer A at a pressure of 700 bar. The column temperature was kept at 60 °C.

For liver tissue samples, MS spectra were acquired using the data-independent acquisition (DIA) mode, enabled by MaxQuant. Live [28], in which the scan protocol was defined. Each acquisition cycle consisted of a survey scan at resolution of 60,000 with an automatic gain control target (AGC) of 3×10^6 and a maximum injection time of 100 ms, followed by 66 DIA cycles at a resolution of 15,000 with an AGC of 3×10^6/22 ms IT at a range of 300–1650 m/z. Higher-energy collisional dissociation (HCD) fragmentation was set to a normalized collision energy of 27%. In all scans, PhiSDM [29] was enabled with 100 iterations, and the spectra type was set to centroid. For adipose tissue samples, the DIA-MS method consisted of an MS1 scan from the 350–1650 m/z range (AGC target of 3×10^6, maximum injection time of 60 ms) at a resolution of 60,000 and 32 DIA segments (Dataset EV1, AGC target of 3×10^6, maximum injection time of 45 ms). The acquisition of samples was randomized to avoid bias.

2.5. Quantification and Statistical Analysis: Raw Data Processing and Analysis

All raw files were analyzed with Spectronaut Pulsar X (version 13.10) with default settings except that the "quantification" data filtering parameter "Q-value" was set to "complete". The DIA hybrid spectra were searched against in-house generated libraries for human liver and adipose tissue using the same LC setup searching against the human FASTA Uniprot database (version 201801, containing 93k entries). Proteins with more than 30% of missing values were discarded. Samples with fewer than 2500 quantified proteins were also discarded. Normalization based on the median protein intensity of each sample was performed. The remaining missing values of the dataset were imputed by drawing random samples from a normal distribution (down-shifted mean by 1.8 standard deviation (SD)) and scaled SD (0.3) relative to that of the proteome abundance distribution, with which we performed the statistical analysis. Statistical and bioinformatics analyses were performed with the Perseus software (version 1.6.5.0) and Python software (version 3.8.2). Specifically, one-way ANOVA was performed using the Python open-source statistical package "pingouin" (https://pingouin-stats.org/) corrected for multiple hypothesis testing by Benjamini-Hochberg at 5% FDR (false discovery rate), followed by Tukey's HSD (honestly significant difference) test. Pair-wise correlation between VAT and liver tissue protein levels was performed with the pingouin. pairwise_correlation module with a significance level of Benjamini-Hochberg-corrected FDR at 5b% (q-value). For the proteomics analyses, a q-value < 0.05 was considered statistically significant.

Before filtering for 70% (meaning that a given protein must be expressed/detectable in 70% of the samples within the specific tissue type), we detected 3200 protein groups (17,570 peptides) in VAT and 5151 protein groups in liver tissue (35,965 peptides).

The following databases were used to characterize the function, cellular compartment, and tissue distribution/expression of the significant proteins: uniprot.org, proteinatlas.org, metabolicatlas.org, genecards.org, and omim.org.

Clinical and anthropometrical data were presented as the mean (SD). p-values were one-way ANOVA with Bonferroni correction or Chi square/Fischer's exact test. $p < 0.05$ was considered statistically significant.

Illustrations were made in Perseus software (version 1.6.5.0) and with the use of biorender.com (accessed on 15 December 2024).

See Figure 1 for a schematic overview of the study workflow.

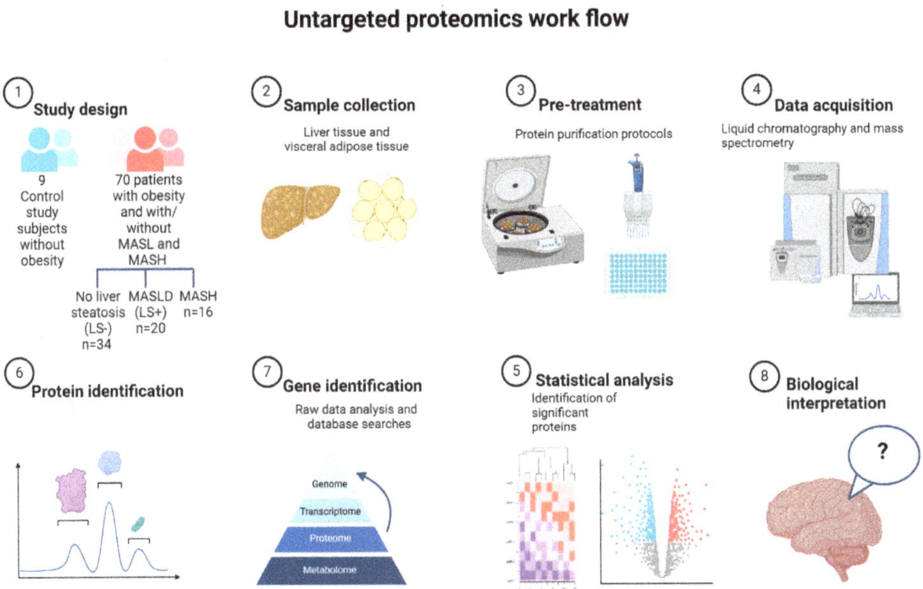

Figure 1. Study workflow. Schematic illustration of the proteomics workflow in liver and visceral adipose tissue sampled from control study subjects and from patients with obesity and increasing severity of MASLD. Created in BioRender. Pedersen, J. (2025) https://www.biorender.com/, accessed on 15 December 2024.

3. Results

Table 1 depicts the clinical characteristics of the three MASLD groups (LS−, $n = 34$; LS+, $n = 20$; and MASH, $n = 16$) and controls (CON, $n = 9$). The number of patients with T2DM in each group was three (LS−), seven (LS+), and nine (MASH). Insulin resistance evaluated by HOMA-IR was progressively worsened from CON to MASH of about four-fold. In the MASLD groups the BMI ranged from 41.8 to 44.6 kg/m^2 compared with 24.4 kg/m^2 in the CON group.

Table 1. Clinical, anthropometrical, and biochemical data at baseline in study subjects with obesity undergoing bariatric surgery and stratified by histological MASLD severity (LS−, LS+, and MASH) and control study subjects without obesity (CON).

Study Subjects with Obesity According to Histology				Subjects Without Obesity
	LS− (n = 34)	LS+ (n = 20)	MASH (n = 16)	CON (n = 9)
Liver histology				
MASLD activity score (NAS)	2.3 (0.9)	3.2 (0.7)	5.1 (0.3)	1.1 (0.9)
Steatosis	0.0 (0.0)	1.1 (0.3)	1.7 (0.6)	0.0 (0.0)
Inflammation	1.1 (0.6)	0.9 (0.3)	1.6 (0.5)	0.9 (0.6)
Ballooning	1.2 (0.5)	1.2 (0.5)	1.9 (0.3)	0.2 (0.4)
Fibrosis	1.0 (0.3)	1.2 (0.4)	1.1 (0.5)	0.9 (0.3)
Age, years	45 (11)	45 (8)	45 (9)	39 (8)
Female (%)	25 (58)	9 (21)	9 (21)	7 (78)
Diabetes, n (%)	3 (16)	7 (37)	9 (47)	NA
Weight, kg	124 (20) *	138 (29) *	125 (17) *	71 (10)
BMI, kg/m^2	41.8 (5.1) *	44.6 (8.4) *	42.4 (5.4) *	24.4 (2.2)
Waist-hip ratio	0.88 (0.11)	0.95 (0.13)	0.98 (0.08) *,†	0.83 (0.10)
Systolic blood pressure, mmHg	126 (12)	130 (14)	131 (16)	117 (11)
Diastolic blood pressure, mmHg	81 (8)	82 (9)	82 (11)	77 (9)
Heart rate (BPM)	72 (12)	76 (13)	76 (14)	69 (7)
ALT, U/L	28 (10)	34 (15)	39 (15) *,†	21 (9)
AST, U/L	24 (6)	25 (9)	27 (7)	21 (4)
Fasting plasma glucose, mmol/L	5.9 (0.7)	6.8 (1.5)	7.0 (2.2)	5.5 (0.4)
C-peptide pmol/L	1162 (343) *	1217 (257) *	1649 (523) *,†,§	791 (204)
Fasting insulin pmol/L	118.8 (47.3)	122.78 (44.6)	208.6 (88.9) *,†,§	63.3 (30.4)
HbA1c	35 (3)	41 (8) *,†	37 (4) *	32 (3)
HOMA-IR	4.4 (1.8)	5.2 (1.7)	9.1 (4.2) *,†,§	2.2 (1.1)
LDL cholesterol, mmol/L	2.79 (0.98)	2.25 (0.56)	2.02 (0.61)	2.59 (0.53)
HDL cholesterol, mmol/L	1.22 (0.27)	1.20 (0.41)	1.09 (0.15)	1.39 (0.23)
VLDL cholesterol, mmol/L	0.58 (0.24)	0.69 (0.43)	0.75 (0.33)	0.50 (0.21)
Triglycerides, mmol/L	1.29 (0.52)	1.53 (0.95)	1.66 (0.74)	1.13 (0.50)
HsCRP (mg/L)	5.2 (4.1)	9.2 (10.7) *	5.1 (3.7)	1.5 (1.3)

Data are presented as mean (SD). p-values are one-way ANOVA with Bonferroni correction or Chi square/Fischer's exact test. LS, liver steatosis; MASH, metabolic dysfunction-associated steatohepatitis; CON, control study subjects; MASLD, metabolic dysfunction-associated steatotic liver disease; BMI, body mass index; mmHg, millimeter mercury; BPM, beats per minute; ALT, alanine aminotransferase; AST, aspartate aminotransferase; HbA1c, glycated hemoglobin; HOMA-IR, homeostatic model assessment for insulin resistance; LDL, low-density lipoprotein; HDL, high-density lipoprotein; VLDL, very-low-density lipoprotein; HsCRP, highly sensitive C-reactive protein; mm, millimeters. * $p < 0.05$ compared with CON. † $p < 0.05$ compared with LS−. § $p < 0.05$ compared with LS+.

3.1. Liver Tissue

In liver tissue we detected 32 differentially expressed proteins (DEPs) with significant upregulation or downregulation between the four groups (Table 2 and Figure 2). Of these, 18 were upregulated, and 14 were downregulated in the MASLD groups when compared with CON.

Table 2. Differentially expressed proteins in liver tissue in CON, LS−, LS+, and MASH identified by untargeted proteomics analyses.

Protein Name	Gene Name	CON Log2 Intensity	LS− Log2 Intensity	LS+ Log2 Intensity	MASH Log2 Intensity	Location in Cell	Tissue Specificity	Main Function(s)
				Upregulated liver proteins in SWO/MASLD groups				
Metabolism								
Isocitrate dehydrogenase 2	**IDH2**	22.57	22.81	22.97 *	23.03 *	M, C, PX	Low	TCA
Glycerol-3-phosphate dehydrogenase 1	**GPD1**	22.12	22.71 *	22.86 *	22.84 *	C	Low	CaM, LiM, LiB
OBG like ATPase 1	**OLA1**	18.86	19.20 *	19.33 *	19.35 *	C	Low	CP, ATPH, GTPH
ATP citrate lyase	**ACLY**	18.40	18.06	18.76 †	18.72 †	C	Low	ACoA, LiM, LiB
Mevalonate kinase	**MVK**	17.99	18.11	18.79	18.92 *,†	C, PX	Low	ChoB, ChoM, LiM, LiB, SterB, SterM
15-hydroxyprostaglandin dehydrogenase	**HPGD**	18.07	18.77	19.37 *,†	19.32 *	C, N	Placenta, liver, GI tract	FAM, LiM, PGM
Perilipin 1	**PLIN1**	14.24	14.99	16.09 *,†	16.25 *,†		Adipose tissue	LiMM, LiBi
Perilipin 2	**PLIN2**	15.09	15.08	16.87 †	17.09 †		Adipose tissue	LiMM, LiBi
Transport and carriers								
Apolipoprotein 3	**APOL3**	15.03	16.21 *	16.51 *	16.64 *	C	Low	LiT
Solute carrier family 25 member 42	**SLC25A42**	15.03	16.31 *	16.51 *	16.57 *	M	Liver	MTC, MTT, ADPT, ATPT, AMPT, ACoAT
Archain 1	**ARCN1**	18.23	18.26	18.38 *,†	18.31	V, ER	Low	ERGT, PT
Protein transport protein Sec24A	**SEC24A**	16.65	16.81	17.00 *,†	17.01 *,†	V	Low	ERGT, PT
Cytoskeleton, ECM and signal transduction								
Collagen type XVIII alpha 1 chain	**COL18A1**	18.62	19.11 *	19.23 *	19.40 *	ECM	Liver	EMO
Radixin	**RDX**	20.70	20.93 *	20.98 *	21.04 *	PM	Adrenal gland	CO, CA, ST
Moesin	**MSN**	20.38	20.96 *	20.93 *	20.76 *	PM	Low	CO, CA, ST
Protein kinase cAMP-dependent type I regulatory subunit alpha	**PRKAR1A**	18.37	18.61 *	18.64 *	18.67 *	C	Low	cAMP, ST
Cell, quality, cell cycle, and apoptosis								
Tumor protein p53 inducible protein 3	**TP53I3**	13.96	15.13 *	15.84 *	16.03 *,†	C	Intestine	Apop(+), SR
Retinoblastoma binding protein 9	**RBBP9**	18.01	18.17	18.31 *	18.28 *	N	Low	SH, TS, CCR

Table 2. *Cont.*

Protein Name	Gene Name	CON Log2 Intensity	LS− Log2 Intensity	LS+ Log2 Intensity	MASH Log2 Intensity	Location in Cell	Tissue Specificity	Main Function(s)
				Downregulated liver proteins in SWO/MASLD groups				
Metabolism								
Glycerate kinase	**GLYCKTK**	19.80	19.36 *	19.09 *	19.15 *	C, G	Liver	FC, SD
Glyoxylate hydroxypyrovate dehydrogenase	**GRHPR**	24.04	23.82	23.59 *,†	23.69 *	C, N	Liver	GlyoxM, PyroM
GTP cyclohydrolase I feedback regulator	**GCHFR**	20.09	19.70 *	19.51 *	19.55 *	C, N	Liver	RP
Methionine adenosyltransferase 1A	**MAT1A**	21.67	21.57	21.38	21.34 *,†	C	Liver	1CM, MT, MetC
Adenosylhomocysteinase	**ACHY**	22.53	22.22 *	22.08 *	22.13 *	C	Low	1CM, MT
Hydroxysteroid 17-beta dehydrogenase 2	**HSD17B2**	19.79	19.32	19.00 *	18.94 *	ER	Liver, intestine, placenta	LiB, LiM, SteB
Hydroxysteroid 17-beta dehydrogenase 11	**HSD17B11**	19.51	19.33	19.98	18.82 *	ER, LD	Immune cells, intestine	LiB, LiM, SterB, AndC, EstB
Cytochrome P450 family 3 subfamily A member 4	**CYP3A4**	21.85	21.71	21.01 *,†	21.19	C, ER	Liver	FAM, CholM, LiM, LiB, SterB, SterM, DrugM
Mitochondrial								
Sideroflexin 2	**SFXN2**	17.88	17.36	17.14 *,†	17.65	M	low	MTTT, AAT
Cytochrome b-c1 complex (CIII)	**CYC1**	19.74	19.35 *	19.35 *	19.23 *	M	low	ET, ATPS, RCP
Intracellular transport and carriers								
VAMP associated protein A	**VAPA**	19.30	19.25	19.14	19.06 *,†	ER, N, PM	Low	ERGT, PT, MF
Cell quality, cell cycle, apoptosis								
Death associated protein	**DAP**	17.97	17.65	17.44	17.24 *,†	V, M, N	Pancreas	Autop(−), Apop(−), NFkaBTF(−)
Heat shock protein family A (Hsp70) member 1B	**HSPA1B**	20.93	20.97	20.65 †	20.78	V, C, N	Vagina	CHA, PF, SR
Cyclin-dependent kinase inhibitor	**CDKN1B**	14.78	14.83	14.40	13.49†	N, V	Low	CCP

Location in cell: C, cytosol; ECM, extra cellular matrix; ER, endoplasmatic reticulum; G, Golgi apparatus; LD, lipid droplets; M, mitochondria; N, nucleus; PM, plasma membrane; PX, peroxisome; V, vesicles. **Main function:** AAT, amino acid transport (serine); ACoA, acetyl CoA; ACoAT, acetyl CoA transport; ADPT, ADP transport; AMPT, AMP transport; AndC, androgen catabolism; Apop(+), positive regulator of cell apoptosis; Apop(−), negative regulator of cell apoptosis; ATPH, ATP hydrolysis; ATPS, ATP synthesis; ATPT, ATP transport; Autop(−), negative regulator of autophagia; CA, cell adhesion; CaM, carbohydrate metabolism; cAMP, cyclic adenosine monophosphate; CCR, cell cycle regulator; CHA, chaperone; ChoB, cholesterol biosynthesis; ChoM, cholesterol metabolism; CO, cytoskeleton organization; CP, cell proliferation; CCP, cell cycle progression; DrugM, drug metabolism; EMO, extracellular matrix organization; ERGT, endoplasmatic reticulum–Golgi apparatus transport; EstB, estrogen biosynthesis; ET, electron transport; FAM, fatty acid metabolism; FC, fructose catabolism; GlyoxM, glyoxylate metabolism; GTPH, GTP hydrolysis; LiB, lipid biosynthesis; LiBi, lipid binding; LiM, lipid metabolism; LiMM, lipid metabolism modulator; LiT, lipid transport; MetC, methionine catabolism; MF, membrane fusion; MT, methylation; MTC, mitochondrial carrier (ACoA transport into mitochondria in exchange for ATP/ADP/AMP); MTTT, mitochondrial transmembrane transport; NFkaBTF(−), negative regulator of NF-Kappa Beta transcription factor; PF, protein folding; PGM, prostaglandin metabolism (interleukins, eicosanoids, etc.); PT, protein transport; PyroM, pyrovate metabolism; RCP, respiratory chain protein; RP, regulatory protein (phenalyalanine metabolism); SD, serine degradation; SH, serine hydrolase (unidentified substrates); SR, stress response; ST, signal transduction; SterB, steroid biosynthesis; SterM, steroid metabolism; TCA, tricarboxylic acid cycle; Ts, tumor suppressor; 1CM, one carbon metabolism. * q-value (FDR adjusted p-value) < 0.05 compared with CON, † q-value (FDR adjusted p-value) < 0.05 compared with LS−.

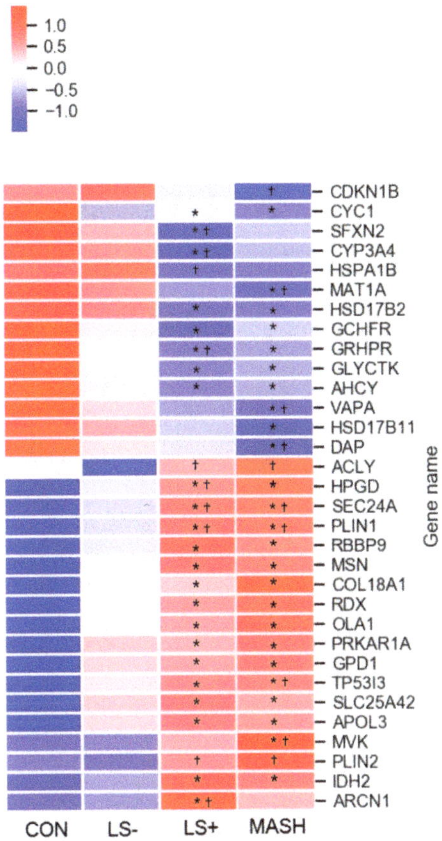

Figure 2. Heat map of significant liver proteins with increasing severity of histological MASLD. The heat map shows the 32 (out of 5151 liver protein groups in total) differentially expressed liver proteins (q value (FDR-adjusted p-value) < 0.05) in CON, LS−, LS+, and MASH. Eighteen proteins were generally upregulated (red color) in MASLD compared with CON, and 14 proteins were downregulated (blue color) in MASLD compared with CON. The specific log2 intensities of a given liver protein and the significance patterns between the four groups for a given protein can be found in Table 3. * q-value (FDR adjusted p-value) < 0.05 compared with CON. † q-value (FDR adjusted p-value) < 0.05 compared with LS−. Created in BioRender. Pedersen, J. (2025) https://BioRender.com/ori5dw6, accessed on 15 December 2024.

Table 3. Differentially expressed proteins in visceral adipose tissue identified by untargeted proteomics analysis in CON, LS−, LS+, and MASH.

Protein Name	Gene Name	CON Log2 Intensity	LS− Log2 Intensity	Ls+ Log2 Intensity	Mash Log2 Intensity	Location in Cell	Tissue Specificity	Main Function(s)
				Upregulated VAT proteins in MASLD				
Metabolism								
L-lactate dehydrogenase B chain	**LDHB**	16.53	17.96 *	18.51 *	18.40 *	C	Heart, kidney	CM, PyrvM, Ferm
Inorganic pyrophosphatase	**PPA1**	13.47	15.30 *	15.28 *	15.68 *	C	Low	PhosM

Table 3. *Cont.*

Protein Name	Gene Name	CON Log2 Intensity	LS− Log2 Intensity	Ls+ Log2 Intensity	Mash Log2 Intensity	Location in Cell	Tissue Specificity	Main Function(s)
Lipid metabolism								
Sulfotransferase 1A1	**SULT1A1**	13.36	14.96 *	14.50	15.36 *	C	Liver	CateM, LiM, SterM, XM
Fatty aldehyde dehydrogenase	**ALDH3A2**	12.41	14.19 *	14.09 *	14.37 *	PXM, ERM	Low	FAM, LiM, SB
Aldo-keto reductase family 1 member C1	**AKR1C1**	16.83	18.12 *	18.28 *	18.47 *	C	Liver	PM, SterM
3-oxo-5-beta-steroid 4-dehydrogenase	**AKR1D1**	14.86	16.97 *	17.16 *	17.85 *	C	Liver	AndM, BAB, ChoC, SterM
Aldo-keto reductase family 1 member B	**AKR1B1**	13.24	14.44	14.42 *	14.45 *	C	Adrenal gland	CM(PP), SteM, PGM, SIG
Aldo-keto reductase family 1 member C3	**AKR1C3**	15.07	16.06 *	16.51 *	16.53 *	C	Liver	M, SteM, ProglM, AndM, CellD(+), Apop(+) ROSM(+)
Liver carboxylesterase 1	**CES1**	17.31	18.45 *	18.95 *	18.94 *	ER	Liver	FAM, XM, ChoB
Epoxide hydrolase 1	**EPHX1**	15.91	17.91 *	17.95 *	17.78 *	ER	Liver, adrenal gland	AHC, DtX
Alkylglycerone phosphate synthase	**AGPS**	7.80	10.68 *	10.68 *	10.16 *	PX	Low	LiB, LiM
Mitochondrial								
Mitochondrial carnitine/acylcarnitine carrier protein	**SLC25A20**	11.57	13.17	13.02 *	13.36 *	M	Low	CarnS
Sulfide:quinone oxidoreductase, mitochondrial	**SQOR**	13.72	12.83	12.89	13.85 †,§	M	Low	H_2SM
Inflammation								
Complement C1q subcomponent subunit C	**C1QC**	15.19	16.37 *	16.61 *	16.26 *	XC (extra cellular)	Lymphoid tissue (monocytes)	ComP, ImR(+)
Complement C1r	**C1QR**	12.93	14.41 *	14.10 *	14.00 *	XC	Lymphoid tissue (monocytes)	ComP, ImR(+)
Alpha-1-microglobulin	**AMBP**	14.86	16.41 *	16.27 *	16.59 *	G, S, XC	Liver	HVI, ImR(−)
Intracellular transport and carriers								
Member RAS oncogene family	**RAB5C**	15.49	16.45 *	16.36 *	16.50 *	EN	Low	PT
VPS35 endosomal protein sorting factor like	**VPS35**	14.76	15.43 *	15.43*	15.69 *	EN, PM	Low	GPMT, PT
Coatomer subunit beta′	**COPB2**	13.56	14.27 *	14.41 *	14.37 *	C	Low	ERGT, PT
ADP-ribosylation factor 3	**ARF3**	15.05	16.11 *	16.11 *	16.13 *	ER	Brain	ERGT, PT
MAL proteolipid protein 2	**MAL2**	11.19	14.12 *	14.23 *	14.42 *	PM	Esophagus	TC (PIGR)

Table 3. *Cont.*

Protein Name	Gene Name	CON Log2 Intensity	LS− Log2 Intensity	Ls+ Log2 Intensity	Mash Log2 Intensity	Location in Cell	Tissue Specificity	Main Function(s)
Cytoskeleton and ECM								
Keratin, type II cytoskeletal 1	**KRT1**	14.85	16.45 *	16.06 *	16.35 *	PM	Skin	CO, ST, ComA
Vimentin	**VIM**	21.16	22.49 *	22.47 *	22.49 *	PM, CS, N	Low	CO, HVI
Collagen alpha-2 (IV) chain	**COL4A2**	18.08	19.55 *	19.90 *	19.92 *	ECM	Placenta	EMO
Tubulin beta-2A chain	**TUBB2A**	14.90	15.41	15.80 *	15.87 *	CS	Brain	CO, MCC
Lipoma-preferred partner	**LPP**							
Signal transduction and regulation, apoptosis								
Tyrosine 3-monooxygenase	**YWHAZ**	18.42	19.21 *	19.28 *	19.44 *	C, N	low	ST, Apop(−), Angio(+)
Phospholysine phosphohistidine inorganic pyrophosphate phosphatase	**LHPP**	12.19	13.88 *	13.90 *	13.71 *	C	Brain	PDP
Annexin A5	**ANXA5**	17.59	18.94 *	19.15 *	19.13 *	NM	Low	ST, BC(−), Apop(−)
Pleckstrin homology-like domain family B member 1	**PHLDB1**	12.23	13.88 *	13.95 *	13.86 *	N, MiS	Brain	Reg
Dual specificity mitogen-activated protein kinase kinase 1	**MAP2K1**	11.92	13.10 *	13.29 *	13.49 *	C, PM	Low	MAPKSC(+), PPARGSC(+)
Receptor-type tyrosine-protein phosphatase S	**PTPRS**	9.16	12.15 *	11.74 *	10.86	C, PM	Low	ST, MAPK(−), ImR(−)
Cell cycle, cell quality, and apoptosis								
Atlastin-3	**ATL3**	12.63	14.00 *	14.24 *	14.21 *	ER	Low	ERQ
Reticulon-4	**RTN4**	13.33	13.90	14.17 *	14.28 *	ER	Low	ERS, Angio(+), Infl(+)
Crystallin alpha B	**CRYAB**	18.29	20.31 *	20.76 *	20.62 *	C, PM	Muscle	CHA
Heat shock protein beta-6	**HSPB6**	16.24	18.22 *	18.23 *	18.35 *	C, G	Muscle	CHA, SR, Angio(+)
Heterogeneous nuclear ribonucleoproteins A2/B1	**HNRNPA2B1**	16.40	17.68 *	17.63 *	17.69 *	N	Low	mRNAp, mRNAs, mRNAt, HVI, ImR(+)
Parkinsonism associated deglycase	**PARK7**	15.51	17.17 *	16.96 *	17.11 *	C, N	Low	CHA, PRep, PDeglyc, OxSS, MtHom
Follistatin-related protein 1	**FSTL1**	10.56	11.50 *	11.67 *	11.98 *	C, V	Low	CP, CD
Coactosin-like protein	**COTL1**	14.19	15.28 *	15.32 *	15.25 *	C	Blood, lymphoid tissue	CHA, LeuS

Table 3. *Cont.*

Protein Name	Gene Name	CON Log2 Intensity	LS− Log2 Intensity	Ls+ Log2 Intensity	Mash Log2 Intensity	Location in Cell	Tissue Specificity	Main Function(s)
Miscellaneous								
Myoglobin	**MB**	9.99	12.72 *	12.05	13.07 *	C	Muscle	OxT, OxR
Cystatin-B	**CSTB**	16.15	17.57 *	17.47 *	17.63 *	C, N	Esophagus, tongue	Pro(−)
Unknown function								
FUN14 domain-containing protein 2	**FUNDC2**	12.99	14.22 *	14.31 *	14.23 *	N, M	Low	MTautop
				Downregulated VAT proteins in MASLD				
Mitochondrial metabolism								
2-oxoisovalerate dehydrogenase subunit alpha, mitochondrial	**BCKDHA**	13.00	12.43	11.32 *	11.04 *	M	Low	BCAAC
Pyruvate dehydrogenase protein X component, mitochondrial	**PDHX**	13.88	12.32 *	12.31 *	11.24 *	M	Low	AcoAB, PyrvM
ATP synthase subunit alpha, mitochondrial	**ATP5A1**	18.58	17.85 *	17.89 *	17:54 *	M	Low	ATPsyn
GTP:AMP phosphotransferase AK3, mitochondrial	**AK3**	16.21	15.25 *	15.08 *	15.51 *	M	Low	NPI
Sulfide:quinone oxidoreductase, mitochondrial	**SQOR**	13.72	12.83	12.89	13.85 †,§	M	Low	H_2SM
Lipid metabolism								
Very-long-chain enoyl-CoA reductase	**TECR**	15.21	14.34 *	14.37 *	14.33 *	ER	Low	FAB, FAE, FAM, LiB, LiM, SteM, SM
Enoyl-CoA delta isomerase 1, mitochondrial	**ECI1**	15.00	14.49	14.13*	13.98 *,†	M	Muscle	FAOX, FAM, LiM
Cytochrome b5	**CYP5A**	17.46	16.51 *	16.47 *	16.00 *	C, V	Liver	ET
Signal transduction								
Calcium/calmodulin-dependent protein kinase II delta	**CAMK2**	14.66	14.04 *	13.70 *	13.92 *	C, PM	Low	CaB, ST
Intracellular transport								
AP-1 complex subunit mu-1	**AP1M1**	15.54	13.93 *	13.93 *	14.36	C, G	Low	PT, HVI
Cytoskeleton, ECM and signaling								
Tight junction protein 2	**TJP2**	12.89	11.71 *	11.22 *	11.05 *	PM, CJ	Low	CA, TJ
Cell cycle, cell quality, and apoptosis								
SH3 domain-containing kinase-binding protein 1	**SH3KBP1**	14.08	12.72 *	12.65 *	13.08	CS	Low	ST, CO, CA
Serine/threonine-protein phosphatase 2A activator	**PTPA**	13.94	13.01 *	13.85 †	13.01	C, N	Low	PF, DNArep, CCP

Table 3. *Cont.*

Protein Name	Gene Name	CON Log2 Intensity	LS− Log2 Intensity	Ls+ Log2 Intensity	Mash Log2 Intensity	Location in Cell	Tissue Specificity	Main Function(s)
Antioxidant defense								
Probable hydrolase PNKD	**PNKD**	13.28	12.41 *	12.26 *	12.22 *	C, M	Low	GlutB(+)
Miscellaneous								
Sperm-associated antigen-17	**SPAG17**	20.56	18.68 *	18.70 *	18.88 *	C, CS	Testis, epididymis, brain	CilB, CilF
Family with sequence similarity member A2	**FAM114A2**	11.54	10.26 *	11.30 †	11.09	V	low	PuNB
Hemoglobin subunit alpha	**HBA1**	25.86	24.55 *	24.36 *	25.02	C	Bone marrow	OxT

Location in cell: C, cytosol; CJ, cell junction; CS, cytoskeleton; ECM, extra cellular matrix; EN, endosome; ER, endoplasmatic reticulum; ERM, endoplasmatic reticulum membrane; G, Golgi apparatus; M, mitochondria; MiS, mitochondrial spindle; N, nucleus; NM, nuclear membrane; PM, plasma membrane; PX, peroxisome; PXM, peroxisome membrane; S, secreted; V, vesicle; XC, extra cellular. **Main function:** ACoAB, acetyl CoA biosynthesis; AHC, aromatic hydrocarbon catabolism; AndM, androgen metabolism; Angio(+), positive regulator of angiogenesis; Apop(+), positive regulator of cell apoptosis; Apop(−), negative regulator of cell apoptosis; ATPsyn, ATP synthesis; BAB, bile acid biosynthesis; BC(−), negative regulator of blood coagulation (anti-coagulant); BCAAC, branched chain amino acid; CA, cell adhesion; CaB, calcium binding; CarnS, carnitine shuttle; CateM, cathecolamin metabolism; CCP, cell cycle progression; CD, cell differentiation; CellD(+), positive regulator of cell death; CHA, chaperone; ChoB, cholesterol biosynthesis; ChoC, cholesterol catabolism; CilB, cilium biosynthesis; CilF, cilium function; CM, carbohydrate metabolism; CM(PP), carbohydrate metabolism (polyol pathway); CO, cytoskeleton organization; ComA, complement activation; ComP, complement pathway; CP, cell proliferation; DNArep, DNA repair; Dtx, detoxification; EMO, extra cellular matrix; ERGT, endoplasmatic reticulum–Golgi apparatus transport; ERS, endoplasmatic reticulum stabilization; ERQ, endoplasmatic reticulum quality; ET, electron transport; FAB, fatty acid biosynthesis; FAE, fatty acid elongation; FAM, fatty acid metabolism; FAOX, fatty acid beta oxidation; Ferm, fermentation; GlutB(+), positive regulator of gluthation biosynthesis; GPMT, Golgi–plasma membrane transport; HVI, host–virus interaction; H2SM, hydrogene sulfide metabolism; ImR(+), positive regulator of immune response; ImR(−), negative regulator of immune response; Infl(+), inflammation; LeuS, leukotriene synthesis; LiB, lipid biosynthesis; LiM, lipid metabolism; MAPK(−), negative regulator of MAP kinase; MAPKSC(+), positive regulator of MAPK signaling cascade; MCC, miotic cell cycle; mRNAp, mRNA processing; mRNAs, mRNA splicing; mRNAt, mRNA transport; MTautop, mitochondrial autophagia; MtHom, mitochondrial homeostasis; NPI, nucleoside phosphate interconversion; OxR, oxygen transport; OxSS, oxygen stress sensor; OxT, oxygen transport; PDeglyc, protein deglucase activity; PDP, protein dephosphorylation; PF, protein folding; PGM, prostaglandin metabolism; PhosM, phosphate metabolism; PM, progesterone metabolism; PPARGSC(+), positive regulator of PPRAG signaling cascade; PRep, protein repair; Pro(−), protease inhibitor; PT, protein transport; PuNB; purine nucleotide binding; PyrvM, pyruvate metabolism; Reg, regulator; ROSM(+), positive regulator of reactive oxygen species; SIG, signaling; SB, sphingolipid biosynthesis; SM, sphingolipid metabolism; SR, stress response; ST, signal transduction; SterM, steroid metabolism; TJ, tight junction; TC, transcytosis; XM, xenobiotic metabolism. * q-value (FDR adjusted p-value) < 0.05 compared with CON, † q-value (FDR adjusted p-value) < 0.05 compared with LS−, § q-value (FDR adjusted p-value) < 0.05 compared with LS+.

Six of the fourteen downregulated proteins and three of the eighteen upregulated proteins were "liver specific", indicating an impaired synthesis of proteins in the liver

The DEPs were grouped primarily in three predominant significance patterns: (1) significant upregulation or downregulation in the MASLD groups (12 proteins) vs. CON with otherwise no significance among the four groups, (2) significant upregulation or downregulation between LS+ or MASH vs. CON and/or LS− (ten proteins), and (3) significant upregulation or downregulation between LS+ and MASH combined vs. CON and/or LS− (seven proteins).

Six proteins were significantly altered in the MASH group compared with LS+, LS−, and CON. One protein was upregulated (mevalonate kinase (MVK)), and five proteins were downregulated (hydroxysteroid 17-beta dehydrogenase 11 (HSD17B11), cyclin-dependent kinase inhibitor 1B (CDKN1B), death associated protein (DAP), methionine adenosyltransferase 1A (MAT1A), and VAMP associated protein A (VAPA)). Four proteins were significantly altered in the LS+ group compared with remaining groups; one was upregulated (archain 1 (ARCN1)), and three were downregulated (cytochrome P450 family 3 subfamily A member 4 (CYP3AB), sideroflexin-2 (SFXN2), and heat shock protein family A (Hsp70) member 1B (HSPA1B)).

3.2. Differentially Expressed Upregulated Liver Proteins (Table 2 and Figure 2)

Among the 18 upregulated proteins, 12 proteins showed the highest intensities in the MASH group, and 6 proteins showed the highest intensities in the LS+ group. None of the proteins expressed the highest intensity in the LS− group.

When we sorted the upregulated proteins according to their main biological functions, the "metabolism" group (proteins associated with primary cellular metabolic functions) comprised the highest number of proteins (eight seven proteins, including isocitrate dehydrogenase 2 (IDH2), Glycerol-3-phosphate dehydrogenase 1 (GPD1), OBG like ATPase 1 (OLA1), ACLY (ATP citrate lyase), (mevalonate kinase (MVK), 15-hydroxyprostaglandin dehydrogenase (HPGD), Perilipin 1 (PLIN1), and perilipin 2 (PLIN2)). As previously mentioned, MVK was the only upregulated DEP in MASH.

The perilipins (PLIN1 and PLIN2) coat lipid droplets and are otherwise known to be highly expressed in adipocytes [30]. Out of the 32 hepatic DEPs, PLIN1 and PLIN2 were the proteins with highest fold changes (around three), whereas PLIN1 was three-fold higher in LS+ and MASH compared with CON (q-value = 0.006); for PLIN2 this three-fold increase was observed between LS+/MASH and LS−, with no statistical significance when compared with CON.

Other liver proteins with significant upregulation were grouped as "intracellular transport proteins" (four proteins) and proteins related to the cytoskeleton, intracellular signal transduction, and extracellular matrix formation (five proteins). In the former group we found apolipoprotein 3 (APOL3), a lipid transporter which showed a 1- to 2.5-fold increase in the MASLD groups. Two proteins from the latter group, moesin (MSN) and radixin (RDX), were significantly upregulated in all three MASLD groups. Together with the protein "ezrin", MSN and RDX were recognized as the "ezrin/radixin/Moesin (ERM) family" [31]. Last, tumor protein p53 inducible protein 3 (TP53I3) was a highly upregulated protein with tripled intensity in MASH and LS+ and doubled intensity in LS− when compared with CON.

3.3. Differentially Expressed Downregulated Liver Proteins (Table 2 and Figure 2)

Among the downregulated DEPs, 50% had the lowest intensities in MASH, and 50% had the lowest intensities in LS+. None of the downregulated proteins had the lowest intensities in LS−.

The largest groups of proteins (eight proteins; Glycerate kinase (GLYCKTK), Glyoxylate hydroxypyrovate dehydrogenase (GRHDR), GTP cyclohydrolase I feedback regulator (GCHFR), Methionine adenosyltransferase 1A (MAT1A), Adenosylhomocysteinase (ACHY), Hydroxysteroid 17-beta dehydrogenase 2 (HSD17B2), Hydroxysteroid 17-beta dehydrogenase 11 (HSD17B11), and Cytochrome P450 family 3 subfamily A member 4 (CYP3A4)) belonged to the "metabolism" group. GLYCKTK, which is involved in the catabolism of serine and the metabolism of fructose, was significantly downregulated in all three MASLD groups. CYP3A4 was significantly downregulated in LS+.

3.4. Visceral Adipose Tissue

In VAT we found 59 DEPs between the four groups (Table 3 and Figure 3). In VAT, 42 proteins (71%) were upregulated, and 17 proteins (29%) were significantly downregulated. Moreover, we observed considerable differences in protein intensities with up to 8.5-fold higher or lower intensities between groups (primarily CON vs. one or more of the MASLD groups) for specific proteins. Significant differences for a given DEP between the groups were predominantly observed between the MASLD groups collectively and CON

(34 upregulated and 9 downregulated), followed by significance between MASH/LS+ and LS−/CON (4 upregulated and 2 downregulated) with the rest of the proteins (4 upregulated and 5 downregulated) showing other significance patterns.

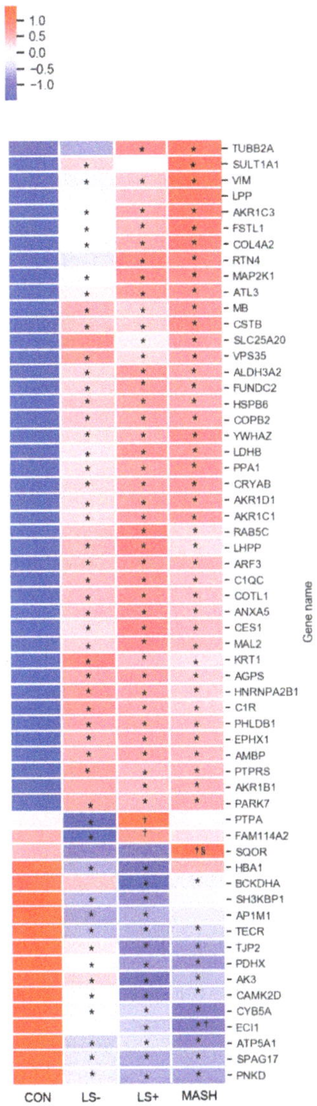

Figure 3. Heat map of significant VAT proteins with increasing severity of histological MASLD. The heat map shows the 59 (out of 3200 VAT protein groups in total) differentially expressed VAT proteins (q-value (FDR adjusted p-value) < 0.05) in CON, LS−, LS+, and MASH. A total of 42 proteins were generally upregulated (red color) in MASLD compared with CON, and 17 proteins were downregulated (blue color) in MASLD compared with CON. The specific log2 intensities of a given VAT protein and the significance patterns between the four groups for a given protein can be found in Table 3. * q-value (FDR adjusted p-value) < 0.05 compared with CON, † q-value (FDR adjusted p-value) < 0.05 compared with LS−, § q-value (FDR adjusted p-value) < 0.05 compared with LS+. Created in BioRender. Pedersen, J. (2025) https://BioRender.com/nbub800, accessed on 15 December 2024.

Only a single protein, the mitochondrial sulfide:quinone oxidoreductase (SQOR), was exclusively downregulated in MASH. LS+ had significant upregulation of the serine/threonine-protein phosphatase 2A activator (PTBA), a chaperone protein governing DNA repair and protein folding.

3.5. *Differentially Expressed Upregulated VAT Proteins (Table 3 and Figure 3)*

Upregulated proteins were grouped according to main function and are depicted in Table 3. Nine of the upregulated proteins were involved in lipid metabolism. Notably, four of these (hydroxysteroid dehydrogenase (AKR1C1), steroid 5β-reductase (AKR1D1), aldose reductase (AKR1B1), hydroxysteroid dehydrogenase (AKR1C3)) belonged to the aldo-keto reductase family.

We found upregulation of the complement system through complement C1 subcomponents C1r and C1q. They assembled with subcomponent C1s to form the C1 complex, which was the first component in the serum complement system and the activator of the classical (antigen–antibody) component pathway.

Other proteins with significant upregulation included intracellular signaling, cytoskeletal, and extracellular matrix proteins and proteins related to cell/organelle quality including several chaperones (heat shock protein beta-6 (HSPB6), crystallin alpha B (CRYAB), parkinsonism associated deglycase (PARK7), and coactosin-like protein (COTL1)). Of these, HSPB6 also functions as a stress sensor [32].

Notably, myoglobin (MB), a protein found primarily in muscle with excellent oxygen binding and reservoir capacities, showed prominent upregulation with four to six times higher expression in MASLD groups than CON. Last, several proteins aiding angiogenesis (e.g., tyrosin-3 monooxygenase (YWHAZ), reticulon 4 (RTN4), and heat shock protein beta-6 (HSPB6)) were upregulated in MASLD groups.

3.6. *Differentially Expressed Downregulated VAT Proteins (Table 3 and Figure 3)*

The 17 downregulated proteins were scattered over several groups.

Five proteins were mitochondrial proteins and included the ATP synthase subunit alpha (ATP5A1), which is one of the core components of the ATP synthase complex in the electron transport chain.

In addition, the mitochondrial 2-oxoisovalerate dehydrogenase subunit alpha (BCKHDA) was also significantly downregulated in LS+ and in MASH by two-fold compared with CON. BCKHDA is the alpha subunit of the decarboxylase component of the branched chain dehydrogenase (BCKD) complex that catalyzes the second and irreversible step in the catabolism of branched chain amino acids valine, leucine, and isoleucine.

3.7. *Associations Between VAT and Liver Tissue in MASLD: Correlation Data (Table 4)*

Twenty-four proteins correlated significantly between VAT and liver tissue (Table 4). Of these, 22 correlated positively, and 2 correlated negatively. The protein with the highest correlation coefficient was Hemoglobin subunit gamma-1 (HBG1), which is the gamma chain of fetal hemoglobin (α2γ2) (Pearson's $r = 0.71$). Interestingly, angiotensinogen (AGT), the precursor of angiotensin, was the protein with the second-strongest correlation coefficient.

Four of the ten proteins with the highest correlation coefficients were related to the immune system; two were immunoglobulins (immunoglobulin heavy constant alpha 2 (IGHA2) and immunoglobulin heavy constant mu (IGHM)), and two belonged to the complement cascade, namely, complement C4-A (C4A) and complement C4-B (C4B). The latter two are the components of the complement component C4, a central component of the classically activated pathway in the complement cascade.

Ribosyldihydronicotinamide dehydrogenase [quinone] (NQO2), glutathione S-transferase theta-1 (GSTT1), and NAD(P)HX epimerase (NAXE), proteins with the third-, fourth-, and fifth-highest correlation coefficients, are all involved in oxidative defense, detoxification, and/or repair mechanisms.

Table 4. The 24 significant FDR-adjusted proteins by correlation analysis between VAT and liver tissue.

Protein Name	Gene Name	*q*-Value	Pearson's *r*	Location in Cell	Tissue Specificity	Main Function(s)
Hemoglobin subunit gamma-1	**HBG1**	0.0000	0.717	C	Placenta	FetalHG, Oxb, OxT
Immunoglobulin heavy constant alpha 2	**IGHA2**	0.0000	0.630	PM, secreted	Low	ImR
Angiotensinogen	**AGT**	0.0000	0.624	Secreted	Liver	RAAS, BPReg
Ribosyldihydronicotinamide dehydrogenase [quinone]	**NQO2**	0.0000	0.603	C	Low	DeTox, OxStress protector
Glutathione S-transferase theta-1	**GSTT1**	0.0001	0.595	C	Breast	GluthB, GluthM
NAD(P)HX epimerase	**NAXE**	0.0001	0.586	C, N	Low	NAD(P)HXrep
Immunoglobulin heavy constant mu	**IGHM**	0.0002	0.557	PM, secreted	Low	ImR
Complement C4-A	**C4A**	0.0005	0.554	Secreted	Liver	CP, ImR(+)
Copine-1	**CPNE1**	0.0006	0.535	N, NM	Low	TNFaSig, TF
Enoyl-CoA hydratase domain-containing protein 3, mitochondrial	**ECHDC3**	0.0006	0.532	M	Liver, muscle	FAM, LiM
Complement C4-B	**C4B**	0.0010	0.521	Secreted	Liver	CP, ImR(+)
Afamin	**AFM**	0.0025	0.5	ECM, Se	Liver	PT, FAB
N-acetylneuraminate lyase	**NPL**	0.0452	0.492	VE, PM	Blood	CM
Epsin-1	**EPN1**	0.0041	0.491	PM, C	Low	Endocytosis
Acyl-coenzyme A thioesterase 1	**ACOT1**	0.0064	0.476	M	Liver	FAM, AcoAM
Phosphoglucomutase-1	**PGM1**	0.0068	0.473	C	Muscle	CM, GluM
Glycogenin-2	**GYG2**	0.0290	0.44	C, N	Adipose tissue, brain, breast	GlycB
Tyrosine-protein kinase CSK	**CSK**	0.0313	0.433	C, V	Lymphoid tissue	Reg, Imm
Heat shock protein HSP 90-alpha	**HSP90AA1**	0.0360	0.428	C	Vagina	Cha, HVI, SR
Interferon-induced protein with tetratricopeptide repeats 1	**IFIT1**	0.0367	0.426	C	Low	HVI, Imm
Histidine-rich glycoprotein	**HRG**	0.0455	0.415	Secreted	Liver	Angio(+), BC, Chem
Tetratricopeptide repeat protein 38	**TTC38**	0.0498	0.411	C, secreted	Liver, intestine	Unknown
60S ribosomal protein L38	**RPL38**	0.0453	−0.416	ER, C	Low	RibP, translation
RAB14 member RAS oncogene family	**RAB14**	0.0450	−0.419	Er, C	Low	RibP, translation

Oxb, oxygen binding; OxT, oxygen transport; ImR, immune response; RAAS, renin–angiotensinogen–aldosterone system; BPReg, blood pressure regulator; DeTox, detoxification process; OxStress, oxidative stress; GluthB, gluthation biosynthesis; GluthM, gluthation metabolism; NAD(P)HXrep, repairs NAD(P)H hydrates (NAD(P)HX); CP, complement pathway; ImR, immune response; TNFaSig, TNF-alpha signaling; TF, transcription factor; FAM, fatty acid metabolism; LiM, lipid metabolism; PT, protein transport; FAB, fatty acid binding; AcoAM, acetyl CoA metabolism; CM, carbohydrate metabolism; GlycB, glycogen breakdown; Imm, adaptive immunity; Cha, chaperone; HVI, host–virus interaction; Angio(+), positive regulator of angiogenesis; BC, blood coagulation; Chem, chemotaxis; RibP, ribosomal protein.

4. Discussion

4.1. No Overlapping DEPs in VAT and Liver Tissue in Subjects with Obesity, MASLD, and MASH

This study presents a comprehensive human investigation analyzing the distinct protein signatures of the liver and VAT in 70 individuals with obesity and varying degrees of MASLD severity. It also explores the relationships between the proteomes of these two tissues. To our knowledge, this represents the largest human MASLD proteomics dataset to date featuring paired liver and VAT biopsies.

We initially hypothesized that certain proteins would be simultaneously and significantly upregulated or downregulated in both tissues; however, no such proteins were identified. We also found no evidence of a MASH-specific proteome in VAT.

These findings challenge our assumption of a unified proteomic signature linking VAT dysfunction with liver pathology in MASLD/MASH and our hypothesis that MASLD progression involves shared proteomic alterations across metabolic tissues such as VAT.

Overall, the protein expression patterns showed minimal differences between the MASLD groups. For instance, we did not find inflammatory proteins in VAT to be generally more upregulated in MASH than in LS+. Surprisingly, we found merely a single VAT protein, which was significantly upregulated in MASH only, namely, SQOR. SQOR catalyzes the primary step in the metabolism of hydrogen sulfide (H_2S) within the mitochondria [33]. H_2S is a gasotransmitter, which is toxic in high concentrations and at low concentrations acts cytoprotectively and is involved in many different biological functions including anti-inflammatory and proinflammatory abilities [34]. We can only speculate if SQOR is upregulated due to high H_2S levels in the VAT of MASH patients, but due to the descriptive nature of this study we can draw no conclusions if this is, in fact, the case.

It is possible that the absence of overlapping DEPs may be due to the inherent heterogeneity between liver and adipose tissues as each exhibits tissue-specific metabolism and protein turnover. It is well established that certain proteins show strong tissue specificity (e.g., adipocytokines in VAT and albumin in the liver). In addition, there are indeed notable metabolic differences between the two tissues, such as the liver being a key site for protein degradation, where hepatocytes break down proteins into amino acids for various liver-specific metabolic pathways, but this study measured intact proteins rather than amino acids or degradation products. Therefore, our data reflect proteins actively synthesized in the tissue, representing gene expression through to translation. However, we cannot from this study determine the ultimate fate of individual proteins—whether they are secreted or rapidly degraded intracellularly.

Although tissue heterogeneity could partly explain the lack of overlapping DEPs between the liver and VAT, it does not explain the lack of a more distinct MASH-specific proteome in VAT. This may instead be attributed to the overall limitations of the study, which are discussed later, or it could be that MASH is not specifically represented in VAT, as the VAT proteome is instead overshadowed by the presence of obesity.

Based on the protein expression patterns, we generally observed the tendency of CON and LS− to group together and LS+ and MASH to group together or that the significance of a given protein (e.g., AKR1B1, SLC25A20, RTN4, BCKDHA, and ECI1) was found between LS+ and MASH vs. CON but not LS− vs. CON. Yet, the log2 intensities for the given protein were often still numerically much higher or lower in LS− compared with CON and thus may indicate a distinct biological difference—probably obesity—between these groups despite the absence of histological liver steatosis in both groups. The observed expression patterns in VAT therefore appear to reflect the metabolic deterioration that is associated with central obesity. The severity of MASLD is linked to the degree of metabolic dysregulation [35]. Our analyses were unable to determine if the observed differences reflected common risk factors or if there was a direct link between metabolic dysfunction in VAT and MASLD severity. Of note, among the included participants, those with MASH and LS+ were more likely to have T2DM, and they had a higher HOMA-IR and had higher levels of plasma liver enzymes. This was, however, not clearly reflected in the VAT DEPs.

Up until very recently [24,36], no human studies had specifically compared VAT and liver tissue proteomics in relation to MASLD severity. In the very recent study by Boel and colleagues [24], 58 liver and 27 VAT samples from an MASLD cohort similar to ours were available for analyses. However, the proteomics data were integrated with liver single-cell analyses and plasma proteomics analyses, making specific comparison with our findings difficult.

Castané et al. [36] performed proteomics analyses of liver and VAT in patients with MASH, but the analyses were also coupled with transcriptomics, plasma, and genetics. Yet, proteomics analyses were only applied in 18 VAT and liver tissue biopsies. Through enrichment analyses of proteomics and lipidomics, they found an association between MASH and mitochondrial dysfunction in VAT. We found similar downregulation of several mitochondrial proteins in VAT, which is discussed in more detail below.

4.2. Changes in the VAT Proteome in Obesity, T2DM, and MASLD

Numerous studies have explored the human obese VAT proteome in relation to T2DM [37–39], in metabolically healthy vs. unhealthy subjects with obesity [40], as well as differences between SAT and VAT from individuals with obesity [41]. Several of the other VAT upregulated DEPs found in our study have been identified in other human obesity/T2DM studies, e.g., annexin (ANXA5) [37,42], liver carboxyl esterase 1 (CES1) [42], Complement C1r C1QC [42], and myoglobin (MB) [43]. Moesin (MSN), which we found upregulated in the liver has similarly been found upregulated in VAT and SAT in subjects with obesity [37]. In addition, we found that C1QC, which is the c-chain of the human complement subcomponent C1q, was significantly upregulated in all three MASLD groups and pointed toward general upregulation of the completement cascade, which is an active innate immune response and promotes inflammation. It is difficult in interpret the latter finding as we have come across no studies for comparison. We also found upregulation of the perilipins PLIN1 and PLIN2 in the liver tissue but not in the VAT. PLIN1 is believed to function as a lipid droplet protector that modulates the action of the hormone sensitive lipase in adipose tissue and thus helps regulate lipid metabolism. In its absence, leanness is promoted at the expense of insulin resistance in PLIN1 knock-out mice [44]. PLIN1 and especially PLIN2 have previously been associated with the development of MASLD in rodent models and human [45,46].

We also note the relative "overrepresentation" of downregulated DEPs related to mitochondrial function and metabolism—e.g., BCKDHA, ATP5A1, PDHX, AK3, and SQOR, the latter being the single VAT DEP significant in MASH only. Prominent downregulation of mitochondrial proteins and proteins related to the respiratory machinery in obesity has recently been recognized in a diet-induced obesity mouse model [47] and in the study by Castañé et al. [36], but more systematic human data are lacking. Our finding of significant downregulation of BCKDHA is interesting as plasma levels of branched chain amino acids (leucine, isoleucine, and valine) have been reported to be increased in insulin resistant individuals with obesity. In addition, adipose tissue is recognized as an important site for BCAA catabolism [48]. Other studies have also reported significant downregulation in obese adipose tissue of the enzymes responsible for BCAA catabolism [49], including the branched chain ketoacid dehydrogenase complex (BCKDHC) of which the BCKDHA is a subunit and that catalyzes the irreversible catabolic step in BCAA breakdown.

4.3. Correlation Analyses Pinpoint Inflammatory and Detoxification Proteins

In the correlation analyses between VAT and liver, the top 10 positive correlations were dominated by inflammatory proteins and proteins involved in oxidative defense mechanisms and detoxification processes. This could point toward simultaneous upregulation and overlapping pathophysiology in the two tissues. It could be argued that the high abundance of secretory proteins (Table 4) among the proteins with high correlation scores represents "contamination" of plasma and blood vessels in the two tissues. However, we would then have expected to see high correlation scores of other plasma proteins with very high abundance in plasma, e.g., albumin or hemoglobin subunit A (normal hemoglobin). But this was not the case. Rather, the finding of IGHA2, IGHM, C4A, and C4B was probably reflective of synergy in intrahepatic and intra-adipose tissue antibody production as a systemic response to regulation of immune homeostasis and inflammation.

The protein with the highest correlation score was fetal hemoglobin gamma chain (HBG1). Under normal physiological conditions (except pregnancy), fetal hemoglobin only exists in very limited amounts in adults, comprising < 0.6% of total hemoglobin [50]. The synthesis of fetal hemoglobin, which has higher oxygen affinity than hemoglobin, is confined to a population of erythrocytes termed the F-cells [50]. The presence of HBG1 and the high correlation score of 0.717 between the two tissues can only be speculative as there are very limited data on adult fetal hemoglobin in conditions other than β-thalassemia and sickle cell anemia. Also, we have not investigated the specific intensities of HBG1 between MASLD groups and CON in VAT and liver. We can only speculate as to whether severe obesity and/or metabolic disease perhaps induce an increase in F-cell erythrocytes that are capable of producing hemoglobin gamma-chains. Further research into this finding is warranted.

4.4. Changes in the Liver Proteome in Relation to Obesity and MASLD

In the liver tissue we found a couple of DEPs that were upregulated or downregulated in MASH and LS+ exclusively, but it was difficult to conclude on any specific patterns as the DEPs were very heterogenous in both function and cellular compartment. However, we did observe a tendency of the upregulated proteins to be related to lipid and cholesterol metabolism (OLA1, ACLY, MVK, HPGD, APOL3, PLIN1, and PLIN2) and to cytoskeleton and ECM reorganization (COL18A1, RDX, and MSN). Upregulation of ECM proteins in MASLD has been recognized in a study by Yuan and colleagues, who analyzed the liver tissue proteome from 12 patients with obesity classified as metabolically healthy but with obesity and 44 patients with obesity and MASLD according to liver histology [23]. By gene ontology analysis, they furthermore report significant downregulation of mitochondrial oxidative phosphorylation through downregulation of components of the complex I (NADH dehydrogenase complex) and complex IV (cytochrome c oxidase) in MASLD subjects. In comparison, we found significant downregulation of complex III (CYC1), but this downregulation was equal in all MASLD groups compared with CON.

We have previously investigated the plasma proteome in a study cohort comprising 48 individuals with and without MASLD and liver cirrhosis and validated a promising panel of plasma proteins in a mouse model [18]. Among the promising proteins we found the polymeric immunoglobin receptor PIGR to be significantly upregulated in MASLD and to increase with increase in liver disease (individuals with obesity but without MASLD, T2DM with MASLD, and patients with cirrhosis). PIGR is a transmembrane glycoprotein, a Fc receptor, that enables transcytosis of immunoglobulins from the basolateral to the apical surface of epithelial cells, thus mediating the secretion of IgA and IgM [51]. We did not confirm the findings of upregulated PIGR in the present data in either liver or adipose tissue. However, we did discover MAL proteolipid protein 2 (MAL2) to be roughly eight-fold increased in all three MASLD groups compared with CON. MAL2 was the protein showing the biggest difference in intensities between groups. This is interesting because MAL2 is an essential component of the transcytotic machinery [52,53] and has previously been implicated in PIGR-mediated transcytosis, where depletion of MAL2 blocked polymeric immunoglobulin receptor transcytosis in liver cells (the hep g2 cell line) [52]. Although data derived from cell lines should be evaluated with some caution, the potential association between MAL2 in VAT and PIGR found in plasma in two different MASLD cohorts is still noteworthy. Adding to this notion, the proteins with the second and the sixth strongest correlations between VAT and liver tissue were the heavy chains of precisely IgA and IgM (IGHA2 and IGHM, respectively).

4.5. Strengths and Limitations

We wanted to explore potential overlapping DEPs in MASH between VAT and liver and to characterize the VAT proteome in MASH. The rationale was to assess common pathophysiological traits in the two tissues. However, this exploratory approach has limitations, which may hinder the true answer(s) to the hypotheses. In addition, as this is a descriptive, cross-sectional study, no causal associations can be made. By stratifying the study cohort based on liver histology and applying one-way ANOVA, we may also have missed interesting and significant proteins.

There are also some inherent drawbacks in proteomics studies in general. For instance, the generated data depend on the subjective threshold set for DEPs. In addition, the analysis discards most of the proteins and as a result focuses on the significant DEPs, which comprise only <0.1% of the analyzed total proteome in the respective tissues. Furthermore, by filtering for 70% (meaning that only proteins that are detectable in 70% of the samples enter the analysis), there is an inherent risk of filtering out proteins that were indeed significant in one group only. We may therefore have missed important proteins in one or more of the groups. Finally, the grouping of the study subjects according to the histopathological MASLD severity may pinpoint the weaknesses of the NAFLD activity score as we observe very little difference in protein expression between the MASLD groups, particularly between LS+ and MASH.

Proteomics studies and the generated data herein are in general difficult to compare due to significant heterogeneity in endpoints, grouping, analytical methodology (e.g., targeted vs. untargeted approach), and data acquisition (use of FDR and considerations regarding significance). In addition, many studies have very low values of n, down to 4 per group [39], but typically, n is around 10 per group. In comparison, our cohort consisted of 79 study subjects, and the applied LC-MS analyses performed were of very high quality and robustness.

5. Conclusions

This study represents the largest human investigation to date evaluating the proteome profiles of visceral adipose tissue (VAT) and liver tissue in individuals with obesity, MASLD, and MASH. Contrary to our hypothesis, we did not identify overlapping DEPs between VAT and liver tissue, nor did we find a VAT-specific proteomic signature that clearly distinguished MASLD severity. Instead, the proteomic patterns in VAT appeared to reflect metabolic dysfunction associated with obesity rather than MASLD progression. Notably, while some inflammatory and metabolic proteins showed significant correlations between VAT and liver, these did not translate into a unified proteomic profile linking the two tissues in MASLD pathology. The identification of proteins such as SQOR and MAL2 raises interesting mechanistic questions, particularly in relation to mitochondrial function and immune regulation, warranting further investigation. Given the heterogeneity of proteomic findings across MASLD groups and the potential influence of methodological constraints, future studies with refined proteomic analyses and larger, more targeted cohorts will be critical for uncovering definitive biomarkers and elucidating the complex metabolic interplay between VAT and liver in MASLD and MASH progression.

Author Contributions: Conceptualization, J.S.P. and N.J.W.A.; formal analysis, J.S.P. and L.N.; funding acquisition, T.H. and F.B.; investigation, J.S.P., V.B.K., I.M.P. and R.R.S.; methodology, J.S.P., L.N., V.B.K., R.R.S., L.L.G. and F.B.; project administration, J.S.P., T.H. and F.B.; resources, L.L.G. and F.B.; software, L.N. and N.J.W.A.; supervision, T.H., L.L.G., S.M. and F.B.; validation, L.N. and N.J.W.A.; visualization, L.N.; writing—original draft, J.S.P.; writing—review and editing, J.S.P., L.N., N.J.W.A., V.B.K., I.M.P., R.R.S., T.H., L.L.G., S.M. and F.B. All authors have read and agreed to the published version of the manuscript.

Funding: This research was funded by a Challenge Grant "MicroBLiver" (grant number NNF15OC 0016692) from the Novo Nordisk Foundation.

Institutional Review Board Statement: The study protocols were approved by the Regional Scientific Ethics Committee (H-16030784 and H-16030782) in the Capital Region of Denmark and the Danish Data Protection Agency.

Informed Consent Statement: The study was conducted in accordance with the Declaration of Helsinki. Oral and written informed consent were obtained from all study participants.

Data Availability Statement: The data presented in this study are available on request from the corresponding author. The data are not publicly available due to restrictions set by the Danish Data Protection Agency.

Acknowledgments: We would like to thank the MicroBLiver Research Consortium and project nurse Karen Lisa Hilsted.

Conflicts of Interest: The authors declare no conflicts of interest.

References

1. Rosen, E.D.; Spiegelman, B.M. What We Talk About When We Talk About Fat. *Cell* **2014**, *156*, 20–44. [CrossRef]
2. Ohlson, L.-O.; Larsson, B.; Svärdsudd, K.; Welin, L.; Eriksson, H.; Wilhelmsen, L.; Björntorp, P.; Tibblin, G. The Influence of Body Fat Distribution on the Incidence of Diabetes Mellitus: 13.5 Years of Follow-up of the Participants in the Study of Men Born in 1913. *Diabetes* **1985**, *34*, 1055–1058. [CrossRef]
3. Nielsen, S.; Guo, Z.; Johnson, C.M.; Hensrud, D.D.; Jensen, M.D. Splanchnic lipolysis in human obesity. *J. Clin. Investig.* **2004**, *113*, 1582–1588. [CrossRef] [PubMed]
4. Tilg, H.; Moschen, A.R. Adipocytokines: Mediators linking adipose tissue, inflammation and immunity. *Nat. Rev. Immunol.* **2006**, *6*, 772–783. [CrossRef] [PubMed]
5. Fontana, L.; Eagon, J.C.; Trujillo, M.E.; Scherer, P.E.; Klein, S. Visceral Fat Adipokine Secretion Is Associated with Systemic Inflammation in Obese Humans. *Diabetes* **2007**, *56*, 1010–1013. [CrossRef] [PubMed]
6. Eckel, R.H.; Grundy, S.M.; Zimmet, P.Z. The metabolic syndrome. *Lancet* **2005**, *365*, 1415–1428. [CrossRef]
7. Vanni, E.; Bugianesi, E.; Kotronen, A.; De Minicis, S.; Yki-Järvinen, H.; Svegliati-Baroni, G. From the metabolic syndrome to NAFLD or vice versa? *Dig. Liver Dis.* **2010**, *42*, 320–330. [CrossRef]
8. Yki-Järvinen, H. Non-alcoholic fatty liver disease as a cause and a consequence of metabolic syndrome. *Lancet Diabetes Endocrinol.* **2014**, *2*, 901–910. [CrossRef]
9. Hotamisligil, G.S.; Shargill, N.S.; Spiegelman, B.M. Adipose expression of tumor necrosis factor-alpha: Direct role in obesity-linked insulin resistance. *Science* **1993**, *259*, 87–91. [CrossRef]
10. Sun, K.; Kusminski, C.M.; Scherer, P.E. Adipose tissue remodeling and obesity. *J. Clin. Investig.* **2011**, *121*, 2094–2101. [CrossRef]
11. Goossens, G.H. The role of adipose tissue dysfunction in the pathogenesis of obesity-related insulin resistance. *Physiol. Behav.* **2008**, *94*, 206–218. [CrossRef]
12. Xu, H.; Barnes, G.T.; Yang, Q.; Tan, G.; Yang, D.; Chou, C.J.; Sole, J.; Nichols, A.; Ross, J.S.; Tartaglia, L.A.; et al. Chronic inflammation in fat plays a crucial role in the development of obesity-related insulin resistance. *J. Clin. Investig.* **2003**, *112*, 1821–1830. [CrossRef] [PubMed]

13. Weisberg, S.P.; McCann, D.; Desai, M.; Rosenbaum, M.; Leibel, R.L.; Ferrante, A.W. Obesity is associated with macrophage accumulation in adipose tissue. *J. Clin. Investig.* **2003**, *112*, 1796–1808. [CrossRef]
14. Younossi, Z.M.; Blissett, D.; Blissett, R.; Henry, L.; Stepanova, M.; Younossi, Y.; Racila, A.; Hunt, S.; Beckerman, R. The economic and clinical burden of nonalcoholic fatty liver disease in the United States and Europe. *Hepatology* **2016**, *64*, 1577–1586. [CrossRef] [PubMed]
15. Item, F.; Konrad, D. Visceral fat and metabolic inflammation: The portal theory revisited: Visceral fat and metabolic inflammation. *Obes. Rev.* **2012**, *13*, 30–39. [CrossRef]
16. Arderiu, G.; Mendieta, G.; Gallinat, A.; Lambert, C.; Díez-Caballero, A.; Ballesta, C.; Badimon, L. Type 2 Diabetes in Obesity: A Systems Biology Study on Serum and Adipose Tissue Proteomic Profiles. *Int. J. Mol. Sci.* **2023**, *24*, 827. [CrossRef]
17. Chen, Z.-Z.; Gao, Y.; Keyes, M.J.; Deng, S.; Mi, M.; Farrell, L.A.; Shen, D.; Tahir, U.A.; Cruz, D.E.; Ngo, D.; et al. Protein Markers of Diabetes Discovered in an African American Cohort. *Diabetes* **2023**, *72*, 532–543. [CrossRef]
18. Niu, L.; Geyer, P.E.; Wewer Albrechtsen, N.J.; Gluud, L.L.; Santos, A.; Doll, S.; Treit, P.V.; Holst, J.J.; Knop, F.K.; Vilsbøll, T.; et al. Plasma proteome profiling discovers novel proteins associated with non-alcoholic fatty liver disease. *Mol. Syst. Biol.* **2019**, *15*, e8793. [CrossRef]
19. Sanyal, A.J.; Williams, S.A.; Lavine, J.E.; Neuschwander-Tetri, B.A.; Alexander, L.; Ostroff, R.; Biegel, H.; Kowdley, K.V.; Chalasani, N.; Dasarathy, S.; et al. Defining the serum proteomic signature of hepatic steatosis, inflammation, ballooning and fibrosis in non-alcoholic fatty liver disease. *J. Hepatol.* **2023**, *78*, 693–703. [CrossRef]
20. Bell, L.N.; Theodorakis, J.L.; Vuppalanchi, R.; Saxena, R.; Bemis, K.G.; Wang, M.; Chalasani, N. Serum proteomics and biomarker discovery across the spectrum of nonalcoholic fatty liver disease. *Hepatology* **2010**, *51*, 111–120. [CrossRef]
21. Govaere, O.; Hasoon, M.; Alexander, L.; Cockell, S.; Tiniakos, D.; Ekstedt, M.; Schattenberg, J.M.; Boursier, J.; Bugianesi, E.; Ratziu, V.; et al. A proteo-transcriptomic map of non-alcoholic fatty liver disease signatures. *Nat. Metab.* **2023**, *5*, 572–578. [CrossRef] [PubMed]
22. Luo, Y.; Wadhawan, S.; Greenfield, A.; Decato, B.E.; Oseini, A.M.; Collen, R.; Shevell, D.E.; Thompson, J.; Jarai, G.; Charles, E.D.; et al. SOMAscan Proteomics Identifies Serum Biomarkers Associated with Liver Fibrosis in Patients With NASH. *Hepatol. Commun.* **2021**, *5*, 760–773. [CrossRef] [PubMed]
23. Yuan, X.; Sun, Y.; Cheng, Q.; Hu, K.; Ye, J.; Zhao, Y.; Wu, J.; Shao, X.; Fang, L.; Ding, Y.; et al. Proteomic analysis to identify differentially expressed proteins between subjects with metabolic healthy obesity and non-alcoholic fatty liver disease. *J. Proteomics* **2020**, *221*, 103683. [CrossRef]
24. Boel, F.; Akimov, V.; Teuchler, M.; Terkelsen, M.K.; Wernberg, C.W.; Larsen, F.T.; Hallenborg, P.; Lauridsen, M.M.; Krag, A.; Mandrup, S.; et al. Deep proteome profiling of metabolic dysfunction-associated steatotic liver disease. *Commun. Med.* **2025**, *5*, 56. [CrossRef]
25. Kakehashi, A.; Stefanov, V.E.; Ishii, N.; Okuno, T.; Fujii, H.; Kawai, K.; Kawada, N.; Wanibuchi, H. Proteome Characteristics of Non-Alcoholic Steatohepatitis Liver Tissue and Associated Hepatocellular Carcinomas. *Int. J. Mol. Sci.* **2017**, *18*, 434. [CrossRef]
26. Nakamura, N.; Hatano, E.; Iguchi, K.; Sato, M.; Kawaguchi, H.; Ohtsu, I.; Sakurai, T.; Aizawa, N.; Iijima, H.; Nishiguchi, S.; et al. Elevated levels of circulating ITIH4 are associated with hepatocellular carcinoma with nonalcoholic fatty liver disease: From pig model to human study. *BMC Cancer* **2019**, *19*, 621. [CrossRef] [PubMed]
27. Younossi, Z.M.; Karrar, A.; Pierobon, M.; Birerdinc, A.; Stepanova, M.; Abdelatif, D.; Younoszai, Z.; Jeffers, T.; Felix, S.; Jeiran, K.; et al. An exploratory study examining how nano-liquid chromatography–mass spectrometry and phosphoproteomics can differentiate patients with advanced fibrosis and higher percentage collagen in non-alcoholic fatty liver disease. *BMC Med.* **2018**, *16*, 170. [CrossRef]
28. Wichmann, C.; Meier, F.; Virreira Winter, S.; Brunner, A.-D.; Cox, J.; Mann, M. MaxQuant.Live Enables Global Targeting of More Than 25,000 Peptides. *Mol. Cell. Proteomics MCP* **2019**, *18*, 982–994. [CrossRef]
29. Grinfeld, D.; Aizikov, K.; Kreutzmann, A.; Damoc, E.; Makarov, A. Phase-Constrained Spectrum Deconvolution for Fourier Transform Mass Spectrometry. *Anal. Chem.* **2017**, *89*, 1202–1211. [CrossRef]
30. Greenberg, A.S.; Egan, J.J.; Wek, S.A.; Garty, N.B.; Blanchette-Mackie, E.J.; Londos, C. Perilipin, a major hormonally regulated adipocyte-specific phosphoprotein associated with the periphery of lipid storage droplets. *J. Biol. Chem.* **1991**, *266*, 11341–11346. [CrossRef]
31. Karvar, S.; Ansa-Addo, E.A.; Suda, J.; Singh, S.; Zhu, L.; Li, Z.; Rockey, D.C. Moesin, an Ezrin/Radixin/Moesin Family Member, Regulates Hepatic Fibrosis. *Hepatology* **2019**, *72*, 1073–1084. [CrossRef] [PubMed]
32. Li, F.; Xiao, H.; Zhou, F.; Hu, Z.; Yang, B. Study of HSPB6: Insights into the Properties of the Multifunctional Protective Agent. *Cell. Physiol. Biochem.* **2017**, *44*, 314–332. [CrossRef]
33. Jackson, M.R.; Melideo, S.L.; Jorns, M.S. Human sulfide: Quinone oxidoreductase catalyzes the first step in hydrogen sulfide metabolism and produces a sulfane sulfur metabolite. *Biochemistry* **2012**, *51*, 6804–6815. [CrossRef]
34. Paul, B.D.; Snyder, S.H. H2S: A novel gasotransmitter that signals by sulfhydration. *Trends Biochem. Sci.* **2015**, *40*, 687. [CrossRef]

35. Younossi, Z.M.; Koenig, A.B.; Abdelatif, D.; Fazel, Y.; Henry, L.; Wymer, M. Global epidemiology of nonalcoholic fatty liver disease—Meta-analytic assessment of prevalence, incidence, and outcomes. *Hepatology* **2016**, *64*, 73–84. [CrossRef]
36. Castañé, H.; Jiménez-Franco, A.; Hernández-Aguilera, A.; Martínez-Navidad, C.; Cambra-Cortés, V.; Onoiu, A.-I.; Jiménez-Aguilar, J.M.; París, M.; Hernández, M.; Parada, D.; et al. Multi-omics profiling reveals altered mitochondrial metabolism in adipose tissue from patients with metabolic dysfunction-associated steatohepatitis. *eBioMedicine* **2025**, *111*, 105532. [CrossRef] [PubMed]
37. Fang, L.; Kojima, K.; Zhou, L.; Crossman, D.K.; Mobley, J.A.; Grams, J. Analysis of the Human Proteome in Subcutaneous and Visceral Fat Depots in Diabetic and Non-diabetic Patients with Morbid Obesity. *J. Proteomics Bioinform.* **2015**, *8*, 133–141. [CrossRef] [PubMed]
38. Kim, S.-J.; Chae, S.; Kim, H.; Mun, D.-G.; Back, S.; Choi, H.Y.; Park, K.S.; Hwang, D.; Choi, S.H.; Lee, S.-W. A Protein Profile of Visceral Adipose Tissues Linked to Early Pathogenesis of Type 2 Diabetes Mellitus. *Mol. Cell. Proteomics MCP* **2014**, *13*, 811–822. [CrossRef]
39. Gómez-Serrano, M.; Camafeita, E.; García-Santos, E.; López, J.A.; Rubio, M.A.; Sánchez-Pernaute, A.; Torres, A.; Vázquez, J.; Peral, B. Proteome-wide alterations on adipose tissue from obese patients as age-, diabetes- and gender-specific hallmarks. *Sci. Rep.* **2016**, *6*, 25756. [CrossRef]
40. Alfadda, A.A.; Masood, A.; Al-Naami, M.Y.; Chaurand, P.; Benabdelkamel, H. A Proteomics Based Approach Reveals Differential Regulation of Visceral Adipose Tissue Proteins between Metabolically Healthy and Unhealthy Obese Patients. *Mol. Cells* **2017**, *40*, 685–695. [CrossRef]
41. Insenser, M.; Montes-Nieto, R.; Vilarrasa, N.; Lecube, A.; Simó, R.; Vendrell, J.; Escobar-Morreale, H.F. A nontargeted proteomic approach to the study of visceral and subcutaneous adipose tissue in human obesity. *Mol. Cell. Endocrinol.* **2012**, *363*, 10–19. [CrossRef] [PubMed]
42. Murri, M.; Insenser, M.; Bernal-Lopez, M.R.; Perez-Martinez, P.; Escobar-Morreale, H.F.; Tinahones, F.J. Proteomic analysis of visceral adipose tissue in pre-obese patients with type 2 diabetes. *Mol. Cell. Endocrinol.* **2013**, *376*, 99–106. [CrossRef]
43. Shang, C.; Sun, W.; Wang, C.; Wang, X.; Zhu, H.; Wang, L.; Yang, H.; Wang, X.; Gong, F.; Pan, H. Comparative Proteomic Analysis of Visceral Adipose Tissue in Morbidly Obese and Normal Weight Chinese Women. *Int. J. Endocrinol.* **2019**, *2019*, 2302753. [CrossRef] [PubMed]
44. Tansey, J.T.; Sztalryd, C.; Gruia-Gray, J.; Roush, D.L.; Zee, J.V.; Gavrilova, O.; Reitman, M.L.; Deng, C.X.; Li, C.; Kimmel, A.R.; et al. Perilipin ablation results in a lean mouse with aberrant adipocyte lipolysis, enhanced leptin production, and resistance to diet-induced obesity. *Proc. Natl. Acad. Sci. USA* **2001**, *98*, 6494–6499. [CrossRef]
45. Orlicky, D.J.; Libby, A.E.; Bales, E.S.; McMahan, R.H.; Monks, J.; Rosa, F.G.; McManaman, J.L. Perilipin-2 promotes obesity and progressive fatty liver disease in mice through mechanistically distinct hepatocyte and extra-hepatocyte actions. *J. Physiol.* **2019**, *597*, 1565–1584. [CrossRef]
46. Straub, B.K.; Stoeffel, P.; Heid, H.; Zimbelmann, R.; Schirmacher, P. Differential pattern of lipid droplet-associated proteins and de novo perilipin expression in hepatocyte steatogenesis. *Hepatology* **2008**, *47*, 1936–1946. [CrossRef]
47. Schöttl, T.; Pachl, F.; Giesbertz, P.; Daniel, H.; Kuster, B.; Fromme, T.; Klingenspor, M. Proteomic and Metabolite Profiling Reveals Profound Structural and Metabolic Reorganization of Adipocyte Mitochondria in Obesity. *Obesity* **2020**, *28*, 590–600. [CrossRef] [PubMed]
48. Newgard, C.B.; An, J.; Bain, J.R.; Muehlbauer, M.J.; Stevens, R.D.; Lien, L.F.; Haqq, A.M.; Shah, S.H.; Arlotto, M.; Slentz, C.A.; et al. A Branched-Chain Amino Acid-Related Metabolic Signature that Differentiates Obese and Lean Humans and Contributes to Insulin Resistance. *Cell Metab.* **2009**, *9*, 311–326. [CrossRef]
49. She, P.; Van Horn, C.; Reid, T.; Hutson, S.M.; Cooney, R.N.; Lynch, C.J. Obesity-related elevations in plasma leucine are associated with alterations in enzymes involved in branched chain amino acid (BCAA) metabolism. *Am. J. Physiol. Endocrinol. Metab.* **2007**, *293*, E1552–E1563. [CrossRef]
50. Rochette, J.; Craig, J.E.; Thein, S.L.; Rochette, J. Fetal hemoglobin levels in adults. *Blood Rev.* **1994**, *8*, 213–224. [CrossRef]
51. Brandtzaeg, P. Transport models for secretory IgA and secretory IgM. *Clin. Exp. Immunol.* **1981**, *44*, 221–232. [PubMed]
52. De Marco, M.C.; Martín-Belmonte, F.; Kremer, L.; Albar, J.P.; Correas, I.; Vaerman, J.P.; Marazuela, M.; Byrne, J.A.; Alonso, M.A. MAL2, a novel raft protein of the MAL family, is an essential component of the machinery for transcytosis in hepatoma HepG2 cells. *J. Cell Biol.* **2002**, *159*, 37–44. [CrossRef] [PubMed]
53. De Marco, M.C.; Puertollano, R.; Martínez-Menárguez, J.A.; Alonso, M.A. Dynamics of MAL2 during glycosylphosphatidylinositol-anchored protein transcytotic transport to the apical surface of hepatoma HepG2 cells. *Traffic Cph. Den.* **2006**, *7*, 61–73. [CrossRef] [PubMed]

livers

MDPI

Article

Useful Predictor for Exacerbation of Esophagogastric Varices after Hepatitis C Virus Eradication by Direct-Acting Antivirals

Yuko Nagaoki [1,*], Kenji Yamaoka [2], Yasutoshi Fujii [2], Shinsuke Uchikawa [2], Hatsue Fujino [2], Atsushi Ono [2], Eisuke Murakami [2], Tomokazu Kawaoka [2], Daiki Miki [2], Hiroshi Aikata [3], C. Nelson Hayes [2], Masataka Tsuge [2,*] and Shiro Oka [2]

1 Department of Gastroenterology, Mazda Hospital, Mazda Motor Corporation, Hiroshima 735-8585, Japan
2 Department of Gastroenterology, Graduate School of Biomedical and Health Science, Hiroshima University, Hiroshima 734-8551, Japan; yamaokak@hiroshima-u.ac.jp (K.Y.); fujiiyas@hiroshima-u.ac.jp (Y.F.); shinuchi@hiroshima-u.ac.jp (S.U.); fujino920@hiroshima-u.ac.jp (H.F.); atsushi-o@hiroshima-u.ac.jp (A.O.); emusuke@hiroshima-u.ac.jp (E.M.); kawaokatomo@hiroshima-u.ac.jp (T.K.); daikimiki@hiroshima-u.ac.jp (D.M.); nelsonhayes@hiroshima-u.ac.jp (C.N.H.); oka4683@hiroshima-u.ac.jp (S.O.)
3 Department of Gastroenterology, Hiroshima Prefectural Hospital, Hiroshima 734-8530, Japan; aikatahiroshi@icloud.com
* Correspondence: nagaoki@mazda.co.jp (Y.N.); tsuge@hiroshima-u.ac.jp (M.T.); Tel.: +81-82-565-5000 (Y.N.); +81-82-257-5192 (M.T.)

Abstract: To clarify the risk factors for the aggravation of esophagogastric varices (EGVs) after hepatitis C virus (HCV) eradication with direct-acting antiviral (DAA) therapy, we enrolled 167 consecutive patients with HCV-related compensated cirrhosis who achieved a sustained virological response (SVR) after DAA therapy. During a median of 69 months, EGVs were aggravated in 42 (25%) patients despite SVR. The cumulative 1-, 3-, 5-, and 10-year aggravated EGV rates were 7%, 23%, 25%, and 27%, respectively. Multivariate analysis identified a platelet count $< 11.0 \times 10^4/\mu L$, LSM ≥ 18.0 kPa, total bile acid ≥ 33.0 µmol/L, and a diameter of left gastric vein (LGV) ≥ 5.0 mm at HCV eradication as independent risk factors for EGV aggravation post-SVR. In groups that met all of these risks, the cumulative EGV aggravation rates at 1, 3, and 5 years were 27%, 87%, and 91%, respectively. However, none of the patients who had only one or none of the risk factors experienced EGV aggravation. Platelet count, LSM, total bile acid, and diameter of LGV at HCV eradication were associated with aggravated EGV post-SVR. EGVs tend to worsen as two or more of these risk factors increase.

Keywords: direct-acting antiviral; sustained virological response; esophagogastric varices; liver stiffness measurement; total bile acid; left gastric vein

1. Introduction

The achievement of sustained virological response (SVR) in patients with chronic hepatitis C virus (HCV) infection reduces the risk of progressing to liver decompensation and hepatocellular carcinoma (HCC), leading to improved survival [1]. Hepatic function in patients with SVR could gradually recover with a long-term maintenance of normalized hepatic enzyme levels and a regression of hepatic liver necrosis, inflammation, and fibrosis [2]. Portal hypertension is a major consequence of cirrhosis and is responsible for its most severe complications, including ascites, bleeding from esophagogastric varices (EGVs), and portosystemic encephalopathy. SVR achievement by direct-acting antiviral (DAA) therapy was reported to decrease portal venous pressures [3–7], which is expected to reduce the risk of portal hypertension in liver cirrhosis patients with HCV infection.

However, if portal hypertension or EGVs have already developed prior to DAA therapy, or if collateral vessels are dilated, symptoms associated with portal hypertension might be difficult to improve even if SVR is achieved. We have previously reported that patients with HCV-related cirrhosis who had already developed collateral vessels may experience an aggravation of EGVs or develop portosystemic encephalopathy after they achieve SVR [8]. Tsuji et al. also reported that even if SVR was achieved with DAA therapy, patients with HCV-related compensated cirrhosis who had already developed portosystemic shunt showed little improvement in liver function [9]. Therefore, careful follow-up is necessary for liver cirrhosis patients with portal hypertension even after achieving SVR. On the other hand, risk factors for complications associated with worsening portal hypertension after SVR remain unclear.

In portal hypertension, it is important to evaluate the status of portal venous pressure, and hepatic venous pressure gradient (HVPG) is used as an estimate [10]. However, the measurement of HVPG is invasive. Therefore, we decided to use non-invasive testing to elucidate the risk factors for worsening portal hypertension after SVR in HCV-related cirrhosis patients. In the present study, in addition to liver stiffness, platelet count, and diameter of portosystemic collateral vessels, we also analyzed autotaxin and bile acid levels as liver fibrosis markers. In particular, although autotaxin has recently been reported as a new liver fibrosis marker that increases from the early stage of fibrosis and has a high diagnostic ability [11], there are few reports on the relationship between bile acid and complications in portal hypertension.

In this study, we retrospectively analyzed the risk factors for worsening portal hypertension in patients with HCV-related cirrhosis after eradicating HCV.

2. Materials and Methods

2.1. Patients

We enrolled 167 patients with HCV-related cirrhosis who achieved SVR following DAA therapy at Hiroshima University Hospital between May 2010 and March 2020. Patients whose serum HCV RNA was undetectable 24 weeks after the end of DAA therapy (EOT) were diagnosed as SVR. All patients underwent regular surveillance via liver function tests, ultrasonography, dynamic computed tomography (CT), and endoscopic examinations. All patients provided written informed consent to participate in the study in accordance with the ethical guidelines of the Declaration of Helsinki and with a program approved by the ethics committee of Hiroshima University Hospital (Approval No. E-873).

2.2. Clinical and Laboratory Assessments

This study included patients with compensated cirrhosis. Cirrhosis was assessed based on liver imaging tests or prior liver biopsy showing F4. Patients with Child–Pugh class A scores without a history of decompensated events were considered to have compensated cirrhosis, and patients with Child–Pugh class B or C or patients with a history of decompensated events were considered to have decompensated cirrhosis. This study did not include patients with decompensated cirrhosis. Laboratory assessment was performed before treatment and at 24 weeks, and 1, 2, and 3 years after the EOT. In addition to general biochemical tests, autotaxin and bile acids were also included, and the albumin–bilirubin (ALBI) score and fibrosis-4 (FIB-4) index, which serve as surrogate markers of hepatic spare ability and liver fibrosis, respectively, were calculated as previously reported [12,13].

2.3. Measurement of Liver Stiffness

We measured the severity of liver stiffness measurement (LSM) before DAA therapy, at 24 weeks (SVR achievement), and 1, 2, and 3 years after DAA therapy using vibration-controlled transient elastography (VCTE). Patients were placed in a supine position with the right hand at the most abducted position for scanning the right lobe of the liver [14]. When at least 10 valid measurements were obtained with valid measurements at $\geq$60% and an interquartile range of <30%, such measurements were considered valid and the median value of these measurements was used for analysis.

2.4. Endoscopic Examination for Assessing EGVs

We evaluated the endoscopic findings of EGVs based on the classification of the Japanese Society for Portal Hypertension and Esophageal Varices [15]. The different forms (F) of EGVs were classified as follows: F0 was treated and completely treated, with no varices; F1 was straight and relatively thin; F2 was beaded and moderately thick; and F3 was thick, nodular, or mass-like. There are three types of red color (RC) sign: red wale marking, cherry red spot, and hematocystic spot. RC1 was observed only in one-line varices, RC2 was observed between RC1 and RC3, and RC3 was observed in all circumferential varices. Endoscopy was performed within 6 months before starting antiviral therapy and was evaluated at least once during each following year. Compared with baseline findings on follow-up endoscopy, a worsening of F and RC signs was defined as an aggravation of EGVs. The endoscopy results were confirmed by two expert endoscopists.

2.5. CT Examination for Portal Hypertension

All patients underwent CT examination 24 weeks after EOT achievement. CT was performed in the high-quality scanning mode. We focused on the left gastric vein (LGV) and splenorenal shunt as portosystemic collateral vessels, and these vessels were evaluated by dynamic CT, measuring the vessel diameter and recording the widest part of the vessel in all cases in this study.

2.6. Statistical Analysis

Continuous variables were expressed as median and range. Continuous variables were analyzed using the Mann–Whitney U-test. Aggravated EGVs were calculated using the Kaplan–Meier method, and differences between groups were assessed using a log-rank test. Multivariate analysis was performed using a Cox proportional hazard model with a stepwise selection of variables or two logistic regression analyses. Receiver operating characteristic curves were used to determine the cutoff values for predicting the aggravated EGV-related events in the patients. All statistical analyses were performed using IBM SPSS version 23.0 and $p < 0.05$ was considered significant.

3. Results

3.1. Baseline Characteristics of the Patients

The baseline characteristics of the 167 patients are shown in Table 1. The present study included 82 men and 85 women, with a median age of 74 (range 48–90) years. The median FIB-4 index was 5.98 (range 3.27–26.09), the ALBI score was −2.56 (range −3.43 to −1.28), and the LSM was 18.9 kPa (range 5.6–44.2). Before initiating DAA therapy, 51 of 167 (31%) patients had complications due to EGVs, classified as F1 in 42 (25%) patients and F2 in 9 (5%) patients. The RC sign was not observed in any of the patients with EGVs.

Table 1. Clinical characteristics of 167 patients with HCV-related compensated cirrhosis who achieved SVR by DAA therapy.

Category	
Age, years	74 (48–90)
Sex, male/female	82/85
Body mass index, kg/m^2	22.3 (14.7–39.1)
Total bilirubin, mg/dL	0.8 (0.3–3.6)
Aspartate aminotransferase, IU/L	49 (12–351)
Alanine aminotransferase, IU/L	37 (82–54)
Albumin, g/dL	3.9 (2.3–5.1)
Total cholesterol, mg/dL	140 (75–256)
Ammonia, μg/dL	40 (10–128)
Platelet count, $\times 10^4/\mu$L	9.8 (3.0–29.5)

Table 1. *Cont.*

Category	
Prothrombin activity, %	83 (31–112)
Alfa-fetoprotein, ng/mL	7.3 (1.1–482.9)
FIB-4 index	5.98 (3.27–26.09)
ALBI score	−2.56 (−3.43–−1.28)
Liver stiffness measurement, kPa	18.9 (5.6–44.2)
Total bile acid, μmol/L	32.3 (1.73–17.7)
Autotaxin, mg/L	1.89 (0.76–43.29)
Past history of HCC treatment *, yes/no	89/78
Diameter of left gastric vein, mm	4.9 (2.8–13.9)
Diameter of splenorenal shunt, mm	8.1 (6.7–23.1)
Esophagogastric varices, F1/ F2	41/7
Gastric varices, F1/F2	1/2
DAA regimen, *n*	
Daclatasvir/asunaprevir	81
Sofosbuvir /ledipasvir	31
Ombitasvir/paritaprevir/ritonavir	16
Elbasvir/grazoprevir	6
Daclatasvir/asunaprevir/beclabuvir	1
Sofosbuvir + ribavirin	19
Glecaprevir/pibrentasvir	16

Continuous data are represented as median and range, and categorical data are represented as counts of patients. *, DAA therapy was received after curative treatment for HCC. FIB-4 index, Fibrosis-4 index; ALBI, albumin-bilirubin grade; HCC, hepatocellular carcinoma.

3.2. Aggravated EGVs after Eradicating HCV

During the median follow-up period of 69 (range 3–127) months, EGVs were aggravated in 42 (25%) patients despite achieving SVR. Twelve patients increased from F0 to F1, two patients from F0 to F3, seventeen patients from F1 to F2 or had an appearance of the RC sign, seven patients from F1 to F3 or had an appearance of the RC sign, and four patients from F2 to F3 or had an appearance of the RC sign. The cumulative 1-, 3-, 5-, and 10-year aggravation rates of EGVs were 7%, 23%, 25%, and 27%, respectively (Figure 1). Although HCC recurred in 53 patients, portal vein tumor thrombosis was not observed in any of them.

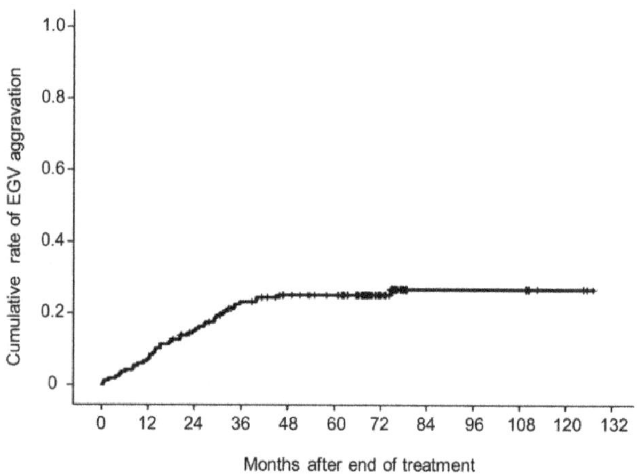

Figure 1. Cumulative rate of esophagogastric varix (EGV) aggravation after the achievement of sustained virological response.

3.3. Changes in Liver Function Test, Serum Fibrosis Markers, and Liver Stiffness after Achieving SVR

Changes in liver function test, serum fibrosis markers, and liver stiffness after SVR depending on the presence or absence of EGV aggravation are shown in Figure 2. In patients without EGV aggravation, the median ALBI score decreased significantly ($p < 0.001$) from −2.59 before treatment to −2.86 at 24 weeks from EOT achievement. One, two, and three years from EOT, the median ALBI score decreased to −2.87, −2.92, and −3.12, respectively, and the improvement in liver function was maintained. The median FIB-4 index decreased significantly ($p < 0.001$) from 5.12 before treatment to 4.19 at 24 weeks from EOT. It decreased to 4.20, 3.86, and 3.14, one, two, and three years from EOT, respectively, and the improvement in liver function was also maintained. The median LSM decreased significantly ($p < 0.001$) from 14.3 kPa before treatment to 12.5 kPa at 24 weeks from EOT, decreasing to 9.2 kPa, 8.9 kPa, and 6.3 kPa, one, two, and three years from EOT, respectively, and the improvement in liver stiffness was maintained. In patients with aggravated EGVs, the median ALBI score decreased significantly ($p < 0.001$) from −2.37 before treatment to −2.72 at 24 weeks from EOT achievement, decreasing to −2.81, −2.81, and −3.12, one, two, and three years from EOT, respectively, and the improvement in liver function was maintained. The median FIB-4 index decreased significantly ($p < 0.001$) from 7.78 before treatment to 6.82 at 24 weeks from EOT achievement and decreased to 5.56, 5.42, and 4.38, one, two, and three years from EOT, respectively. The improvement in liver function was maintained. On the other hand, no significant improvement in LSM was observed, decreasing only slightly from 27.5 kPa before treatment to 27.4 kPa at 24 weeks from EOT and 26.2 kPa even one year from EOT. However, LSM decreased significantly to 22.5 kPa two years from EOT ($p < 0.001$).

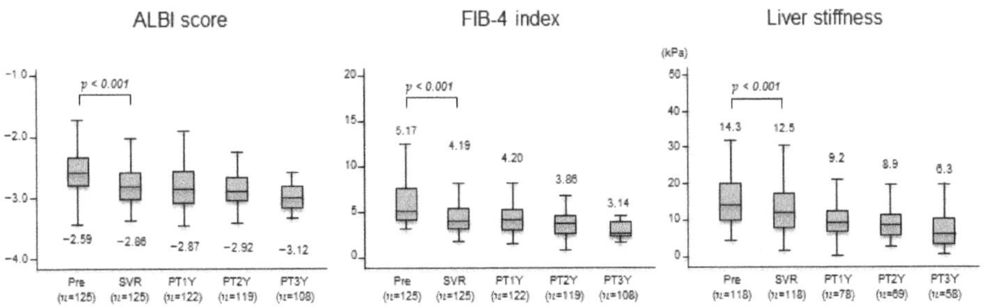

(**a**) without EGV aggravation

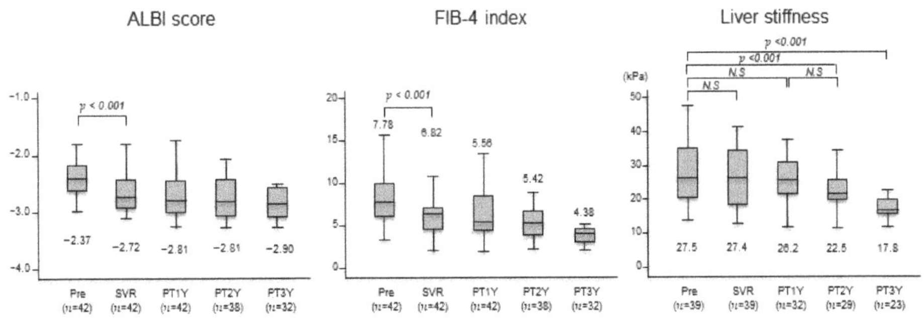

(**b**) with EGV aggravation

Figure 2. Changes in liver function and liver fibrosis following achievement of sustained virological response. Changes in ALBI score, FIB-4 index, and liver stiffness at baseline (Pre), SVR, and one year (PT1Y), two years (PT2Y), and three years (PT3Y) post-treatment in patients with and without aggravation of esophagogastric varices (EGVs). In these box-and-whisker plots, lines within the boxes represent median values. The upper and lower lines of the boxes represent the 75th and 25th percentiles, respectively, and the upper and lower bars outside the boxes represent the 90th and 10th percentiles, respectively.

3.4. Changes in Liver Stiffness after Achieving SVR and Aggravated EGVs after Eradicating HCV by Pretreatment LSM

Because LSM seems to be associated with aggravated EGVs, we analyzed changes in LSM after SVR based on the pretreatment LSM level. In the group of patients with a pretreatment LSM of 15–20 kPa, the median LSM decreased significantly from 18.5 at pretreatment to 13.6 when SVR was achieved ($p < 0.05$) and further reduced to 9.6 and 9.4 kPa at 1 and 2 years from EOT, respectively (Figure 3a). In the group with an LSM of 20–30 kPa, the median LSM decreased significantly from 25.2 at pretreatment to 21.8 when SVR was achieved ($p < 0.05$) and further reduced to 16.9 and 12.6 kPa at 1 and 2 years from EOT, respectively. By contrast, in the group with pretreatment LSM ≥ 30 kPa, the median LSM decreased only slightly from 34.7 at pretreatment to 33.2 when SVR was achieved and 31.6 kPa at 1 year from EOT. These findings indicate that LSM is less likely to improve despite eliminating HCV when pretreatment LSM ≥ 30 kPa. We analyzed the association between aggravated EGVs and pretreatment LSM. The cumulative aggravated EGV rates at 1, 3, and 5 years were 14%, 63%, and 74% for the group with a pretreatment LSM ≥ 30 kPa; 10%, 31%, and 31% for the group with an LSM of 20–30 kPa; 4%, 16%, 16% for the group with an LSM of 15–20 kPa; and 0%, 0%, and 7% for the group with an LSM of 10–15 kPa, respectively (Figure 3b). By contrast, no patients with a pretreatment LSM < 10 kPa had aggravated EGVs ($p < 0.001$).

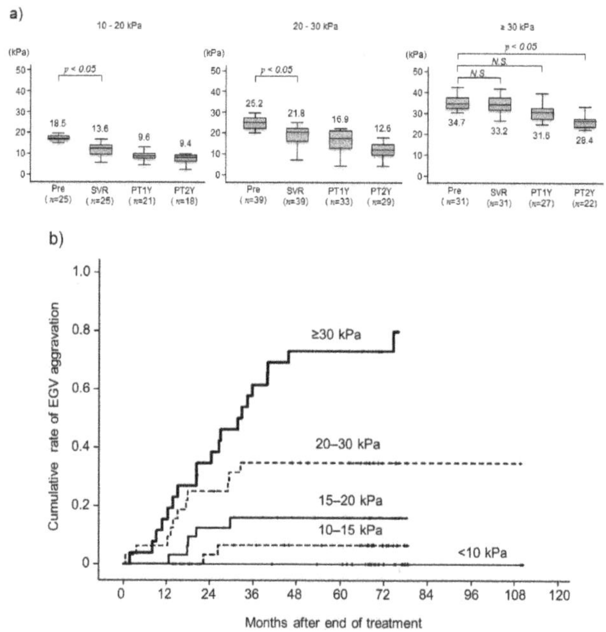

Figure 3. (**a**) Changes in liver stiffness measurement (LSM). Patients were classified into three groups with respect to LSM at the start of antiviral therapy 15–20 kPa, 20–30 kPa, and ≥30 kPa. LSM was measured at baseline (Pre), SVR, one year (PT1Y), and two years (PT2Y). (**b**) Cumulative rate of esophagogastric varix (EGV) aggravation after end of treatment according to liver stiffness measurement (LSM) at the start of antiviral therapy.

3.5. Serum Bile Acid and Predictive Factors Associated With Aggravated EGVs

The total serum bile acid level at 24 weeks from EOT was significantly correlated with LGV diameters (Figure 4). We then analyzed predictors for post-SVR aggravated EGVs, including serum total bile acid. Univariate analysis showed that platelet count, LSM, total bile acid level, autotaxin level, history of HCC, and the diameter of the LGV at 24 weeks from EOT were significantly associated with aggravated EGVs (Table 2). Multivariate analysis identified platelet count < $11.0 \times 10^4/\mu L$ (hazard ratio [HR] 3.769 for $\geq 11.0 \times 10^4/\mu L$, $p = 0.008$), LSM $\geq$ 18.0 kPa (HR 4.834 for <18.0 kPa; $p = 0.006$), total bile acid $\geq$ 33.0 μmol/L (HR 3.341 for <33.0 μmol/L, $p = 0.009$), and the diameter of LGV $\geq$ 5.0 mm when HCV was eradicated (HR 5.891 for <5.0 mm, $p < 0.001$) as independent risk factors for aggravated EGVs after achieving SVR. On the other hand, although the correlation between the LGV diameters at 24 weeks from EOT and autotaxin level is shown in Figure S1, autotaxin level was not a significant factor in multivariate analysis. Receiver operating characteristic curves were generated for both values, and the optimal cutoff values were identified as $11.0 \times 10^4/\mu L$ for platelet count at SVR, with an area under the curve (AUC) of 0.786 ($p < 0.001$), 18.0 kPa for liver stiffness at SVR with an AUC of 0.883 ($p < 0.001$), 5.0 mm for the maximal diameters of the LGV with an AUC of 0.901 ($p < 0.001$), and 33 μmol/L for total bile acid at SVR with an AUC of 0.767 ($p < 0.001$) (Figure 5).

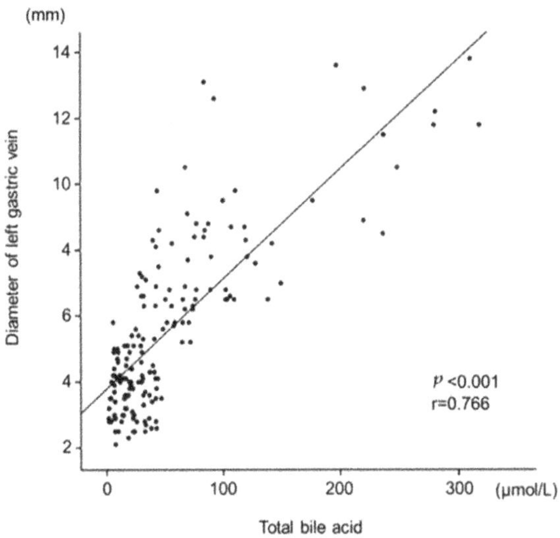

Figure 4. Correlation between the diameter of the left gastric vein and total bile acid at the end of treatment.

Table 2. Univariate and multivariate analyses of risk factors associated with aggravation of esophagogastric varices after eradicating HCV.

Category	Univariate Analysis *p*-Value	Multivariate Analysis HR (95% CI) *p*-Value	
Age, <70/70≤ years	0.559	–	–
Sex, male/female	0.649	–	–
Body mass index, <23/23≤ kg/m^2	0.562	–	–
Total bilirubin, <1.0/1.0≤ mg/dL	0.656	–	–
Aspartate aminotransferase, <30/30≤ IU/L	0.317	–	–

Table 2. *Cont.*

Category	Univariate Analysis *p*-Value	Multivariate Analysis HR (95% CI)	 *p*-Value
Alanine aminotransferase, <20/20≤ IU/L	0.258	–	–
Albumin, <4.2/4.2≤ g/dL	0.086	–	–
Total cholesterol, <170/170≤ mg/dL	0.382	–	–
Ammonia, <40/40≤ μg/dL	0.426	–	–
Platelet count, <11.0/11.0≤ ×10⁴/μL	<0.001	3.769 (1.424–9.977)	0.008
Prothrombin activity, <80/80≤ %	0.351	–	–
Alfa-fetoprotein, <5.0/5.0≤ ng/mL	0.763	–	–
FIB-4 index, <4.39/4.39≤	0.482	–	–
ALBI score, <−2.82/−2.82≤	0.095	–	–
Liver stiffness measurement, <18.0/18.0≤ kPa	<0.001	4.834 (1.706–10.794)	0.006
Total bile acid, <33.0/33.0≤ μmol/L	<0.001	3.341 (1.350–8.173)	0.009
Autotaxin, <1.9/1.9≤ mg/L	0.008	1.921 (0.685–5.832)	0.286
Past history of HCC treatment *, yes/no	0.022	1.532 (0.523–4.386)	0.485
Diameter of left gastric vein, <5.0/5.0≤ mm	<0.001	5.891(2.596–14.228)	<0.001
Diameter of splenorenal shunt, <8.0/8.0≤ mm	0.051	–	–

FIB-4 index, Fibrosis-4 index; ALBI, albumin–bilirubin; HCC, hepatocellular carcinoma; HR, hazard ratio; CI, confidence interval. *, DAA therapy was received after curative treatment for HCC.

We analyzed the cumulative rate of aggravated EGVs according to the number of risk factors. In patients who had all four risk factors, LGV diameter $\geq$ 5.0 mm, LSM $\geq$ 18.0 kPa, platelet count < 11.0 $\times$ $10^4/\mu$L, and total bile acid $\geq$ 33.0 μmol/L, the cumulative EGV aggravation rates at 1, 3, and 5 years were 27%, 87%, and 91%, respectively. In patients with three risk factors, the cumulative aggravation rates at 1, 3, and 5 years were 7%, 40%, and 53%, respectively. In patients with two risk factors, the cumulative aggravation rates at 1, 3, and 5 years were 0%, 12%, and 12%, respectively. By contrast, none of the patients who had zero or one risk factors experienced aggravated EGVs during the observation period (p < 0.001) (Figure 6).

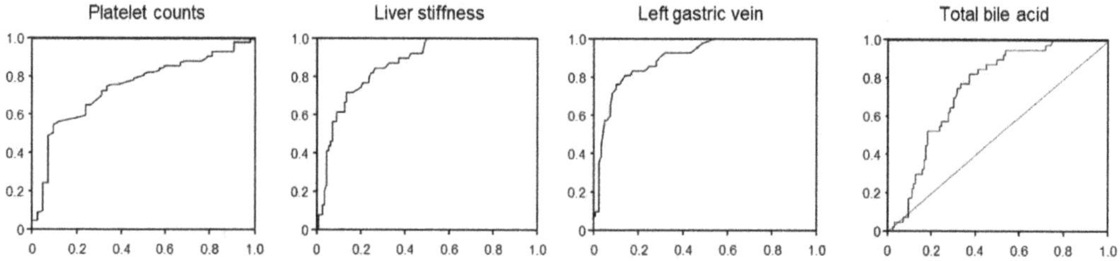

Figure 5. Receiver operating characteristic curves for platelet count, liver stiffness measurement (LSM), diameter of the left gastric vein (LGV), and total bile acid at SVR.

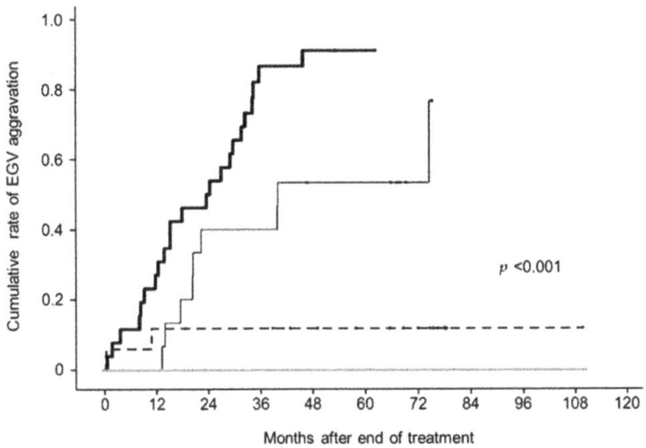

Figure 6. Cumulative rate of esophagogastric varix (EGV) aggravation after the end of treatment. Patients were divided into four groups based on risk factors (the diameter of left gastric vein $\geq$ 5.0 mm, liver stiffness measurement > 18.0 kPa, platelet count < 11.0 $\times$ 10^4/μL, and total bile acid $\geq$ 33.0 μmol/L). Patients having all four risk factors (thick solid line), three risk factors (thin solid line), two risk factors (long dotted line), and with one or no risk factors (gray solid line).

4. Discussion

During the median observation period of 69 months, 42 (25%) patients with HCV-related liver cirrhosis experienced an aggravation of their EGVs despite achieving SVR. This finding is consistent with previous reports that EGVs were aggravated in 13–58% of patients with HCV-related cirrhosis who achieved SVR [16,17].

Liver function and liver fibrosis estimates based on the ALBI score and FIB-4 index improved after SVR regardless of whether EGVs were aggravated. However, the median LSM failed to improve for the first two years when LGV worsened. Moreover, in patients who had LSM $\geq$ 30 kPa before treatment, the median LSM did not decrease until one year from EOT, and subsequently improved by two years from EOT. Furthermore, the cumulative aggravated EGV rates at 1, 3, and 5 years were 14%, 63%, and 74% for the group with a pretreatment LSM $\geq$ 30 kPa, and aggravation rates were significantly higher in the LSM $\geq$ 30 kPa group. Liver stiffness obtained by elastography has been reported to be useful not only for diagnosing liver fibrosis but also for diagnosing portal hypertension, especially clinically significant portal hypertension [18]. LSM is widely used as a non-invasive test for liver cirrhosis and portal hypertension [19]. In this study, the LSM cutoff in Figure 3 was used as a criterion for liver stiffness, and the analysis was performed using the LSM presented in the Baveno VII guideline as a reference [20]. Previously, according to the Baveno VI criteria, if liver stiffness by VCTE is LSM $\leq$ 15.0 kPa and platelet count $\geq$ 15 $\times$ 104/μL, clinically significant portal hypertension is excluded. However, in compensated cirrhosis patients whose liver stiffness with VCTE is LSM $\geq$ 20 kPa and platelet count $\leq$ 15 $\times$ 104 /μL, the presence of clinically significant portal hypertension cannot be ruled out, and upper gastrointestinal endoscopy is proposed [10]. Indeed, as shown in Figure 3a, when liver stiffness is already elevated before DAA therapy, a drastic reduction in liver stiffness is not expected after SVR because a long time is needed to improve liver stiffness, suggesting a high risk of EGV worsening. Furthermore, the aggravation of EGVs has been observed even when LSM was 10–15 kPa, so liver stiffness and platelets alone may not be sufficient; therefore, it is necessary to combine several risk factors to identify the conditions that aggravate EGVs.

Recently, spleen stiffness has been measured in the same way as liver stiffness and is reported to relate to EGV thickness and HVPG [21]. Furthermore, liver stiffness is positively correlated with EGVs in HCV-related cirrhosis patients [22]. Ogasawara et al. reported that liver stiffness 24 weeks after EOT is associated with aggravated EGVs in HCV-related cirrhosis patients after SVR [23]. Based on these observations, we believe it is important to evaluate EGV status before DAA therapy in patients with HCV-related cirrhosis.

This study newly found that total bile acids were associated with the diameter of LGV and were an independent factor for predicting EGV aggravation after SVR. Bile acids are produced in the liver and stored in the gallbladder. After meals, the stored bile acids are released into the small intestine. Approximately 95% of the bile acids in the intestinal tract are reabsorbed and return to the liver through the portal vein as part of the bile acid enterohepatic circulation [24]. Other than that, bile acid concentrations are influenced by absorption from the intestine [25], as well as uptake by hepatocytes [26], hepatic blood flow [27], and renal clearance [28]. Serum total bile acids are elevated in patients with liver cirrhosis [29,30], and portosystemic shunts are associated with elevated serum bile acid in peripheral blood [31,32]. Hayashi et al. measured portal pressure in patients who underwent percutaneous transhepatic portal vein puncture and showed that bile acid levels were positively associated with portal pressure [33]. Certainly, in portal hypertension, it is necessary to understand the status of portal venous pressure, and HVPG is used as a substitute for portal venous pressure [10]. However, since HVPG measurement is invasive and is not currently covered by insurance in Japan, non-invasive tests are needed for evaluating portal hypertension. In this study, we demonstrated the usefulness of total bile acids for indicating the changes in portal hypertension and its progress.

As mentioned above, several cases showed a worsening of EGVs after SVR even though LSM was low at the start of treatment. Therefore, we believe that it is necessary to use multiple factors, including other fibrosis markers, to identify cases with EGV aggravation. Here, we identified the following independent risk factors for post-SVR aggravated EGVs: platelet count $< 11.0 \times 10^4/\mu L$; LSM $\geq$ 18.0 kPa; total bile acid $\geq$ 33.0 μmol/L; and LGV diameter $\geq$ 5.0 mm. These findings are consistent with the Baveno VII guidelines [20], which recommends a surveillance of EGVs based on platelet count and LSM. The existence of EGVs or portosystemic collateral vessels increases the risk of aggravated EGVs and the incidence of portosystemic encephalopathy in patients with HCV-related cirrhosis, even after successfully eradicating HCV through DAA therapy [7–9]. By adding serum bile acid levels to these previously reported factors, the risk of aggravated EGVs can be stratified with higher accuracy. Patients with all four risk factors had a significantly higher risk of aggravated EGVs; thus, strict surveillance by dynamic CT and endoscopic examination is warranted for such patients. By contrast, no patients with one or none of these risk factors developed aggravated EGVs. These patients seem to have an extremely low risk of aggravated EGVs after SVR, suggesting that the surveillance of EGVs is not needed for such patients.

5. Conclusions

In conclusion, we found that even among patients who successfully achieved SVR following DAA therapy, portal hypertension did not immediately improve in patients with compensated liver cirrhosis, particularly those with at least two of the following risk factors: LGV diameter $\geq$ 5.0 mm, LSM > 18.0 kPa, platelet count $< 11.0 \times 10^4/\mu L$, and total bile acid $\geq$ 33.0 μmol/L. These patients may require monitoring for aggravated EGVs after SVR is achieved.

Supplementary Materials: The following supporting information can be downloaded at: https://www.mdpi.com/article/10.3390/livers4030025/s1, Figure S1. Correlation between the diameter of left gastric vein and autotaxin at the end of treatment.

Author Contributions: Conception and design: Y.N., M.T., H.A. and S.O.; Acquisition of data: Y.N., K.Y., Y.F., S.U., H.F., A.O., E.M., T.K., D.M., M.T., H.A. and S.O.; Analysis and interpretation of data: Y.N.; Drafting of the manuscript: Y.N.; Statistical analysis: Y.N.; Study supervision: C.N.H., M.T., H.A. and S.O.; Critical revision of the manuscript: M.T., H.A., C.N.H. and S.O. All authors have read and agreed to the published version of the manuscript. All authors agreed to be accountable for all aspects of the work in ensuring that questions related to the accuracy or integrity of any part of the work are appropriately investigated and resolved.

Funding: This study did not receive any funding.

Institutional Review Board Statement: All patients provided written informed consent to participate in the study in accordance with the ethical guidelines of the Declaration of Helsinki and in accordance with a program approved by the ethics committee of Hiroshima University Hospital.

Informed Consent Statement: All patients provided written informed consent to participate in the study in accordance with the ethical guidelines of the Declaration of Helsinki.

Data Availability Statement: All data generated or analyzed during this study are included in the published article.

Acknowledgments: The authors thank Emi Nishio for clerical assistance.

Conflicts of Interest: All authors declare no competing interests. Yuko Nagaoki is an employee of Mazda Motor Corporation. This paper did not receive support in the design of the experiment of this manuscript, provide materials and equipment, or funding support.

References

1. Carrat, F.; Fontaine, H.; Dorival, C.; Simony, M.; Diallo, A.; Hezode, C.; De Ledinghen, V.; Larrey, D.; Haour, G.; Bronowicki, J.; et al. Clinical outcomes in patients with chronic hepatitis C after direct-acting antiviral treatment: A prospective cohort study. *Lancet* **2019**, *393*, 1453–1464. [CrossRef] [PubMed]
2. Mauro, E.; Crespo, G.; Montironi, C.; Londoño, M.C.; Hernández-Gea, V.; Ruiz, P.; Lombardo, J.; Mariño, Z.; Díaz, A.; Colmenero, J.; et al. Portal pressure and liver stiffness measurements in the prediction of fibrosis regression after sustained virological response in recurrent hepatitis C. *Hepatology* **2018**, *67*, 1683–1694. [CrossRef] [PubMed]
3. Mandorfer, M.; Kozbial, K.; Schwabl, P.; Freissmuth, C.; Schwarzer, R.; Stern, R.; Chromy, D.; Stättermayer, A.F.; Reiberger, T.; Beinhardt, S.; et al. Sustained virologic response to interferon-free therapies ameliorates HCV-induced portal hypertension. *J. Hepatol.* **2016**, *65*, 692–699. [CrossRef] [PubMed]
4. Afdhal, N.; Everson, G.T.; Calleja, J.L.; McCaughan, G.W.; Bosch, J.; Brainard, D.M.; McHutchison, J.G.; De-Oertel, S.; An, D.; Charlton, M.; et al. Effect of viral suppression on hepatic venous pressure gradient in hepatitis C with cirrhosis and portal hypertension. *J. Viral Hepatol.* **2017**, *24*, 823–831. [CrossRef] [PubMed]
5. Lens, S.; Alvarado-Tapias, E.; Mariño, Z.; Londoño, M.C.; LLop, E.; Martinez, J.; Fortea, J.I.; Ibañez, L.; Ariza, X.; Baiges, A.; et al. Effects of all-oral anti-viral therapy on HVPG and systemic hemodynamics in patients with hepatitis C virus-associated cirrhosis. *Gastroenterology* **2017**, *153*, 1273–1283. [CrossRef] [PubMed]
6. Mandorfer, M.; Kozbial, K.; Schwabl, P.; Chromy, D.; Semmler, G.; Stättermayer, A.F.; Pinter, M.; Hernández-Gea, V.; Fritzer-Szekeres, M.; Steindl-Munda, P.; et al. Changes in hepatic venous pressure gradient predict hepatic decompensation in patients who achieved sustained virologic response to interferon-free therapy. *Hepatology* **2020**, *71*, 1023–1036. [CrossRef] [PubMed]
7. Nagaoki, Y.; Aikata, H.; Kobayashi, T.; Fukuhara, T.; Masaki, K.; Tanaka, M.; Naeshiro, N.; Nakahara, T.; Honda, Y.; Miyaki, D.; et al. Risk factors for the exacerbation of esophageal varices or portosystemic encephalopathy after sustained virological response with IFN therapy for HCV-related compensated cirrhosis. *J. Gastroenterol.* **2013**, *48*, 847–855. [CrossRef] [PubMed]
8. Nagaoki, Y.; Imamura, M.; Teraoka, Y.; Morio, K.; Fujino, H.; Ono, A.; Nakahara, T.; Murakami, E.; Yamauchi, M.; Kawaoka, T.; et al. Impact of viral eradication by direct-acting antivirals on the risk of hepatocellular carcinoma development, prognosis, and portal hypertension in hepatitis C virus-related compensated cirrhosis patients. *Hepatol. Res.* **2020**, *50*, 1222–1233. [CrossRef] [PubMed]
9. Tsuji, S.; Uchida, Y.; Uemura, H.; Kouyama, J.I.; Naiki, K.; Nakao, M.; Motoya, D.; Sugawara, K.; Nakayama, N.; Imai, Y.; et al. Involvement of portosystemic shunts in impaired improvement of liver function after direct-acting antiviral therapies in cirrhotic patients with hepatitis C virus. *Hepatol. Res.* **2020**, *50*, 512–523. [CrossRef]
10. de Franchis, R. Expanding consensus in portal hypertension: Report of the Baveno VI Consensus Workshop: Stratifying risk and individualizing care for portal hypertension. *J. Hepatol.* **2015**, *63*, 743–752. [CrossRef]
11. Shao, X.; Uojima, H.; Setsu, T.; Okubo, T.; Atsukawa, M.; Furuichi, Y.; Arase, Y.; Hidaka, H.; Tanaka, Y.; Nakazawa, T.; et al. Usefulness of autotaxin for the complications of liver cirrhosis. *World J. Gastroenterol.* **2020**, *26*, 97–108. [CrossRef]
12. Johnson, P.J.; Berhane, S.; Kagebayashi, C.; Satomura, S.; Teng, M.; Reeves, H.L.; O'Beirne, J.; Fox, R.; Skowronska, A.; Palmer, D.; et al. Assessment of liver function in patients with hepatocellular carcinoma: A new evidence-based approach-the ALBI grade. *Clin. Oncol.* **2015**, *33*, 550–558. [CrossRef]
13. Sterling, R.K.; Lissen, E.; Clumeck, N.; Sola, R.; Correa, M.C.; Montaner, J.; Sulkowski, M.S.; Torriani, F.J.; Dieterich, D.T.; Thomas, D.L.; et al. Development of a simple noninvasive index to predict significant fibrosis in patients with HIV/HCV coinfection. *Hepatology* **2006**, *43*, 1317–1325. [CrossRef] [PubMed]

14. Sandrin, L.; Fourquet, B.; Hasquenoph, J.M.; Yon, S.; Fournier, C.; Mal, F.; Christidis, C.; Ziol, M.; Poulet, B.; Kazemi, F.; et al. Transient elastography: A new noninvasive method for assessment of hepatic fibrosis. *Ultrasound Med. Biol.* **2003**, *29*, 1705–1713. [CrossRef] [PubMed]
15. The Japan Society for Portal Hypertension. *The General Rules for Study of Portal Hypertension*, 3rd ed.; Kanehara: Tokyo, Japan, 2013; pp. 37–38.
16. Puigvehí, M.; Londoño, M.C.; Torras, X.; Lorente, S.; Vergara, M.; Morillas, R.M.; Masnou, H.; Serrano, T.; Miquel, M.; Gallego, A.; et al. Impact of sustained virological response with DAAs on gastroesophageal varices and Baveno criteria in HCV-cirrhotic patients. *J. Gastroenterol.* **2020**, *55*, 205–216. [CrossRef] [PubMed]
17. Di Marco, V.; Calvaruso, V.; Ferraro, D.; Bavetta, M.G.; Cabibbo, G.; Conte, E.; Cammà, C.; Grimaudo, S.; Pipitone, R.M.; Simone, F.; et al. Effects of eradicating hepatitis C virus infection in patients with cirrhosis differ with stage of portal hypertension. *Gastroenterology* **2016**, *151*, 130–139. [CrossRef] [PubMed]
18. You, M.W.; Kim, K.W.; Pyo, J.; Huh, J.; Kim, H.J.; Lee, S.J.; Park, S.H. A Meta-analysis for the Diagnostic Performance of Transient Elastography for Clinically Significant Portal Hypertension. *Ultrasound Med. Biol.* **2017**, *43*, 59–68. [CrossRef] [PubMed]
19. Berzigotti, A. Non-invasive evaluation of portal hypertension using ultrasound elastography. *J. Hepatol.* **2017**, *67*, 399–411. [CrossRef] [PubMed]
20. de Franchis, R.; Bosch, J.; Garcia-Tsao, G.; Reiberger, T.; Ripoll, C. Baveno VII—Renewing consensus in portal hypertension. *J. Hepatol.* **2022**, *76*, 959–974. [CrossRef]
21. Tseng, Y.; Li, F.; Wang, J.; Chen, S.; Jiang, W.; Shen, X.; Wu, S. Spleen and liver stiffness for noninvasive assessment of portal hypertension in cirrhotic patients with large esophageal varices. *J. Clin. Ultrasound* **2018**, *46*, 442–449. [CrossRef]
22. Vizzutti, F.; Arena, U.; Romanelli, R.G.; Rega, L.; Foschi, M.; Colagrande, S.; Petrarca, A.; Moscarella, S.; Belli, G.; Zignego, A.L.; et al. Liver stiffness measurement predicts severe portal hypertension in patients with HCV-related cirrhosis. *Hepatology* **2007**, *45*, 1290–1297. [CrossRef] [PubMed]
23. Ogasawara, N.; Saitoh, S.; Akuta, N.; Sezaki, H.; Suzuki, F.; Fujiyama, S.; Kawamura, Y.; Hosaka, T.; Kobayashi, M.; Suzuki, Y.; et al. Advantage of liver stiffness measurement before and after direct-acting antiviral therapy to predict hepatocellular carcinoma and exacerbation of esophageal varices in chronic hepatitis C. *Hepatol. Res.* **2020**, *50*, 426–438. [CrossRef] [PubMed]
24. Liu, X.; Wang, Y. An overview of bile acid synthesis and its physiological and pathological functions. *Yi Chuan* **2019**, *41*, 365–374. [PubMed]
25. LaRusso, N.F.; Hoffman, N.E.; Korman, M.G.; Hofmann, A.F.; Cowen, A.E. Determinants of fasting and postprandial serum bile acid levels in healthy man. *Am. J. Dig. Dis.* **1978**, *23*, 385–391. [CrossRef]
26. Ahlberg, J.; Angelin, B.; Björkhem, I.; Einarsson, K. Individual bile acids in portal venous and systemic blood serum of fasting man. *Gastroenterology* **1977**, *73*, 1377–1382. [CrossRef]
27. Gilmore, I.T.; Thompson, R.P.H. Kinetics of 14C-glycocholic acid clearance in normal man and in patients with liver disease. *Gut* **1978**, *19*, 1110–1115. [CrossRef]
28. Lindblad, L.; Lundholm, K.; Schersten, T. Bile acid concentrations in systemic and portal serum in presumably normal man and in cholestatic and cirrhotic conditions. *Scand. J. Gastroenterol.* **1977**, *12*, 395–400. [CrossRef]
29. Tarantino, G.; Cambri, S.; Ferrara, A.; Marzano, M.; Liberti, A.; Vellone, G.; Ciccarelli, A.F. Serum concentration of bile acids and portal hypertension in cirrhotic patients. Possible correlations. *Riv. Eur. Sci. Med. Farmacol.* **1989**, *11*, 195–205.
30. Siciliano, M.; Milani, A.; Marra, L.; Rossi, L. Serum bile acids in cirrhosis: Correlation with liver function parameters and with the severity of the disease. *Quad. Sclavo Diagn. Clin. Lab.* **1986**, *22*, 355–361.
31. Poupon, R.E.; Poupon, R.Y.; Grosdemouge, M.L.; Erlinger, S. Effect of portacaval shunt on serum bile acid concentration in patients with cirrhosis. *Digestion* **1977**, *16*, 138–145. [CrossRef]
32. Ohkubo, H.; Okuda, K.; Lida, S.; Ohnishi, K.; Ikawa, S.; Makino, I. Role of portal and splenic vein shunts and impaired hepatic extraction in the elevated serum bile acids in liver cirrhosis. *Gastroenterology* **1984**, *86*, 514–520. [CrossRef] [PubMed]
33. Hayashi, H.; Beppu, T.; Okabe, H.; Nitta, H.; Imai, K.; Doi, K.; Chikamoto, A.; Baba, H. Combined measurements of serum bile acid level and splenic volume may be useful to noninvasively assess portal venous pressure. *J. Gastroenterol.* **2012**, *47*, 1336–1341. [CrossRef] [PubMed]

livers

MDPI

Review

Cutaneous Manifestations of Liver Cirrhosis: Clinical Significance and Diagnostic Implications

Rita Kamoua [1], Rebecca Reese [1], Risha Annamraju [1], Tian Chen [1], Colleen Doyle [1], Adriana Parella [1], Amelia Liu [1], Yazan Abboud [2], Craig Rohan [3] and Jeffrey B. Travers [3,*]

1 Boonshoft School of Medicine, Wright State University, Dayton, OH 45324, USA; kamoua.2@wright.edu (R.K.); reese.95@wright.edu (R.R.); risha.annamraju@wright.edu (R.A.); chen.227@wright.edu (T.C.); doyle.67@wright.edu (C.D.); parella.2@wright.edu (A.P.); liu.173@wright.edu (A.L.)

2 Department of Internal Medicine, Rutgers New Jersey Medical School, Newark, NJ 07103, USA; yazanabboud.md@gmail.com

3 Department of Dermatology, Boonshoft School of Medicine, Wright State University, Dayton, OH 45324, USA; craig.rohan@wright.edu

* Correspondence: jeffrey.travers@wright.edu

Abstract: Liver cirrhosis, a progressive and often irreversible condition, exerts widespread systemic effects, with the skin frequently serving as a visible window into the extent of hepatic dysfunction. Cutaneous manifestations, such as spider angiomas, palmar erythema, jaundice, and pruritus, not only reflect underlying pathophysiologic changes but also serve as important, non-invasive diagnostic and prognostic markers of disease severity. Early detection of such cutaneous findings may allow for early treatment, optimize patient management, and improve outcomes. This review addresses the various cutaneous manifestations of liver cirrhosis, their pathogenesis, and their prognostic and diagnostic importance, emphasizing the need for heightened clinical awareness of the improvement in patient care.

Keywords: liver cirrhosis; cutaneous manifestations; spider angiomas; palmar erythema; jaundice; pruritus; dermatologic signs; hepatic dysfunction

1. Introduction

Liver cirrhosis represents the end stage of chronic liver injury from a variety of etiologies, including alcohol use, viral hepatitis, and metabolic-dysfunction-associated steatotic liver disease (MASLD), and other etiologies [1,2]. As the liver progressively fails, systemic manifestations emerge, often offering the clinician early and critical clues to the underlying disease [3]. Among these, dermatologic signs are especially valuable, providing a non-invasive and accessible means for detecting hepatic dysfunction [4].

There are several etiologies that can lead to liver cirrhosis. These include but are not limited to metabolic-dysfunction-associated steatotic liver disease (MASLD), alcohol-associated liver disease, hepatitis C virus (HCV), hepatitis B virus (HBV), autoimmune hepatitis, primary biliary cholangitis (PBC), primary sclerosing cholangitis (PSC), drug-induced liver injury, and genetic syndromes, such as hemochromatosis, Wilson's disease, and alpha-1 antitrypsin deficiency. Among these etiologies, MASLD is currently the fastest-growing indication of liver transplantation in Western countries, with high prevalence in the United States.

Cutaneous manifestations, such as spider angiomas, palmar erythema, jaundice, and pruritus, are common in cirrhotic patients and often precede more severe clinical deterioration. These signs reflect a complex interplay between vascular, hormonal, and metabolic disturbances resulting from impaired liver function [5]. Furthermore, the presence and severity of certain skin findings have been correlated with disease progression and prognosis, making them essential components of the clinical assessment [6].

Despite their diagnostic significance, the recognition of these cutaneous clues is frequently overlooked or underestimated, delaying appropriate intervention [7]. In order to address this gap in the literature, we provide this review article after conducting a comprehensive PubMed search to identify original and review articles discussing skin manifestations of cirrhosis, with a focus on their pathophysiology and prognostic significance. Relevant studies were screened to ensure inclusion of the most current and clinically meaningful evidence. This review aims to explore the spectrum of skin manifestations in liver cirrhosis, delve into their underlying pathophysiological mechanisms, and highlight their clinical implications in diagnosis, disease staging, and management.

The current review article summarizes up-to-date data on various skin manifestations of liver cirrhosis. It offers a one-stop shop for hepatologists and dermatologists to review current evidence on the pathophysiology of different cutaneous manifestations in patients with liver cirrhosis. Furthermore, it summarizes the diagnostic and prognostic value of various skin findings in liver cirrhosis.

2. Overview of Liver Cirrhosis and Systemic Manifestations

Cirrhosis is due to chronic liver inflammation that leads to diffuse fibrosis [8]. Three main cell types contribute to the progression of fibrosis and alteration of the hepatic architecture, as follows: hepatic stellate cells (HSCs), myofibroblasts, and liver sinusoidal endothelial cells (LSECs). HSCs and myofibroblasts secrete extracellular matrix, while LSECs lose their permeability and undergo new capillary formation and vasoconstriction. Another major component of the development of fibrosis is the presence of inflammatory cells, such as macrophages and neutrophils, that release pro-inflammatory cytokines and produce reactive oxygen species [9]. The combination of inflammation and vasoconstriction leads to high resistance and pressure in the portal vasculature. As a result, there is increased production of nitric oxide and vasodilation in the splanchnic circulation as an attempt to increase portal blood flow. Increased resistance and blood flow lead to the development of portal hypertension, a sign of cirrhosis that is associated with a high risk of complications, such as ascites, gastrointestinal bleeding, hepatic encephalopathy, and renal dysfunction [8]. A compensatory mechanism in response to portal hypertension is the creation of alternate pathways for blood to travel between the portal and systemic circulation. The most clinically relevant examples are esophageal or gastric varices, which are prone to bleeding if the pressure exceeds the capacity of the vessel wall [10].

Portal hypertension and hepatic insufficiency lead to the distinctive clinical manifestations of cirrhosis. One of the most common symptoms of cirrhosis is ascites, the accumulation of fluid in the peritoneal cavity. Ascites fluid formation is due to a downstream effect of hypoperfusion of the renal system, leading to activation of the renin–angiotensin–aldosterone system and retention of fluid. The rise in blood volume causes more filtration out of mesenteric vessels into the peritoneum [10]. Another common complication of cirrhosis is hepatic encephalopathy (HE), which is reported in 30% of patients with cirrhosis. While its pathophysiology is not entirely understood, HE is a spectrum of neuropsychiatric abnormalities that is thought to be due to decreased metabolism of ammonia by the liver. Ammonia is capable of crossing the blood–brain barrier and precipitates encephalopathy by causing swelling of astrocytes, altering pH, and disrupting cellular metabolism [11]. Acute kidney injuries (AKIs) are also prevalent in patients with cirrhosis and manifest as a rise in serum creatinine greater than 50% from baseline and a decrease in glomerular filtration rate. Other manifestations include hepatorenal syndrome, which is a specific type of renal failure in patients with cirrhosis [8]. Other non-specific systemic manifestations of cirrhosis include fatigue, weakness, and weight loss. Cirrhosis can also present asymptomatically, and laboratory findings can aid in establishing a diagnosis, such as elevated liver enzymes, thrombocytopenia, anemia, and coagulopathy [9].

3. Cutaneous Manifestations: Clinical Features

- *Spider Angiomas/Telangiectasias*

Telangiectasias refer to dilated small blood vessels visible on the surface of skin or mucous membranes. Spider angiomas, also referred to as spider telangiectasias, are the most common telangiectatic lesion seen in patients with cirrhosis. They appear as a central erythematous to violaceous brown macule surrounded by clusters of web-like vessels (Figure 1A,B). They are vascular dermatologic lesions which arise when the sphincteric muscle surrounding a cutaneous arteriole fails, resulting in dilation of the arteriole and its associated numerous thin-walled capillary branches, resulting in their spider-leg-like appearance. They are blanchable and most commonly observed on the face, neck, upper chest, and arms in adults, possibly due to the proximity to the superior vena cava. It is estimated that one-third of patients with liver cirrhosis present with spider angiomas, and they are more common in women than men [12].

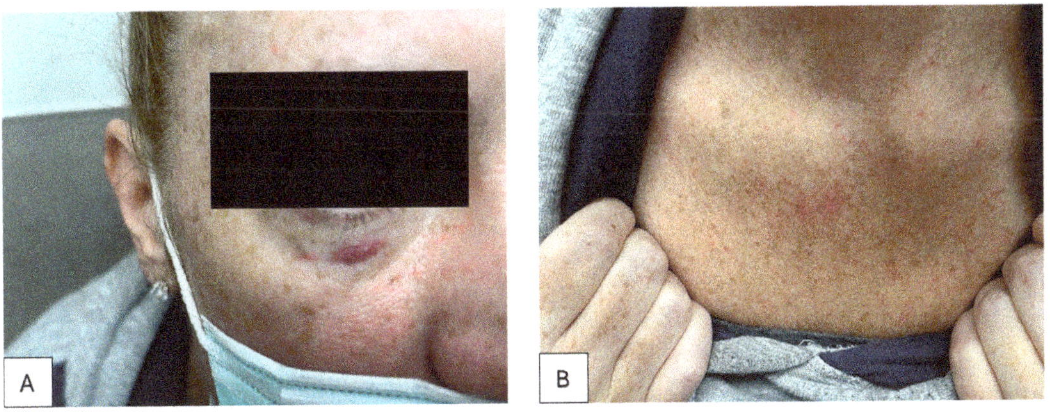

Figure 1. Telangiectasises overlying erythematous patches on the right lower eyelid (**A**) and upper chest (**B**).

While the exact pathogenesis is still unknown, neovascularization is a likely contributor of spider angioma formation through vascular endothelial growth factor (VEGF) and basic fibroblast growth factor (bFGF), which stimulate endothelial cell proliferation and angiogenesis (Figure 2). Elevated levels of both VEGF and bFGF were found in the plasma of cirrhotic patients compared to healthy controls, and the elevation of VEGF was correlated with the size of patients' spider angiomas [13]. Elevated levels of substance P have also been detected in patients with MASLD cirrhosis [14]. However, spider angiomas can also be observed in non-cirrhotic conditions, including pregnancy and patients taking oral contraceptives, which are thought to occur due to increased estrogen levels, resulting in increased dilation, permeability, and proliferation of vessels, which often resolve spontaneously following childbirth or cessation of birth control [12]. The impaired ability of the liver to metabolize estrogen in a cirrhotic state thus also likely contributes to the formation of spider angiomas in cirrhosis.

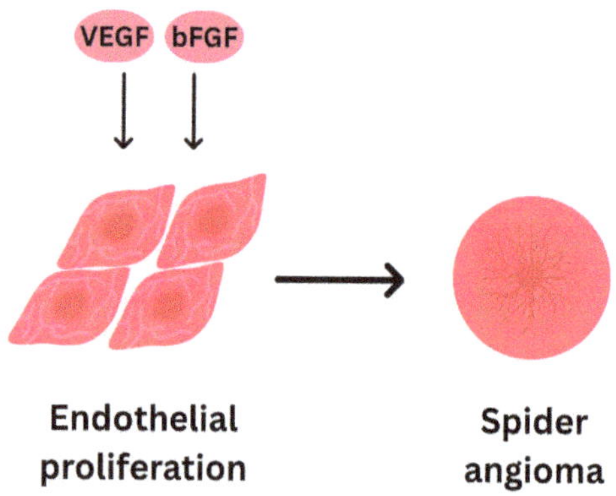

Figure 2. Simplified figure illustrating the pathophysiology of spider angioma in liver cirrhosis. VEGF: vascular endothelial growth factor; bFGF: basic fibroblast growth factor.

The presence of spider angiomas has been shown to correlate with and can act as skin markers for hepatopulmonary syndrome and esophageal varices, two serious complications of cirrhosis [12,15]. While a prior study suggested that the total number of spiders angiomas and their locations could be associated with the severity of chronic liver disease, more research is needed to determine the overall prognostic importance [16].

While spider angiomata is the most common telangiectatic lesion seen in patients with cirrhosis, diffuse cutaneous telangiectasias, including acquired bilateral telangiectatic macules (ABTMs), and telangiectasia macularis eruptiva perstans (TMEP) have also been described in the setting of chronic liver disease [17].

ABTM refers to a pattern of red brown macules with telangiectasia along the upper arms, notably, the telangiectatic nature of the macules is typically only visible via dermoscopy. In a study characterizing the etiology of these lesions, Kim et al. found that 54% of patients had hepatic disease, including alcoholic cirrhosis. Treatment for ABTM involves addressing the underlying liver disease [17]. Differential diagnoses for ABTM include erythematotelangiectatic rosacea, generalized essential telangiectasia, spider angiomata, hereditary hemorrhagic telangiectasia, and pigmented purpuric dermatoses (PPD).

TMEP is a type of cutaneous mastocytosis that presents with pruritic erythematous to brownish macules seen with telangiectasia, typically distributed on the trunk and upper extremities [18]. Unlike other mast-cell-mediated disorders, TMEP has a negative Darier's sign, meaning physical disruption of lesions do not result in swelling and urticaria. Histopathology traditionally shows perivascular mast cell infiltrate. A case report by Huang et al. describes a patient with cirrhosis and TMEP and highlights the importance of consideration of telangiectatic disorders in cirrhosis outside of the predominant spider angiomata. TMEP is managed with antihistamines and avoidance of hepatotoxic substances. Differential diagnoses for TMEP include urticaria pigmentosa (presents without telangiectasia), spider angiomata (presents with spiraling vessels extending from central arteriole and without increased mast cells on biopsy), and systemic mastocytosis [18]

- *Palmar Erythema*

Another cutaneous manifestation of cirrhosis is palmar erythema (Figure 3). Palmar erythema presents as bilateral and symmetric, non-pruritic, and non-painful erythema along the palmar surface, most commonly along both the thenar and hypothenar eminences. It has been estimated that about 23% of cirrhotic patients present with palmar erythema [19]. It is thought to occur most frequently in the palms due to the higher density of arteriovenous shunts and microscopic evaluation in patients with palmar erythema has shown an increase in the dilation of capillaries and increased palmar superficial arterial and venous plexi [20].

Again, increased estrogen levels are thought to be the mechanism associated with the vasodilation leading to palmar erythema, as estradiol stimulates the production of nitric oxide via nitric oxide synthase which induces vasodilation [15,20].

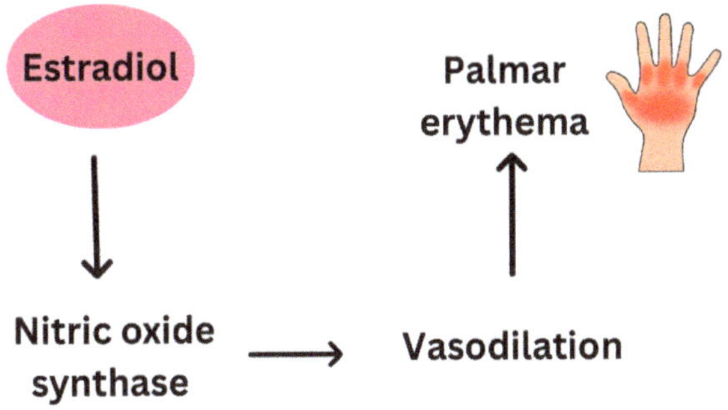

Figure 3. Simplified figure illustrating the pathophysiology of palmar erythema in liver cirrhosis.

As palmar erythema is associated with increased free estrogen levels, it can be a physiologic change observed in pregnancy. Palmar erythema is also associated with autoimmune diseases, including rheumatoid arthritis, Kawasaki disease, diabetes, and sarcoidosis. In addition, palmar erythema can be drug-induced with normal liver function, with offending medications including albuterol and topiramate or other medications that induce hepatic damage, such as amiodarone, statins, fibric acid derivatives, and biologics [19,21].

- *Jaundice*

Jaundice refers to yellow to green discoloration of skin caused by the deposition of bilirubin and its precursors. Jaundice is typically seen when serum bilirubin exceeds between 2 and 3 mg/dL. The face, sclera, and mucous membranes (tissues with high elastin content) are most often affected, though discoloration can be seen throughout the body [5].

The liver is the primary organ involved in bilirubin metabolism as part of the hemoglobin breakdown process. The conjugation state of the bilirubin allows for differentiation of jaundice etiologies, as follows: prehepatic, with unconjugated hyperbilirubinemia, intrahepatic, with conjugated and unconjugated hyperbilirubinemia, and post hepatic, with conjugated hyperbilirubinemia. Jaundice in cirrhosis is classified as intrahepatic, and the degree of jaundice generally correlates with advancement of liver disease [5]. Jaundice is an extremely clinically significant sign. It is a poor prognostic marker and indicates an increased risk of complications. New-onset jaundice in a patient with cirrhosis warrants evaluation for acute-on-chronic causes of hepatic decompensation, including drug-induced hepatitis, infection, or biliary stricture. Treatment of jaundice involves treatment of the underlying pathology. In the case of intrahepatic causes, treatment should prioritize appropriate volume status and prevention of infection or gastrointestinal bleeding. In cases where biliary obstruction is noted, endospcoical or surgical drainage may be necessary [22,23].

- *Pruritus*

Pruritus is a common symptom and often an early symptom of chronic liver disease. Pruritus typically affects the palms and soles, though it can become generalized throughout the back, abdomen, and legs [24]. It is often chronic, though periodic, as it has been matched to circadian rhythm and shown to be worse in the evenings. Warm weather can trigger itching and advanced age, concomitant diabetes, and worsening liver disease are risk factors for development of pruritus [25]. Associated excoriation, lichenification, and secondary infection can mimic prurigo nodularis, lichen simplex chronicus, and contact dermatitis.

Pruritus is most prevalent in patients with cholestatic pathologies, affecting 70% of those with primary biliary cirrhosis (PBC). Further, patients with hepatitis B and C, intrahepatic cholestasis of pregnancy (ICP), sclerosing cholangitis, bile duct carcinoma, and biliary obstructions have been shown to be affected at greater levels [24]. The mechanism of cholestatic pruritus is multifaceted and likely involves bile acid accumulation, various cytokine release, endogenous opioids, and activation of specific sensory receptors. Prior research has established that bile salts can cause mast cell degranulation, which leads to itching [26].

T-cell involvement is likely, as when bile acids activated farnesoid X receptor, a nuclear regulator of bile acid metabolism, increased release of IL-31, a cytokine known to induce itching, was seen. Further, when patients with cholestatic liver pathologies were given Cilefexor, a nonsteroidal FXR agonist, they had increased levels of IL-31 and pruritus [27]. Notably, not all patients with pruritus and chronic liver disease have elevated bile acids; thus, newer theories implicate the release of other pruritogens lysophosphatidic acid (LPA) and autotaxin due to hepatocyte injury in the pathogenesis. Endogenous opioids are thought to be involved in cholestatic pruritus, as impaired clearance leads to subsequent systemic elevation of compounds such as enkephalins and b-endorphin. These compounds act on the known pruritis inducing mu-opioid receptor (MOR) and may downregulate the kappa opioid receptor (KOR), an inhibitor of itch. Studies have investigated MOR inhibitors naloxone and naltrexone for the treatment of cholestatic pruritus and showed a decrease in scratching activity [28,29]. Recent research has shown that bile acids activate sensory neuron receptor Mas-related G protein-coupled receptor X4 (MRGPRX4), and murine studies have demonstrated that upregulation of MRGPRX4 results in increased pruritus (Figure 4) [30].

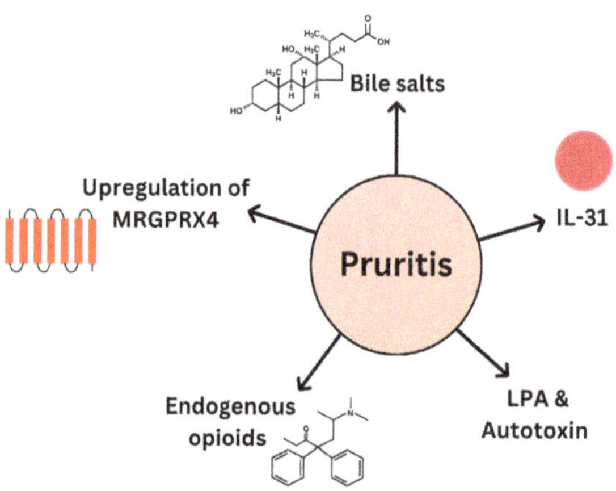

Figure 4. Simplified figure illustrating the pathophysiology of pruritus in liver cirrhosis.

Treatment of pruritis in hepatic disease focuses on removal of bile acids from systemic circulation. Cholestyramine, an anion exchange resin, which binds bile acids in the gut lumen, is the first-line treatment [26]. Alternate therapies focus on disrupting metabolism of potential pruritogens or blockage of the itch response and include rifampicin, naltrexone, and sertraline [26].

- ***Stasis ulcers***

Stasis ulcers, also referred to as venous ulcers, occur in cirrhotic patients secondarily to portal hypertension, resulting in edema and swelling from venous incompetency.

Most commonly, the skin will initially experience statis dermatitis due to fluid leakage from the venous capillaries, causing inflammation and thickening of the skin. The edematous fluid has impaired immune cell trafficking, resulting in chronic inflammation with mononuclear cells, fibroblast proliferation and collagen deposition, and progressive lymphatic duct obliteration. As inflammation and interstitial edema progresses, open ulcers may arise (Figure 5). Most commonly, the ulcers are shallow and flat, with irregular borders that may be surrounded by discoloration [31].

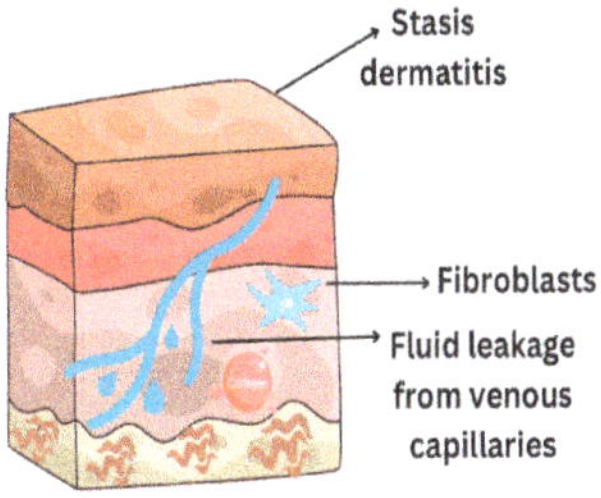

Figure 5. Simplified figure illustrating the pathophysiology of stasis dermatitis in liver cirrhosis.

Stasis ulcers are most common on the lower legs due to the effects of gravity on the microcirculation [31]. Classically, these lower leg ulcers are often refractory and difficult to treat, but a case series revealed that decompression of the portal circulation via the placement of a transjugular intrahepatic portosystemic shunt (TIPS) leads to complete and sustained ulcer healing [32]. While cirrhosis is a known cause of stasis ulcers, venous hypertension resulting in stasis ulcers can also arise secondary to heart failure, renal failure, use of vasodilator drugs such as amlodipine, and with diseases of the lymph vessels [31]. More research is needed to better elucidate the relationship and prevalence between cirrhosis and statis ulcer development (Figure 6).

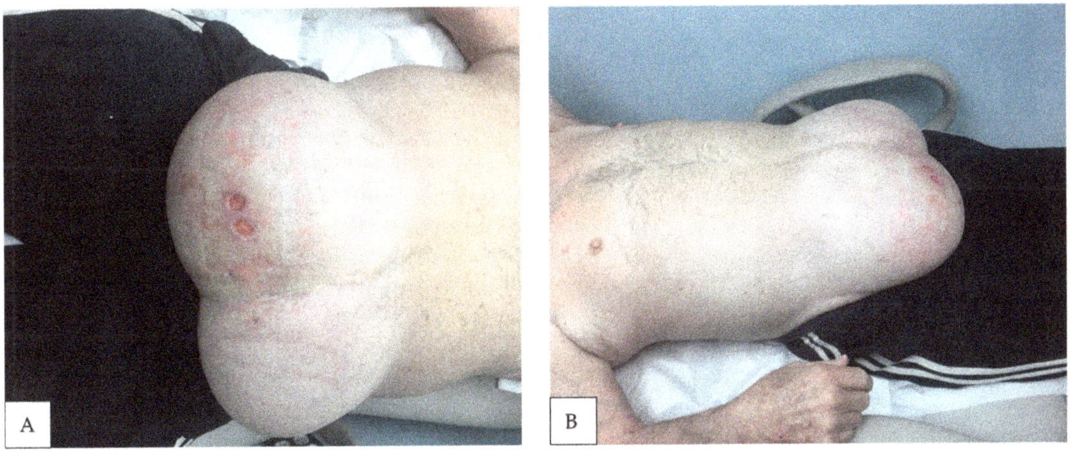

Figure 6. A well-demarcated venous stasis ulcer on the lower abdominal wall (**A**) and chronic ascites in the lower abdomen (**B**).

- ***Other Skin and Nails Findings:***
    - **Terry's nails**

Terry's nails, coined in 1954, refers to proximal whitish discoloration of the nail bed with a narrow (0.5–3 mm) brown to red band at the onychodermal region, seen in patients with alcoholic cirrhosis [33].

Prevalence of Terry's nails in cirrhosis is approximately 25% and is hypothesized to be caused by telangiectatic changes in the nail and hypoalbuminemia [34,35]. Though initially discovered in cirrhosis, Terry's nails have been described in patients with congestive heart failure, renal disease, diabetes, tuberculosis, reactive arthritis, and as an age-related phenomenon [34]. (Notably, when identified in younger patients, Terry's nails are more likely to be caused by hepatic disease, thus a high degree of clinical suspicion must be maintained in these individuals [34].) Key differential diagnoses of Terry's nails include Lindsay's nails, proximal white discoloration of approximately 50% of the nails with blanchable distal red-brown discoloration (half and half nails) strongly associated with chronic kidney disease and thought to be caused by azotemia. Both Terry's and Lindsay's nails are a form of proximal apparent leukonychia (whitish discoloration due to disruption of the nail plate), and one study found that 43.8% of patients at a liver disease treatment center had leukonychia, predominantly Terry's nails type though Lindsay's nail type was noted [36]. Degree of distal discoloration and whether it is blanchable (Terry's nails are typically non-blanching) are useful differentiating features. Treatment for Terry's nails involves treatment of underlying hepatic disease, though visible nail changes may take months and lag behind resolution of other symptoms.

○ **Clubbing**

Clubbing refers to rounded, bulging growth of the distal nail with a loss or increase in the nail bed angle associated with chronic systemic disease.

In the case of cirrhosis, long standing hypoxia with subsequent increased blood flow and growth factor release result in the spongy, bulbous appearance of fingernails (Figure 7). One study found clubbing in 35% of patients with liver cell failure [37]. Clubbing has been noted in cirrhosis in cases of advanced disease and thought to be connected to release of hepatocyte growth factor [38]. Differential diagnoses for etiology of clubbing include pulmonary, cardiac, and gastrointestinal pathologies. Other nail changes seen in cirrhosis include brittle nails, onychorrhexis, and increased longitudinal striations [37]. The myriad nail changes described in association with cirrhosis warrant comprehensive nail examination for patients with suspected hepatic dysfunction.

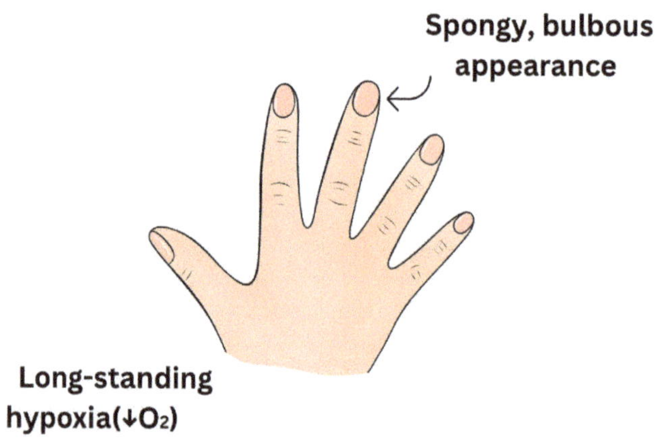

Figure 7. Simplified figure illustrating the pathophysiology of clubbing in liver cirrhosis.

○ **Xanthomas/xanthelasma**

Xanthomas refer to yellow to orange papules, plaques, or nodules, which are cutaneous cholesterol deposits. Pathogenesis involves impaired hepatic clearance of lipoproteins, leading to deposits of lipid-laden macrophages in the dermis (Figure 8). Lesions are typically soft, fluctuant in growth, and asymptomatic, though they can be pruritic in the setting of cholestatic disease [5]. Xanthomas can occur throughout the body and in any pathology with hypercholesterolemia, as well as secondary dyslipidemia in the setting of hepatic disease. In patients with cirrhosis, lesions are noted to appear as eruptive xanthomas, clusters of papules typically distributed on extensor surfaces, which appear and resolve in the course of weeks, xanthelasma, and tendinous or planar xanthomas [39]. Xanthelasma refers to the distribution of xanthomas along the medial upper eyelid and is associated with PBC [40]. Tendinous xanthomas (the Achilles tendon is often affected) and xanthoma striatum palmare, in which the creases of the palms and digits appear with soft yellow deposits, are also associated with PBC [41].

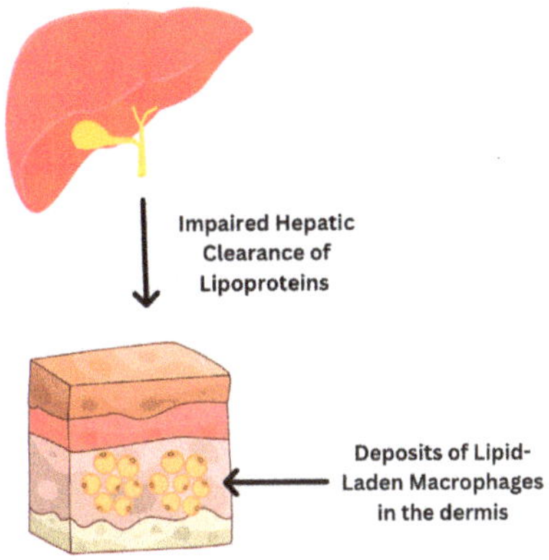

Figure 8. Simplified figure illustrating the pathophysiology of xanthomas in liver cirrhosis.

Treatment of xanthomas involves addressing hyperlipidemia; therapeutic options that have shown success in cirrhosis-associated lesions include cholestyramine and ursodeoxycholic acid (UDCA), as well as plasmapheresis in severe cases [42]. Xanthelasma may not be refractory to pharmacological therapy, and surgical excision and laser treatment may be necessary [43]. Differential diagnoses for xanthomas include but are not limited to syringoma, sebaceous gland hyperplasia, milia, cutaneous sarcoidosis, and necrobiotic xanthogranuloma [44].

○ **Caput medusae**

Caput medusae refers to engorgement of superficial periumbilical veins and formation of collateral vessels in response to severe portal hypertension and rerouting through portocaval anastomoses.

The name is derived from the tortuous and snake-like appearance of the vessels and is a cutaneous sign of severe portal hypertension; studies have shown the presence of caput medusa in patients with hepatic dysfunction to have a positive likelihood ratio of 9.5 for cirrhosis [45]. It is associated with increased risk of complications including gastrointestinal bleeding and hepatic encephalopathy. When evaluating caput medusae, blood flow toward the head and limbs is indicative of portal hypertension. General enlargement of abdominal wall venous structures is not seen as often as caput medusa but is also a highly specific cutaneous sign of cirrhosis [46]. Treatment for caput medusae typically includes non-selective beta blockers carvedilol or propranolol to address portal hypertension. Intractable cases may necessitate transjugular intrahepatic portosystemic shunt (TIPS), and liver transplantation is definitive therapy in cirrhosis with severe portal hypertension [47]. Differential diagnoses for caput medusae encompass any pathology that elevates portal venous pressure, including portal vein thrombosis, right-sided heart failure, abdominal mass or malignancy, inferior vena cava obstruction, schistosomiasis, and Budd-Chiari syndrome [48].

- **Pellagra**

Pellagra refers to the syndrome caused by deficiency of niacin (vitamin B3), an important co-factor in metabolism. The triad of pellagra involves skin manifestations and neurological and gastrointestinal symptoms. Cutaneous manifestations are often marked photosensitivity and symmetrical erythematous-to-hyperpigmented plaques in sun-exposed areas. Classically, there is involvement of the C3–C4 dermatome with a "collar-like" distribution. Neurologic and gastrointestinal symptoms associated with pellagra include irritability, insomnia, general cognitive decline, encephalopathy, diarrhea, and glossitis. Pellagra is relevant in the context of alcoholic cirrhosis, as alcohol interferes with hepatic metabolism of B3 and with the absorption of the precursor to niacin—tryptophan. Further, alcoholic cirrhosis is often associated with malnutrition, and, thus, insufficient intake of vitamin B3 further predisposes individuals to deficiencies. Pellagra may present as altered mental status, and the triad of symptoms may be subtle, and, thus, clinicians must have a high degree of suspicion to identify this syndrome.

- **Acanthosis Nigricans**

Acanthosis nigricans (AN) presents as hyperpigmented, velvety plaques in intertriginous regions, including the axilla, groin, and neck. The pathophysiology of AN, which is strongly associated with metabolic syndrome and T2DM, is likely due to hyperinsulinemia and subsequent activation of various fibroblast growth factors. MASLD involves insulin resistance, and, thus, AN is a potential cutaneous manifestation of this disease. A recent cross-sectional study demonstrated that AN correlated to a greater degree of steatosis in individuals with MASLD cirrhosis.

- **Erythema Nodosum and Pyoderma Gangrenosum**

Inflammatory bowel disease (IBD), with or without primary sclerosing cholangitis (PSC), is associated with erythema nodosum or pyoderma gangrenosum. Erythema nodosum presents as red, tender nodules on the lower extremities. Pyoderma gangrenosum manifests first as erythematous pustules or nodules and then spreads to adjacent skin and develops into burrowing ulcers. Both of these skin manifestations are extrahepatic complications of PSC, and when seen clinically, should raise suspicion for underlying cirrhotic disorders.

4. Pathophysiological Mechanisms Linking Liver Dysfunction to Skin Changes

The liver plays a vital role in numerous physiological processes, including the synthesis of hormone-transporting proteins, conjugation of bilirubin, detoxification of drugs and toxins like alcohol, and the metabolism of lipids, carbohydrates, and other nutrients [43]. Hepatic injury can impair any of these functions, potentially leading to systemic effects that can involve the skin [43].

Hormonal imbalances resulting from liver cirrhosis have widespread effects, particularly on sex hormone regulation. In the bloodstream, both testosterone and estradiol are bound to albumin and sex-hormone-binding globulin (SHBG), with testosterone having a higher affinity for SHBG [49]. Damage from cirrhosis results in impaired hepatic clearance of estrogen secondary to portal hypertension, decreased testosterone production, elevated SHBG levels, and dysfunction of the hypothalamic–pituitary axis [50]. Increased SHBG levels are thought to result from upregulated hepatic synthesis, driven by excess estrogen and diminished testosterone-mediated suppression [50]. Because SHBG preferentially binds testosterone, free testosterone levels are further disproportionately reduced [51,52]. Excessive estrogen contributes to several dermatological manifestations commonly seen in cirrhosis, such as spider angiomas and palmar erythema [52].

Dysfunction of the bilirubin cycle due to liver cirrhosis can cause elevation of both unconjugated and conjugated bilirubin [53]. Fibrosis of hepatic parenchyma from liver cirrhosis disrupts liver structure and function. Damage to hepatocytes results in decreased hepatic intake of unconjugated bilirubin and decreased conjugation [54]. Hepatocellular dysfunction and scar tissue compression of bile ducts also result in impairment of excretion of conjugated bilirubin into bile [54]. The elevation of bilirubin levels beyond 2.5–3.0 mg/dL leads to jaundice [5].

Fat malabsorption due to hyperbilirubinemia from liver cirrhosis can lead to nutritional deficiencies in fat-soluble vitamins A, D, E, and K [55]. Damage to hepatic parenchyma also contributes to decreased storage and impairment of the conversion of vitamins to their metabolically active forms [55]. In the skin, vitamin A is integral to maintaining the specialized epithelial surfaces of the body and deficiency can cause inappropriate keratinization of stratified squamous epithelium [56]. Low vitamin D has been associated with alopecia areata [15]. Collagen cross-linking was accelerated in rats with vitamin E deficiency [57]. Vitamin K is necessary for the formation of clotting factors in the coagulation cascade; deficiency can present as purpura, ecchymoses, and gingival bleeding [58].

Autoimmune liver conditions, including primary biliary cholangitis (PBC), primary sclerosing cholangitis (PSC), and autoimmune hepatitis (AIH), have also been associated with dermatologic conditions. For example, PBC causes destruction of intrahepatic bile ducts leading to cholestasis and resultant dyslipidemia, which can lead to the formation of cutaneous xanthomas. Xanthomas often appear as soft yellow-brown papules/plaques and are commonly found on the eyelids (referred to as xanthelasma) or skin folds, such as on the palmar creases and are most commonly described in patients with familial hypercholesterolemia. Interestingly, xanthomas in PBC have been associated with an abnormal lipoprotein called lipoprotein X (Harris). Additionally, AIH has been associated with a variety of additional autoimmune-mediated cutaneous disorders, including vitiligo; psoriasis; alopecia; autoimmune bullous diseases such as pemphigus vulgaris/dermatitis herpetiform; neutrophilic dermatoses such as pyoderma gangrenosum; and lichen planus. As patients with AIH often receive immunosuppressive treatment, they are also at an increased risk of non-melanoma skin cancer.

Additional cutaneous manifestations of liver cirrhosis include cyanosis and digital clubbing, typically only seen in patients with pulmonary complications, such as hepatopulmonary syndrome (HPS) and portopulmonary hypertension (POPH). Though the exact pathophysiology remains unclear, the occurrence of intrapulmonary vascular dilatations in advanced hepatic disease disrupts pulmonary gas exchange, which can lead to ventilation–perfusion mismatch. In patients presenting with vague pulmonary symptoms, the presence of cyanosis and digital clubbing, in conjunction with other cutaneous findings of advanced liver disease, can aid in identification of HPS or POPH in advanced stages of cirrhosis. Identification of these complications is critical, particularly in evaluation for liver transplantation.

5. Diagnostic and Prognostic Value of Skin Signs

Cutaneous skin findings are one of the earliest indicators of hepatic dysfunction that leads clinicians to suspect a diagnosis of cirrhosis. The presence of multiple cutaneous skin manifestations, such as jaundice, pruritus, palmar erythema, and spider angiomas, further suggests cirrhosis [5]. Understanding these dermatologic manifestations and using them as critical diagnosis and prognostic indicators allows clinicians to help optimize patient care and improve clinical outcomes in cirrhotic patients. Jaundice stems from hepatocyte failure or biliary obstruction that causes the elevation of bilirubin accumulation reflecting advanced-stage cirrhosis [8]. Cholestasis and bile acid deposition on the skin leads to pruritus, which is also associated with advanced cirrhosis and worse quality of life measures [59]. Palmer erythema with symmetric redness on the hands due to elevated nitric oxide and estrogen levels reflects peripheral vasodilation [60]. Portal hypertension and impaired hepatic metabolism of estrogen in advanced stages of cirrhosis lead to spider angiomas on the face, neck, upper chest, and arms [16]. A large area, a significant number, or atypical locations of spider angiomas are correlated with higher severity of chronic liver disease [61].

Distinguishing skin findings that occur in patients with liver cirrhosis from those that can also occur in patients without liver cirrhosis can be challenging. It requires a holistic approach, assessing the patient's clinical picture while integrating the skin manifestations with other physical exam findings and diagnostic modalities. While certain findings, such as Terry nails, spider angiomata, palmar erythema, jaundice, and caput medusae, can be more specific in cirrhosis, they can also occur in other diseases. However, their presence should prompt a comprehensive liver evaluation. In contrast, there are many other less specific findings, such as pruritus and xerosis, that may be seen in various systemic conditions. An astute clinician should utilize physical exam findings along with other data to evaluate for different etiologies that may be causing those skin manifestations to improve early diagnosis.

Although pruritus and other skin manifestations of cirrhosis may have limited diagnostic value, they play a crucial role in assessing patients' quality of life. These symptoms hold significant clinical importance, particularly for symptom management and improving patient outcomes. Having said that, there have been data showing some association of certain skin manifestations with advanced disease. Prior studies have showed that patients who have more spider angiomas tend to have higher serum bilirubin and longer prothrombin time, both of which are markers of more advanced liver disease. Furthermore, there have been reports suggesting that the severity of cutaneous manifestations often parallels that of hepatic dysfunction which is measured by Model for End-Stage Liver Disease (MELD) scores and Child–Pugh classifications. Serum bilirubin quantifies jaundice and directly contributes to both MELD and Child–Pugh calculations. Pruritus intensity shows a positive association with bilirubin levels and MELD scores in cholestatic cirrhosis [59]. When spider angiomas appear on the chest or abdomen, it is associated with a higher MELD score (10.77 ± 6.76 versus 7.68 ± 5.42, $p = 0.003$), indicating a higher mortality [16]. Child–Pugh classification can be integrated with cutaneous manifestations to assess disease severity. These data, while scarce, suggest a possible role of cutaneous manifestations in evaluating the degree of cirrhosis. Thus, clinicians need to recognize and identify the presence of these characteristic skin changes and their associations with the stage of cirrhosis. Further research is warranted to better elucidate the diagnostic and prognostic value of different skin manifestations in liver cirrhosis.

The following table summarizes the key dermatologic manifestations, their prevalence in liver cirrhosis, and their clinical relevance based on available literature (Table 1).

While the data evaluating the prognostic and diagnostic value of cutaneous entities in cirrhosis are limited, there is a growing body of literature showing the impact of skin symptoms on patients' quality of life. For instance, pruritus is associated with poor sleep and psychological impairment, which lead to worse quality of life. Skin manifestations in cirrhosis impose a significant burden, negatively impacting physical comfort, sleep, mental well-being, and social life. Regular evaluation and focused treatment of these symptoms are vital to enhancing quality of life and patient-centered outcomes.

Table 1. Key skin findings in liver cirrhosis, their prevalence, and clinical relevance.

Skin Manifestation	Prevalence in Cirrhosis	Clinical Relevance
Spider Angiomas	33–40%	More specific for cirrhosis; associated with advanced disease and portal hypertension
Palmar Erythema	23–30%	More specific for cirrhosis; reflects hyperestrogenism and advanced disease
Jaundice	28–47%	Indicates impaired bilirubin metabolism; maker of decompensation
Pruritus	39%	Nonspecific; common in cholestatic liver disease; impacts quality of life
Stasis Ulcers	<5%	Nonspecific; may indicate severe hypoalbuminemia or venous insufficiency
Terry's Nails	25.6%	Highly specific for cirrhosis; associated with advanced disease
Clubbing	5–15%	Nonspecific
Xanthomas	<5%	Nonspecific
Caput Medusae	1–5%	More specific for portal hypertension and advanced cirrhosis

6. Management Implications

The management of cutaneous manifestations of cirrhosis relies on addressing the underlying hepatic dysfunction. Antiviral therapies that treat hepatitis B and C reduce liver inflammation and, thus, reduce spider angiomas and pruritis. Abstinence from alcohol and nutritional support can resolve palmer erythema in alcoholic cirrhosis [62]. Liver transplantation remains a definitive treatment for end-stage cirrhosis, which can lead to the resolution of these cutaneous symptoms [61]. Management of pruritis relies on the traditional first-line treatment of cholestyramine, which is a bile acid sequestrant that can decrease the amount of bile acid in the serum [63]. However, other studies have suggested a transition of first-line treatment to fibrates, as it provides a safer profile and anticholestatic properties [64]. Antihistamines and topical corticosteroids remain as other options for the symptomatic management of pruritis. Jaundice treatment primarily follows treating the underlying liver dysfunction. Monitoring cutaneous signs provides a simple, non-invasive method to assess the disease progression and treatment response. At baseline, these cutaneous signs should be identified and continually documented throughout to establish any systemic improvement or worsening of hepatic function.

7. Overall Importance of Recognizing and Addressing Cutaneous Manifestations of Liver Cirrhosis

Cutaneous signs of advanced liver disease may provide some insight into the severity of hepatic dysfunction and overall prognosis. For example, one study determined that the presence of at least one of four characteristic skin findings (spider naevi, palmar erythema, nail changes, or bleeding) was associated with the presence of severe fibrosis or cirrhosis. Conversely, only a low percentage of patients were found to have advanced liver disease in the absence of these findings [6]. Patients with spider nevi in particular were more than four times more likely to have severe liver disease [65]. Furthermore, the presence of subcutaneous collateral vessels upon physical exam predicted worse outcomes in patients with cirrhosis [66].

Skin findings may serve as early non-invasive indicators of advanced liver disease. Given their potential prognostic significance, they could provide a more accessible and cost-effective tool in the assessment of advanced liver disease. Therefore, dermatologists may play an important role in the multidisciplinary care team for these patients. For one, early identification of characteristic skin findings by dermatologists can prompt further testing, facilitate more rapid diagnosis, and improve long-term outcomes [60,67]. Additionally, in patients with pre-existing liver disease, dermatologists can play a role in monitoring for findings suggestive of illness progression.

Despite the potential clinical utility of cutaneous findings in characterization of severe liver disease, there are still significant limitations to its application. Variation among individual patients may impact the prognostic value of skin findings. Moreover, many of these findings lack sensitivity for advanced liver disease, thus limiting their usefulness for screening otherwise asymptomatic individuals without a high suspicion for advanced liver disease. For example, spider angiomas have a high association with pregnancy due to the hormonal changes that take place during gestation [5]. Lastly, the identification of any cutaneous lesion can vary widely based on skin tone, further necessitating the incorporation of diversity in research and medical education materials.

One of the essential components to provide a holistic approach to patient care is the collaboration between dermatologists and hepatologists for patients with skin manifestations of liver cirrhosis. Early recognition of the skin presentations of liver cirrhosis by dermatologists can lead to timely referral and early diagnosis, potentially preventing disease progression and improving patient outcomes. On the other hand, hepatologists should also consider prompt dermatology referrals that can help in further addressing patients' symptoms and improving quality of life. A multidisciplinary collaborative approach can help in improving patient education and understanding of their disease and even adherence to treatment and follow-up.

8. Future Directions

The integration of dermatologic screening into the routine clinical care of patients suspected to have cirrhosis can facilitate earlier diagnosis. Cirrhosis management reduces the risk of serious complications and liver decompensation if initiated early, while significantly improving a patient's quality of life [62]. Further research is needed to establish how specific cutaneous manifestations correlate to the severity and progression of cirrhosis. For example, spider angiomas can be seen in one-third of patients with cirrhosis and correlates with the frequency of esophageal varices, a complication of liver cirrhosis that can lead to hemorrhage [15,62]. Additionally, examining the psychosocial impact of cutaneous manifestations could help determine if dermatological interventions should be incorporated as part of the standard of care for cirrhosis patients.

Integrating the skin manifestations of liver cirrhosis and their underlying pathophysiology, diagnostic significance, and prognostic value into medical curricula and training programs offers a valuable opportunity to enhance early recognition among healthcare trainees. Educating medical students and residents on these cutaneous signs and their clinical implications can build clinical skills needed for the detection of liver disease at an earlier stage, prompting timely referrals, diagnosis, and management. Understanding the pathophysiology behind these disorders can also help in fostering further research studies to explore these biochemical pathways. This can also foster a collaborative multidisciplinary approach between hepatology and dermatology, providing a more holistic approach to patient care.

9. Conclusions

Cutaneous manifestations of liver cirrhosis reflect the underlying systemic dysfunction and can serve as early indicators of hepatic pathology. Non-specific signs such as spider angiomas, palmar erythema, jaundice, and pruritus may precede more overt clinical symptoms and offer valuable diagnostic and prognostic insights. Given their accessibility during physical examination, these dermatologic features should be routinely assessed in patients at risk for chronic liver disease. Regular skin evaluations can facilitate earlier detection of liver cirrhosis, allowing for timely diagnostic workup, initiation of management strategies, and improved patient outcomes. A thorough dermatological examination can aid in the assessment of liver cirrhosis by identifying skin manifestations that are more specific to liver disease, such as spider angioma, palmar erythema, and Terry's nails. These findings, when interpreted in the context of other clinical and laboratory data, are often associated with advanced liver disease and clinically significant portal hypertension, and their presence should prompt a comprehensive evaluation for signs of decompensation. Increasing clinician awareness and education regarding the dermatologic signs of liver cirrhosis is essential. By recognizing these cutaneous clues, healthcare providers can intervene earlier, mitigating complications and enhancing the quality of care for individuals with or at risk for liver cirrhosis.

Author Contributions: Conceptualization, R.K., Y.A., and J.B.T.; methodology, R.K., Y.A., and J.B.T.; software, R.K.; validation, C.R., and J.B.T.; formal analysis, R.K.; investigation, R.K., and J.B.T.; resources, R.K.; data curation, R.K.; writing—original draft preparation, R.K., R.R., R.A., T.C., C.D., A.P., and A.L.; writing—review and editing, C.R., and J.B.T.; visualization, C.R., and J.B.T.; supervision, C.R., and J.B.T.; project administration, R.K. All authors have read and agreed to the published version of the manuscript.

Funding: This research received no external funding.

Institutional Review Board Statement: Our review article involved only two patients and was limited to descriptive reporting without hypothesis testing or systematic investigation. As such, it does not meet the definition of human subjects research per institutional guidelines and was exempt from IRB/ethics committee review. Informed consent was obtained from both patients for the publication of their clinical information and images. No identifiable personal information was included in the manuscript. All other data included in the manuscript were based on available medical literature.

Informed Consent Statement: Informed consent was obtained from the patients to share deidentifed data.

Data Availability Statement: No new data were created or analyzed in this study. Data sharing is not applicable to this article.

Conflicts of Interest: The authors declare no conflicts of interest.

References

1. Tsochatzis, E.A.; Bosch, J.; Burroughs, A.K. Liver cirrhosis. *Lancet* **2014**, *383*, 1749–1761. [CrossRef] [PubMed]
2. Schuppan, D.; Afdhal, N.H. Liver cirrhosis. *Lancet* **2008**, *371*, 838–851. [CrossRef] [PubMed]
3. Horvatits, T.; Drolz, A.; Trauner, M.; Fuhrmann, V. Liver Injury and Failure in Critical Illness. *Hepatology* **2019**, *70*, 2204–2215. [CrossRef] [PubMed]
4. Martínez Jiménez, S. Cutaneous Manifestations of Liver Disease: A Narrative Review. *Cureus* **2024**, *16*, e70357. [CrossRef] [PubMed]
5. Liu, Y.; Zhao, Y.; Gao, X.; Liu, J.; Ji, F.; Hsu, Y.-C.; Li, Z.; Nguyen, M.H. Recognizing skin conditions in patients with cirrhosis: A narrative review. *Ann. Med.* **2022**, *54*, 3016–3028. [CrossRef] [PubMed]
6. Niederau, C.; Lange, S.; Frühauf, M.; Thiel, A. Cutaneous signs of liver disease: Value for prognosis of severe fibrosis and cirrhosis. *Liver Int.* **2008**, *28*, 659–666. [CrossRef]

7. Runyon, B.A. A Primer on Detecting Cirrhosis and Caring for These Patients without Causing Harm. *Int. J. Hepatol.* **2011**, *2011*, 801983. [CrossRef]
8. Ginès, P.; Krag, A.; Abraldes, J.G.; Solà, E.; Fabrellas, N.; Kamath, P.S. Liver cirrhosis. *Lancet* **2021**, *398*, 1359–1376. [CrossRef]
9. Somnay, K.; Wadgaonkar, P.; Sridhar, N.; Roshni, P.; Rao, N.; Wadgaonkar, R. Liver Fibrosis Leading to Cirrhosis: Basic Mechanisms and Clinical Perspectives. *Biomedicines* **2024**, *12*, 2229. [CrossRef]
10. Jagdish, R.K.; Roy, A.; Kumar, K.; Premkumar, M.; Sharma, M.; Rao, P.N.; Reddy, D.N.; Kulkarni, A.V. Pathophysiology and management of liver cirrhosis: From portal hypertension to acute-on-chronic liver failure. *Front. Med.* **2023**, *10*, 1060073. [CrossRef]
11. Fallahzadeh, M.A.; Rahimi, R.S. Hepatic Encephalopathy: Current and Emerging Treatment Modalities. *Clin. Gastroenterol. Hepatol.* **2022**, *20*, S9–S19. [CrossRef]
12. Samant, H.; Kothadia, J.P. Spider Angioma. In *StatPearls [Internet]*; StatPearls Publishing: Treasure Island, FL, USA, 2023. [PubMed]
13. Li, C.P. Spider angiomas in patients with liver cirrhosis: Role of vascular endothelial growth factor and basic fibroblast growth factor. *World J. Gastroenterol.* **2003**, *9*, 2832. [CrossRef]
14. Li, C.P.; Lee, F.Y.; Hwang, S.J.; Chang, F.-Y.; Lin, H.-C.; Lu, R.-H.; Hou, M.-C.; Chu, C.-J.; Chan, C.-C.; Luo, J.-C.; et al. Role of Substance P in The Pathogenesis of Spider Angiomas in Patients with Nonalcoholic Liver Cirrhosis. *Am. J. Gastroenterol.* **1999**, *94*, 502–507. [CrossRef]
15. Bhandari, A.; Mahajan, R. Skin Changes in Cirrhosis. *J. Clin. Exp. Hepatol.* **2022**, *12*, 1215–1224. [CrossRef] [PubMed]
16. Terp, K.; Izquierdo-Pretel, G. Spider Angioma Number and Location as Potential Prognostic Indicators in Chronic Liver Disease: A Case Report. *Cureus* **2023**, *15*, e34193. [CrossRef] [PubMed]
17. Kim, G.-W.; Shin, K.; Kim, T.-W.; Kim, T.-W.; You, H.-S.; Jin, H.-J.; Shim, W.-H.; Kim, H.-S.; Ko, H.-C.; Kim, B.-S.; et al. The importance of dermoscopy for the diagnosis of acquired bilateral telangiectatic macules: The angioid streak pattern reveals underlying chronic liver disease. *J. Eur. Acad. Dermatol. Venereol.* **2018**, *32*, 1597–1601. [CrossRef] [PubMed]
18. Huang, A.; Desai, A.; Brinster, N.; Marmon, S. Telangiectasia macularis eruptiva perstans in the presence of liver cirrhosis. *JAAD Case Rep.* **2020**, *6*, 438–440. [CrossRef] [PubMed]
19. Serrao, R.; Zirwas, M.; English, J.C. Palmar Erythema. *Am. J. Clin. Dermatol.* **2007**, *8*, 347–356. [CrossRef]
20. Nautiyal, A.; Chopra, K.B. Liver Palms (Palmar Erythema). *Am. J. Med.* **2010**, *123*, 596–597. [CrossRef]
21. Milam, P.; Berger, M.; Ramaswamy, B.; Reinbolt, R.; Wesolowski, R.; Kaffenberger, B.H. Spider Telangiectases and Palmar Erythema as Harbingers of Structural Liver Changes in Three Breast Cancer Patients on Ado-trastuzumab Emtansine. *J. Clin. Aesthet Dermatol.* **2019**, *12*, 23.
22. Gustot, T.; Stadlbauer, V.; Laleman, W.; Alessandria, C.; Thursz, M. Transition to decompensation and acute-on-chronic liver failure: Role of predisposing factors and precipitating events. *J. Hepatol.* **2021**, *75*, S36–S48. [CrossRef]
23. Harrison, P.M. Management of patients with decompensated cirrhosis. *Clin. Med.* **2015**, *15*, 201–203. [CrossRef] [PubMed]
24. Selim, R.; Ahn, J. Pruritus in Chronic Liver Disease. *Clin. Liver Dis.* **2023**, *27*, 47–55. [CrossRef]
25. Bassari, R. Jaundice associated pruritis: A review of pathophysiology and treatment. *World J. Gastroenterol.* **2015**, *21*, 1404. [CrossRef]
26. Düll, M.M.; Kremer, A.E. Newer Approaches to the Management of Pruritus in Cholestatic Liver Disease. *Curr. Hepatol. Rep.* **2020**, *19*, 86–95. [CrossRef]
27. Xu, J.; Wang, Y.; Khoshdeli, M.; Peach, M.; Chuang, J.; Lin, J.; Tsai, W.; Mahadevan, S.; Minto, W.; Diehl, L.; et al. IL-31 levels correlate with pruritus in patients with cholestatic and metabolic liver diseases and is farnesoid X receptor responsive in NASH. *Hepatology* **2023**, *77*, 20–32. [CrossRef]
28. Terg, R.; Coronel, E.; Sordá, J.; Muñoz, A.E.; Findor, J. Efficacy and safety of oral naltrexone treatment for pruritus of cholestasis, a crossover, double blind, placebo-controlled study. *J. Hepatol.* **2002**, *37*, 717–722. [CrossRef]
29. Bergasa, N.V.; Talbot, T.L.; Alling, D.W.; Schmitt, J.M.; Walker, E.C.; Baker, B.L.; Korenman, J.C.; Park, Y.; Hoofnagle, J.H.; Jones, E. A controlled trial of naloxone infusions for the pruritus of chronic cholestasis. *Gastroenterology* **1992**, *102*, 544–549. [CrossRef] [PubMed]
30. Meixiong, J.; Vasavda, C.; Snyder, S.H.; Dong, X. MRGPRX4 is a G protein-coupled receptor activated by bile acids that may contribute to cholestatic pruritus. *Proc. Natl. Acad. Sci. USA* **2019**, *116*, 10525–10530. [CrossRef] [PubMed]
31. Naschitz, J.E. Stasis Ulcers—The Unifying Concept. *J. Clin. Res. Rep.* **2021**, *9*, 1–5. [CrossRef]
32. El Younis, C.M.; Bergasa, N.V. Healing of leg ulcers associated with transjugular intrahepatic portosystemic shunt in decompensated cirrhosis: Case series of a possible hepatodermal syndrome. *Gastroenterol Hepatol.* **2008**, *4*, 211.
33. Terry, R. White nails in hepatic cirrhosis. *Lancet* **1954**, *263*, 757–759. [CrossRef] [PubMed]
34. Nia, A.M.; Ederer, S.; Dahlem, K.M.; Gassanov, N.; Er, F. Terry's Nails: A Window to Systemic Diseases. *Am. J. Med.* **2011**, *124*, 602–604. [CrossRef] [PubMed]

35. Sack, J.S.; Liu, A.F.; Gray, M.; Roat, J.; Zucker, S.D. Association of Terry Nails with Liver Cirrhosis. *Am. J. Gastroenterol.* **2021**, *116*, 2455–2458. [CrossRef]
36. Fernandez-Somoza, J.-M.; Ginarte, M.; Otero, E.; Tomé, S.; Soutullo, C.; Martínez-Ulloa, A.; Gonzalez-Quintela, A.; Sepehrimanesh, M. Clinical and capillaroscopic findings in patients with liver disease and proximal apparent leukonychia (Terry nails and its variants). *Medicine* **2021**, *100*, e26207. [CrossRef]
37. Salem, A.; Al Mokadem, S.; Attwa, E.; Abd El Raoof, S.; Ebrahim, H.; Faheem, K. Nail changes in chronic renal failure patients under haemodialysis. *J. Eur. Acad. Dermatol. Venereol.* **2008**, *22*, 1326–1331. [CrossRef] [PubMed]
38. Hojo, S.; Fujita, J.; Yamadori, I.; Ezaki, T.; Watanabe, S.; Yamanouchi, H.; Miyawaki, H.; Yamaji, Y.; Nishioka, M.; Takahara, J. Hepatocyte Growth Factor and Digital Clubbing. *Intern. Med.* **1997**, *36*, 44–46. [CrossRef]
39. Baila-Rueda, L.; Mateo-Gallego, R.; Lamiquiz-Moneo, I.; Cenarro, A.; Civeira, F. Severe hypercholesterolemia and phytosterolemia with extensive xanthomas in primary biliary cirrhosis: Role of biliary excretion on sterol homeostasis. *J. Clin. Lipidol.* **2014**, *8*, 520–524. [CrossRef]
40. Al Aboud, A.M.; Shah, S.S.; Blair, K.; Al Aboud, D.M. Xanthelasma Palpebrarum. In *StatPearls [Internet]*; StatPearls Publishing: Treasure Island, FL, USA, 2025. Available online: https://www.ncbi.nlm.nih.gov/books/NBK531501/ (accessed on 1 July 2025).
41. Sexton, F.; Shanahan, W.; Ryan, J.D. Xanthoma striatum palmare: Getting a handle on hyperlipidaemia in primary biliary cholangitis. *Clin. Res. Hepatol. Gastroenterol.* **2024**, *48*, 102255. [CrossRef]
42. Suzuki, L.; Hirayama, S.; Fukui, M.; Sasaki, M.; Hiroi, S.; Ayaori, M.; Terai, S.; Tozuka, M.; Watada, H.; Miida, T. Lipoprotein-X in cholestatic patients causes xanthomas and promotes foam cell formation in human macrophages. *J. Clin. Lipidol.* **2017**, *11*, 110–118. [CrossRef]
43. Hazin, R.; Tamimi, T.I.A.R.; Abuzetun, J.Y.; Zein, N.N. Recognizing and treating cutaneous signs of liver disease. *Cleve Clin. J. Med.* **2009**, *76*, 599–606. [CrossRef] [PubMed]
44. Van Alfen, B.; Hatch, J.; Conley, M.; Seeliyur Duraiswamy, S. A Case Report of Xanthelasma and the Associated Differential Diagnosis. *Cureus* **2025**, *17*, e81971. [CrossRef]
45. Saunders Elsevier. *Evidence-Based Physical Diagnosis*; Saunders Elsevier: Philadelphia, PA, USA, 2012.
46. Wilson, R.; Williams, D.M. Cirrhosis. *Med. Clin. N. Am.* **2022**, *106*, 437–446. [CrossRef]
47. Abraldes, J.G.; Caraceni, P.; Ghabril, M.; Garcia-Tsao, G. Update in the Treatment of the Complications of Cirrhosis. *Clin. Gastroenterol. Hepatol.* **2023**, *21*, 2100–2109. [CrossRef]
48. Simonetto, D.A.; Liu, M.; Kamath, P.S. Portal Hypertension and Related Complications: Diagnosis and Management. *Mayo Clin. Proc.* **2019**, *94*, 714–726. [CrossRef] [PubMed]
49. Nelson, L.R.; Bulun, S.E. Estrogen production and action. *J. Am. Acad. Dermatol.* **2001**, *45*, S116–S124. [CrossRef] [PubMed]
50. Neong, S.F.; Billington, E.O.; Congly, S.E. Sexual Dysfunction and Sex Hormone Abnormalities in Patients with Cirrhosis: Review of Pathogenesis and Management. *Hepatology* **2019**, *69*, 2683–2695. [CrossRef]
51. Sinclair, M.; Grossmann, M.; Gow, P.J.; Angus, P.W. Testosterone in men with advanced liver disease: Abnormalities and implications. *J. Gastroenterol. Hepatol.* **2015**, *30*, 244–251. [CrossRef]
52. Patel, A.D.; Katz, K.; Gordon, K.B. Cutaneous Manifestations of Chronic Liver Disease. *Clin. Liver Dis.* **2020**, *24*, 351–360. [CrossRef]
53. Roche, S.P.; Kobos, R. Jaundice in the adult patient. *Am. Fam. Phys.* **2004**, *69*, 299–304.
54. Berumen, J.; Baglieri, J.; Kisseleva, T.; Mekeel, K. Liver fibrosis: Pathophysiology and clinical implications. *WIREs Mech Dis.* **2021**, *13*, e1499. [CrossRef] [PubMed]
55. Dogra, S.; Jindal, R. Cutaneous Manifestations of Common Liver Diseases. *J. Clin. Exp. Hepatol.* **2011**, *1*, 177–184. [CrossRef]
56. Roche, F.C.; Harris-Tryon, T.A. Illuminating the Role of Vitamin A in Skin Innate Immunity and the Skin Microbiome: A Narrative Review. *Nutrients.* **2021**, *13*, 302. [CrossRef]
57. Igarashi, A.; Uzuka, M.; Nakajima, K. The effects of vitamin E deficiency on rat skin. *Br. J. Dermatol.* **1989**, *121*, 43–49. [CrossRef]
58. Ballal, S.; Prathibha, J.P.; Pinto, A.V.; Srinivasa, S.; Augustine, M. Unusual Manifestation of Vitamin K Deficiency, Nodular Purpura: A Case Series. *Indian Dermatol. Online J.* **2025**, *16*, 132–136. [CrossRef]
59. Mayo, M.J.; Carey, E.; Smith, H.T.; Mospan, A.R.; McLaughlin, M.; Thompson, A.; Morris, H.L.; Sandefur, R.; Kim, W.R.; Bowlus, C.; et al. Impact of Pruritus on Quality of Life and Current Treatment Patterns in Patients with Primary Biliary Cholangitis. *Dig. Dis. Sci.* **2023**, *68*, 995–1005. [CrossRef] [PubMed]
60. Schwarz, M.; Schwarz, C.; Burghart, L.; Pfisterer, N.; Bauer, D.; Hübl, W.; Mandorfer, M.; Gschwantler, M.; Reiberger, T.; Elbahrawy, A. Late-stage presentation with decompensated cirrhosis is alarmingly common but successful etiologic therapy allows for favorable clinical outcomes. *PLoS ONE* **2023**, *18*, e0290352. [CrossRef] [PubMed]
61. Jindal, A.; Gupta, A.; Bhadoria, A.S. Resolution of Multiple Large Spider Angiomas After Liver Transplantation in Severe Alcoholic Hepatitis. *Indian J. Dermatol.* **2022**, *67*, 837. [CrossRef]
62. Fadlallah, H.; El Masri, D.; Bahmad, H.F.; Abou-Kheir, W.; El Masri, J. Update on the Complications and Management of Liver Cirrhosis. *Med. Sci.* **2025**, *13*, 13. [CrossRef]

63. Ebhohon, E.; Chung, R.T. Systematic review: Efficacy of therapies for cholestatic pruritus. *Therap. Adv. Gastroenterol.* **2023**, *16*. [CrossRef]
64. Bolier, R.; de Vries, E.S.; Parés, A.; Helder, J.; Kemper, E.M.; Zwinderman, K.; Elferink, R.P.O.; Beuers, U. Fibrates for the treatment of cholestatic itch (FITCH): Study protocol for a randomized controlled trial. *Trials* **2017**, *18*, 230. [CrossRef]
65. Udell, J.A.; Wang, C.S.; Tinmouth, J.; FitzGerald, J.M.; Ayas, N.T.; Simel, D.L.; Schulzer, M.; Mak, E.; Yoshida, E.M. Does This Patient with Liver Disease Have Cirrhosis? *JAMA* **2012**, *307*, 832. [CrossRef] [PubMed]
66. Li, H.; Wang, R.; Méndez-Sánchez, N.; Peng, Y.; Guo, X.; Qi, X. Impact of spider nevus and subcutaneous collateral vessel of chest/abdominal wall on outcomes of liver cirrhosis. *Arch. Med. Sci.* **2019**, *15*, 434–448. [CrossRef] [PubMed]
67. Ginès, P.; Castera, L.; Lammert, F.; Graupera, I.; Serra-Burriel, M.; Allen, A.M.; Wong, V.W.; Hartmann, P.; Thiele, M.; Caballeria, L.; et al. Population screening for liver fibrosis: Toward early diagnosis and intervention for chronic liver diseases. *Hepatology* **2022**, *75*, 219–228. [CrossRef] [PubMed]

livers

Review

Low Hepatic CEACAM1 Tethers Metabolic Dysfunction Steatohepatitis to Atherosclerosis

Sacha El Khoury [1,†], Sami N. Al Harake [1,†], Tya Youssef [1], Carl E. Risk [1], Naim G. Helou [2], Natalie M. Doumet [3], Karl Aramouni [4], Sami Azar [1], Sonia M. Najjar [5,6,*] and Hilda E. Ghadieh [1,*]

1 Department of Biomedical Sciences, Faculty of Medicine and Medical Sciences, University of Balamand, Al-Koura, Tripoli P.O. Box 100, Lebanon; sacha.khoury@std.balamand.edu.lb (S.E.K.); sami.harake@std.balamand.edu.lb (S.N.A.H.); tya.youssef@std.balamand.edu.lb (T.Y.); carl.rizk@std.balamand.edu.lb (C.E.R.); sami.azar@balamand.edu.lb (S.A.)
2 Gilbert and Rose-Marie Chagoury School of Medicine, Lebanese American University, Byblos P.O. Box 36, Lebanon; naim.helou@lau.edu
3 Center for Diabetes and Endocrine Research, University of Toledo College of Medicine, Toledo, OH 43614, USA; natalie.doumet@rockets.utoledo.edu
4 Department of Medicine, Faculty of Medicine, American University of Beirut, Riad El-Solh, P.O. Box 11-0236, Beirut 1107-2020, Lebanon; kma56@mail.aub.edu
5 Department of Biomedical Sciences, Heritage College of Osteopathic Medicine, Ohio University, Athens, OH 45701, USA
6 Diabetes Institute, Heritage College of Osteopathic Medicine, Ohio University, Athens, OH 43614, USA
* Correspondence: najjar@ohio.edu (S.M.N.); hilda.ghadieh@balamand.edu.lb (H.E.G.)
† These authors contributed equally to this work.

Abstract: Metabolic dysfunction-associated steatohepatitis (MASH) and atherosclerosis are cardiometabolic twin disorders with shared underlying pathophysiological mechanisms such as insulin resistance and chronic inflammation. This review explores the salient role of carcinoembryonic antigen-related cell adhesion molecule 1 (CEACAM1) in linking hepatic dysfunction to cardiovascular disease. Findings in mice with genetic modulation of *Ceacam1* gene established a critical role for CEACAM1 protein in regulating insulin and lipid metabolism and endothelial integrity and modulating immune response. Loss of CEACAM1 in hepatocytes impairs insulin clearance, causing chronic hyperinsulinemia, a process that ultimately leads to insulin resistance and hepatic and extra-hepatic fat accumulation, which in turn causes inflammatory infiltration. This prompts a paradigm shift that positions impaired hepatic CEACAM1 function as a mechanistic underpinning of the link between insulin resistance, MASH, and atherosclerosis.

Keywords: atherosclerosis; endothelial injury; MASH; hepatic fibrosis; CEACAM1; insulin resistance; hyperinsulinemia; metabolic syndrome

1. Introduction

The rampant increase in the prevalence of obesity and insulin resistance worldwide has precipitated an alarming rise in metabolic disorders, including metabolic dysfunction-associated steatohepatitis (MASH) and atherosclerosis. Modern medicine is redefining these abnormalities of the hepatic and vascular systems as twin manifestations of a broader systemic metabolic dysregulation. Atherosclerosis, characterized by intimal plaque accumulation, remains the principal cause of cardiovascular mortality worldwide [1,2]. Concurrently, MASH, an advanced stage of metabolic dysfunction-associated steatotic liver disease (MASLD) afflicts approximately 30% of the adult population and represents a major risk factor for liver cirrhosis and hepatocellular carcinoma [3,4]. Characterization of shared pathophysiological mechanisms is emerging to bridge hepatic dysfunction and vascular injury. These include chronic low-grade inflammation, oxidative stress, and aberrant lipid metabolism [5,6]. Moreover, epidemiological analysis provides evidence of a two-to-threefold increase in cardiovascular risk among patients with MASLD, independent of traditional risk factors such as type 2 diabetes (T2D) and dyslipidemia. In parallel, patients with established atherosclerotic disease also present with comorbid hepatic steatosis [7–9]. Furthermore, these analyses frame insulin resistance, a critical hallmark of multisystem metabolic derangements, as a unifying disease driver [10,11]. For instance, insulin resistance promotes de novo lipogenesis and impairs fatty acid β-oxidation (FAO) in the liver, ultimately leading to hepatic steatosis and hepatocellular injury [12]. Similarly, insulin resistance diminishes nitric oxide (NO) bioavailability and compromises endothelial integrity, contributing to the development of an atherogenic milieu in the vasculature [13,14]. Thus, hepatic and cardiovascular pathophysiology resides at the crossroad of hyperinsulinemia, aberrant lipid metabolism, endothelial dysfunction, and chronic proinflammatory signaling.

Recent findings have established a regulatory role for carcinoembryonic antigen-related cell adhesion molecule 1 (CEACAM1) in hepatic metabolism and vascular integrity [15,16]. CEACAM1, expressed predominantly in hepatocytes, promotes insulin clearance via receptor-mediated endocytosis [10,17]. Interestingly, obesity and metabolic syndrome (MetS) are associated with low hepatic CEACAM1 levels and impaired insulin clearance with resultant persistent hyperinsulinemia and insulin resistance [18,19]. Moreover, murine models with global null deletion or hepatocyte-specific deletion of *Ceacam1* gene emulate cardinal features of human MetS, including insulin resistance, steatohepatitis, visceral adiposity, and endothelial dysfunction [20,21]. CEACAM1 deficiency promotes hepatic inflammation via the activation of nuclear factor kappa B (NF-κB) and attenuates endothelial NO synthase (eNOS) activity, producing a proinflammatory atherogenic milieu with oxidative stress in mice. CEACAM1 loss serves therefore as a molecular bridge between hepatic insulin resistance endothelial injury and oxidative stress [15,22,23].

It is becoming increasingly apparent that efficient therapeutic management of MetS requires an integrated multisystem molecular approach, targeting shared mediators such as CEACAM1, that is particularly relevant in addressing the role of the liver in systemic metabolic dysfunction. This review aims to discuss the impact of the loss of hepatic CEACAM1 in the broader spectrum of metabolic disorders by providing evidence of its function in hepatic metabolism and vascular physiology. Furthermore, it posits CEACAM1′s potential as a therapeutic target in MetS-associated clinical presentations, namely atherosclerosis and MASH.

2. Pathophysiology of Atherosclerosis: Mechanisms and Cardiovascular Implications

2.1. *Atherosclerosis: Prevalence and Clinical Significance*

Atherosclerosis is the major indicator of cardiovascular disease (CVD), which represents the most common cause of death worldwide [1]. The World Health Organization (WHO) has estimated that ~18 million people die from CVD annually, accounting for ~32% of all deaths worldwide [2]. The salient rise in CVD incidence is tethered to a global epidemic of obesity and T2D [5]. Although atherosclerotic lesions may begin at an early age, the timeline of clinical manifestations and related complications remains poorly characterized [24,25]. Initially raised as an obstruction process of the arteries, atherosclerosis is mostly caused by accumulation of cholesterol plaques in the intima, the innermost layer of blood vessels, and hardening of elastic (i.e., aorta) and muscular arteries, such as coronary and cerebral arteries [26,27]. The pathogenesis and progression of atherosclerosis are best described as an insidious process slowly unfolding over the span of several decades, often with minimal symptomatic manifestation. Ultimately, this culminates in critical vessel narrowing and plaque accumulation, thereby instigating life-threatening complications such as angina pectoris, acute coronary syndrome, and sudden cardiac death [28]. Atherosclerosis is now recognized as part of MetS, a constellation of metabolic and vascular conditions such as obesity, hypertension, and T2D. Lifestyle modification such as smoking cessation, physical activity, and healthy diet can mitigate atherosclerosis progression, further corroborating the recognition of atherosclerosis as a lifestyle disease [1].

2.2. *The Pathophysiological Hallmarks of Atherosclerosis*

It is crucial to delineate the fundamental pathophysiological processes in atherosclerosis to gain a better understanding of pathways and molecular events that could constitute therapeutic targets.

2.2.1. Endothelial Dysfunction

The luminal surface of all blood vessels is lined by a layer of endothelium [29]. Together with collagen and elastic fibers, the endothelium comprises the intima, which is wrapped up mostly by the vascular smooth muscle layer of the tunica media, followed by the adventitia, a dense connective tissue matrix, which provides robust structural support [29]. Endothelium is essential in preserving the structural integrity and regulating the physiological function of blood vessels. This includes maintaining the equilibrium between vasodilation and vasoconstriction, as well as orchestrating the migration and multiplication of vascular smooth muscle cells [30,31].

Endothelial dysfunction, an early sign of atherogenesis [32,33], often starts at the branching points and orifices of the arteries. These sites experience disturbed blood flow and shear stress, which leads to the accumulation of low-density lipoproteins (LDL) and lipoprotein buildup [14,34–37]. Endothelial dysfunction is further exacerbated by altered expression of specific endothelial genes, often as a direct consequence of disturbed blood flow and abnormal hemodynamic forces [38,39]. To date, more than 40 atherogenic genes linked to endothelial dysfunction have been identified [40,41]. In fact, these genes are upregulated in endothelial cells and are implicated in different steps of plaque formation. For example, monocyte chemoattractant protein 1 (MCP-1) that attracts monocytes to the vessel wall [42,43] and platelet-derived growth factor (PDGF) that promote vascular smooth muscle migration [44,45].

Conversely, NO, an endothelium-derived vasodilator, plays a critical athero-protective role in the maintenance of vascular homeostasis and endothelial integrity [46]. NO has multiple beneficial effects: Besides its role in smooth muscle relaxation and vasodilation, it also enhances cardiovascular and metabolic outcomes. NO slows down the development of atherosclerosis by reducing inflammation and oxidative stress and inhibiting platelet aggregation. Furthermore, NO promotes insulin secretion, facilitates glucose clearance, and reduces hepatic steatosis and triglyceride levels, thereby offering protection against the broader metabolic dysfunction [47,48]. However, the protective effects of NO are weakened by cardiovascular risk factors. For example, hyper-cholesterolemic and hypertensive patients often have reduced NO levels [49,50]. In fact, cardiovascular risk factors—namely hypertension, hyperlipidemia, obesity, and diabetes—potentiate NF-κB downstream proinflammatory signaling and cytokine production, in addition to the vasoconstrictor Endothelin-1, which in turn inhibits the activity of the endothelial nitric oxide synthase (eNOS) [51,52]. Even aside from its impact on eNOS, the oxidative stress linked to these risk factors directly contributes to endothelial dysfunction and atherosclerosis [13,14,53].

2.2.2. Lipid Accumulation and Plaque Formation

Atherosclerosis arises from an interplay between endothelial dysfunction and lipoprotein accumulation, which promotes a chronic inflammatory environment that drives disease progression [54]. Cholesterol, a major structural component of the cell membrane, is carried in the blood by lipoproteins. Among the five types of plasma lipoproteins, LDL, intermediate density lipoproteins (IDL), and very low-density lipoproteins (VLDL) are most strongly linked to plaque formation [55]. LDL particles cross the endothelium through a process called caveolae-mediated transcytosis, which involves receptors like SR-B1 and ALK1 [56–58]. The proatherogenic role of caveolae-facilitated LDL transcytosis is evidenced by the higher levels of the structural protein caveolin 1 in atherosclerotic plaques [59]. Once inside the vessel wall, LDL is oxidized by enzymes like phospholipase and lipoxygenase and by reactive oxygen species (ROS) [60]. Additionally, the depletion of antioxidants, such as alpha-tocopherol and carotenoids, further exacerbates LDL oxidation. Oxidized LDL (oxLDL) triggers proinflammatory signaling cascades in endothelial cells and drives macrophage chemotaxis, constituting key pathogenic events in atherosclerosis [60]. Activation of NF-κB in endothelial cells promotes the expression of its transcriptional targets such as VCAM-1 and ICAM-1 adhesion molecules and MCP-1 and IL-8 chemokines, as well as other prothrombotic factors [61]. After endothelial cells are activated, monocyte recruitment occurs through a multistep process: rolling, adhesion, activation, and transmigration [62]. This entire process is mediated by the interaction between monocyte integrins and endothelial adhesion molecules. Chemokines such as CXCL1, CXCL2, CXCL4, and CCL5 coordinate these events [63]. While monocyte infiltration in atherosclerosis primarily occurs through paracellular migration across endothelial junctions, the transcellular route can also be implicated [64]. The chemokine MCP-1 plays a crucial role in facilitating monocyte trans-endothelial migration [65]. Once in the subintimal space, monocytes differentiate into macrophages, which can either adopt a proinflammatory M1 phenotype or an anti-inflammatory M2 phenotype, dictated by the cytokine milieu [66,67]. M1-polarized macrophages produce NO and inflammatory cytokines, which further increase endothelial permeability and promote inflammation [68]. These macrophages take up oxLDL via different scavenger receptors such as CD36, SRA-l, and LOX-I, which are upregulated in response to high oxLDL levels, promoting further lipid internalization [69,70]. Under homeostatic conditions, the ABCA1 transporter system facilitates cholesterol efflux from macrophages, thereby preventing excessive lipid accumulation [69]. However, when exposed to a continuous inflammatory stimulus, the macrophage's lipid efflux mechanism is disrupted, leading to the transformation of M1 macrophages into foam cells that play a direct role in atherosclerotic plaque formation [71,72]. This self-perpetuating process continues as the lipid-laden macrophages and oxLDL trigger NF-κB pathway activation, which in turn promotes further monocyte recruitment, differentiation and oxLDL internalization, marking the formation of a fatty streak—an early phase of atherosclerosis [71,72]. Additional pathways, such as NLRP3 inflammasome activation and consequent caspase-1 activation in macrophages, also contributes to atherosclerotic plaque progression and cholesterol crystal formation [73].

2.2.3. Vascular Smooth Muscle Cell Migration and Proliferation

Monocytes are not the only cells that internalize oxLDL and contribute to the foam cell population. In fact, vascular smooth muscle cells (VSMC) constitute up to 50% of the foam cell population in atherosclerotic plaques [74]. These VSMCs, typically located in the tunica media, migrate to the subendothelial space in response to epidermal growth factor (EGF), fibroblast growth factor (FGF), insulin-like growth factor (IGF), PDGF, transforming growth factor-β (TGF-β), and vascular endothelial growth factor (VEGF) secreted by foam cells and endothelial cells. Once in the subendothelial space, VMSCs begin to proliferate and secrete extracellular matrix (ECM) components such as collagen and elastin, contributing to the formation of the fibrous cap that covers the atherosclerotic plaque [75]. Additionally, plaque-residing macrophages produce IL-1, which promotes VSMC proliferation [71,72]. Progressively, microcalcifications form within the plaque driven by the osteogenic trans-differentiation of pericytes and VSMCs in response to the high calcium orthophosphate microenvironment. These cells acquire an osteoblast-like phenotype, like processes taking place in bone tissue formation. This calcification event produces a hardened fibrous atherosclerotic lesion, which promotes plaque stability and reduces the risk of complications such as rupture and thrombus formation.

2.3. Risk Factors and Their Impact on Atherosclerosis Progression

There are several well-recognized risk factors for atherosclerosis, including obesity, hypercholesterolemia, hypertension, diabetes, and smoking. These risk factors share overlapping and interrelated pathophysiological pathways that lead to the development of atherosclerotic disease. In fact, atherosclerosis is now considered a state of chronic vascular inflammation, triggered by the effects of these risk factors on the arterial wall. Identifying the role of these risk factors and implementing targeted lifestyle modifications is an effective way to halt atherosclerosis progression [76]. For instance, toxic chemical constituents of cigarettes are potent dose-dependent risk factors for the development of calcified atherosclerotic plaques. Moreover, smoking cessation is strongly recommended to slow atherosclerosis progression and reduce mortality risk [77]. As mentioned earlier, oxidative stress plays a central role in the development of atherosclerotic lesions. Diabetes, hypertension, obesity, dyslipidemia, and smoking are all known inducers of ROS generation that lower NO bioavailability. Among these factors, hypertension is the most significant contributor to endothelial dysfunction and can be worsened by other comorbidities, such as obesity, diabetes, insulin resistance, hyperinsulinemia, hypercholesterolemia, and renal disease. For instance, obesity stimulates the renin–angiotensin–aldosterone system, promoting sodium retention and hypertension [78,79]. Hypercholesterolemia is strongly linked to atherosclerosis development. In fact, mounting evidence of this association have supported the "lipid hypothesis" of atherosclerosis. The advent of statins (HMG-CoA reductase inhibitors)—the most potent lipid-lowering agents thus far—provided definitive evidence that reducing plasma cholesterol levels can prevent atherosclerosis [80]. Elevated levels of LDL, due to hypercholesterolemia, not only trigger aberrant endothelial activation but also upregulate adhesion molecules on the endothelial cell surface, facilitating monocyte and lymphocyte adherence to the intima [81]. Hyperglycemia also has a strong association with cardiovascular disease, leading to sorbitol accumulation via the aldose reductase pathway, which contributes to endothelial dysfunction [82]. Moreover, elevated glucose levels induces post-translational modifications in myocardial ECM proteins and impairs the expression and function of intramyocellular calcium channels, resulting in systolic and diastolic dysfunction [83]. Additionally, platelet aggregation plays a crucial role in the ensuing micro- and macrovascular complications of diabetes mellitus and atherogenesis [72]. Non-enzymatic glycation leads to the formation of advanced glycation end products (AGEs), which modify LDL and cause damage to the endothelium. AGEs also interact with the receptor for advanced glycation end products (RAGE), present on vascular smooth muscle cells, to accelerate atherosclerosis [84,85]. Another contributing pathway is hyperglycemia-induced polyol pathway activation, which further exacerbates vascular damage in patients with diabetes [86]. Activation of protein kinase C (PKC) and hexosamine flux pathways have also been reported to contribute to atherosclerotic plaque initiation. The complex crosstalk between adipose tissue and the cardiovascular system has been extensively documented. In 1847, an autopsy report on an obese man described the presence of a large, fibrous heart filled with fat. Subsequent studies revealed that severely obese individuals often exhibit increased cardiac output and pulmonary hypertension and eventually develop heart failure [87]. Abdominal obesity subjects the heart to high afterload pressures, leading to increased cardiac output, which leads to left ventricular (LV) remodeling, wall thickening, and left ventricular hypertrophy (LVH). Furthermore, obesity in patients with T2D is strongly associated with heart failure [87,88]. In metabolic abnormal states marked by high levels of fatty acids and carbohydrates, such as obesity and insulin resistance, lipids accumulate in the myocardium, a process known as cardiac steatosis. Lipid deposition in cardiomyocytes is largely due to an imbalance between lipid uptake and fatty acid β-oxidation [89]. Furthermore, the accumulation of visceral adipose tissue in pericardial and epicardial fat depots produces inflammatory cytokines and adipokines, which can affect myocardial contractility. In addition, free fatty acid-mediated potentiate macrophage-associated inflammation, disrupting cardiac electric modeling [90]. The NF-κB signaling pathway also contributes to the pathogenesis of heart failure owing to its involvement in cardiac remodeling [91].

2.4. Rising Incidence of HFpEF and LV Diastolic Dysfunction in Women Suggests a Potential Link to Hyperinsulinemia

Left ventricular diastolic dysfunction (LVDD) is defined as functional and metabolic instability during myocardial relaxation, leading to insufficient filling of the left ventricle. This condition can result from impaired cardiac relaxation, increased myocardial stiffness, and left atrial dysfunction [92]. LVDD is diagnosed using echocardiographic measurements and can range from mild, asymptomatic condition to progression into heart failure, with symptoms such as dyspnea and chest discomfort. While the prevalence of LVDD in the general population ranges between 3.1% and 35%, contingent on factors such as age, lifestyle, and discrepancies in diagnostic criteria, the global prevalence of heart failure is ~1–2.5% worldwide [93]. Subsequently, management of risk factors and a robust understanding of the preclinical disease stages are essential for prevention. Although there is no significant difference in the prevalence of heart failure between men and women, women are more likely to develop heart failure with preserved ejection fraction (HFpEF). In one study, 67% of women with heart failure exhibited HFpEF, compared to only 42% of men [93]. For non-modifiable risk factors, sex-related differences in cardiac function and structure accounts for such statistical disparities. In fact, women typically have lower left ventricular mass and volume, along with a higher left ventricular ejection fraction and a greater Global Longitudinal Strain compared to men [94–96]. As women age, they experience an abrupt increase in left ventricular mass and slower cardiomyocyte compared to men, predisposing them to a greater concentric LV remodeling and evolving HFpEF [97]. When LVDD progresses to HFpEF, clinical symptoms become apparent despite a preserved ejection fraction (EF > 50%) [98]. To date, the pathophysiology of HFpEF remains poorly understood, and accordingly, adequate treatment is lacking. In the context of confounding comorbidities, such as chronic obstructive pulmonary disease (COPD) and atrial fibrillation, the diagnosis of HFpEF becomes challenging, as it can mimic other presentations resembling exercise-induced dyspnea. HFpEF seems to be underdiagnosed in elderly women [99], in particular in patients with diabetes [100]. Failure to diagnose HFpEF is detrimental to patient's quality of life. Obesity, on the other hand, is an established risk factor for heart failure, with women having 4% to 29% higher prevalence of obesity compared to men [101]. Persistent hypercholesterolemia and insulin resistance adversely affect the cardiovascular system, since insulin receptors are abundantly expressed on myocardial, endothelial, and vascular smooth muscle cells [102]. Moreover, insulin signaling is important for the maintenance of cardiac integrity, mitochondrial metabolism, and substrate uptake for β-oxidation. Impairment of these processes may manifest themselves as left ventricular remodeling to contribute to HFpEF emergence. Downstream insulin signaling stimulates phosphoinositide-3 kinase (PI3K/Akt) and Shc/Ras/mitogen-activated protein kinase (MAPK) pathways [103]. Insulin resistance and hyperinsulinemia overstimulate the MAPK pathway, leading to increased production of the vasoconstrictor Endothelin-1, in turn enhancing the hypertensive effects of the sympathetic nervous system, eventually progressing to cardiac hypertrophy and atherosclerosis [104]. Concurrently, hyperinsulinemia inhibits the PI3K/Akt pathway, which regulates the metabolic effects of insulin and the production of NO by vascular smooth muscle cells and endothelial cells [104,105]. The cumulative effects of disrupted insulin signaling and the growth-promoting effects of chronic hyperinsulinemia on vascular smooth muscle cells lead to increased left ventricular mass with a concentric remodeling pattern that worsens HFpEF. Early efforts in reducing hyperinsulinemia and insulin resistance could mitigate their adverse cardiovascular co-morbidities and halt progression to HFpEF [106].

3. Pathophysiology of MASH

3.1. Overview, Prevalence, and Clinical Significance of MASH

MASLD has been recognized as the hepatic manifestation of MetS. MASLD encompasses a broad spectrum of clinical stages ranging from hepatic steatosis to more severe presentations, such as steatohepatitis, MASH, fibrosis, and cirrhosis, that could eventually culminate in hepatocellular carcinoma (HCC) and end-stage liver disease that necessitates liver transplantation [107,108]. The global prevalence of MASLD exceeds 30% of the adult population, rendering it a worldwide health threat [3,4,109]. Alarmingly, approximately 20 million people are projected to die from complications of steatotic liver disease worldwide. Data from the Global Burden of Disease database indicates that MASLD is the fastest-growing cause of liver cirrhosis, liver failure, and liver cancer. It is important to note that MASLD is not merely a liver-specific disorder but a component of concomitant systemic conditions associated with multi-organ metabolic dysfunction. The diagnosis of MASLD requires the detection of steatosis in more than 5% of hepatocytes, associated with a defined metabolic abnormality, such as obesity, T2D, or dyslipidemia [110–112]. Unfortunately, MASLD imposes a growing economic and public health burden on society, highlighting the urgent need for targeted therapies that depend on further exploration of its underlying mechanisms [113,114].

3.2. Key Mechanisms in the Development of MASH

3.2.1. Hepatic Steatosis and Lipid Accumulation

Lipid levels in hepatocytes are tightly regulated via a delicate balance between lipid uptake and de novo synthesis on one hand and FAO and fatty acid export on another. Disruption of hepatic lipid homeostasis results in lipid accumulation, primarily in the form of triglycerides within hepatocytes. Lipid uptake is mediated by various proteins, including fatty acid-binding protein 1 (FABP1), which is predominantly expressed in the liver. FABP1 is an important regulator of lipid metabolism that participates in fatty acid transport, β-oxidation, and incorporation into triglycerides [12]. In fact, higher levels of FABP1 correlate with increased hepatic lipid accumulation and steatosis [115]. However, the utilization of FABP1 serum levels as a diagnostic biomarker of hepatic steatosis remains challenging, as it is co-expressed by renal tubules [116].

Additionally, cluster of differentiation 36 (CD36) and fatty acid transport protein 5 (FATP5) are also implicated in lipotoxicity. For instance, CD36 expression is upregulated in response to a high-fat diet and correlates with liver fat content of MASLD patients [117,118]. Similarly, FATP 5 expression is also increased, particularly in males with MASLD, reflecting a higher degree of hepatic steatosis in these patients [119]. CD36 and FATP5 serve as important therapeutic targets for halting the progression of MASLD into MASH. Aberrant triglyceride synthesis via de novo lipogenesis is also implicated in the development of hepatic steatosis [120]. De novo lipogenesis is mediated by three enzymes: acetyl-CoA carboxylase (ACC), which converts acetyl-CoA to malonyl-CoA; fatty acid synthase (FASN), which transforms malonyl-CoA into palmitate; and stearoyl-CoA desaturase-1 (SCD1), which generates oleate and palmitoleate [121]. In fact, higher levels of oleate and palmitoleate are associated with increased hepatic steatosis [121]. Moreover, activation of the transcription factors sterol regulatory element-binding protein 1c (SREBP-1c) by insulin and carbohydrate regulatory element-binding protein (ChREBP) upregulate lipogenic enzymes, thereby enhancing hepatic lipid accumulation [122–124]. Notably, ChREBP knock out mice display reduced expression of ACC and FASN in response to a carbohydrate-rich diet, highlighting its pro-steatotic role [125].

Conversely, impaired FAO and defective export of lipids from hepatocytes also leads to lipid accumulation. FAO occurs mainly in the mitochondria, facilitated by the outer mitochondrial membrane (OMM) enzyme carnitine palmitoyl transferase 1 (CPT1), which is in turn regulated by peroxisome proliferator-activated receptor-α (PPARα) [121,126–129]. PPARα activation induces transcription of lipolytic genes in the mitochondria (CPT1), peroxisomes (acyl-CoA oxidase, ACOX), and cytochromes (Cyp4A family) [126,130,131]. Reciprocally, hepatic PPARα levels are regulated by glycogen synthase kinase 3β (GSK3β) via phosphorylation at its serine-73 residue (Ser73) [129]. GSK3β-mediated phosphorylation of PPARα promotes its ubiquitination and subsequent degradation, thereby decreasing its lipolytic activity [129]. This is consistent with the observation that patients with MASLD exhibit a diminished activity and expression of PPARα, which accounts for its involvement in diet-induced hepatic steatosis [130,132]. Triglyceride export is another mechanism that may contribute to intrahepatic lipid buildup. Apolipoprotein B100 (apoB100) and microsomal triglyceride transfer protein (MTTP) are key regulators of this process. MTTP facilitates lipid loading onto apoB100, enabling the maturation and secretion of VLDL. VLDL particles are generated in the endoplasmic reticulum (ER) and are subsequently sent to the Golgi apparatus, where they undergo maturation before being released into the bloodstream through an ApoB100-dependent mechanism. However, excessive fatty acid levels overwhelm ApoB100 secretion capacity, inducing endoplasmic reticulum (ER) stress and promoting steatosis. This underscores the implication of genetic defects in MTTP, and the ensuing alteration in triglyceride export, that account for the onset of MASLD and the pathophysiological mechanisms responsible for aberrant intrahepatic lipid accumulation [133]. Studies in the Han Chinese population demonstrated that MTTP polymorphisms influence MASLD development. In a genetic murine MASLD model, high MTTP expression reduces hepatic triglyceride levels via enhancing VLDL secretion. Similarly, diminished ApoB100 levels results in decreased secretion of VLDL and promotes lipid accumulation in hepatocytes. Additionally, patients with MASH exhibit lower ApoB100 synthesis, indicative of a lower lipid transport rate, which could contribute significantly to advanced steatosis and lipotoxicity in these patients [134]. Furthermore, buildup of saturated fatty acids generates lipotoxic intermediates, such as diacylglycerols, which induce ER stress and ROS production, recognized for their direct participation in MASH pathogenesis [135–137]. In addition, SFAs bind to Toll-like receptor 4 (TLR4), triggering pro-inflammatory NF-κB signaling and exacerbating mitochondrial dysfunction [136]. Delineating the physiological derangements in pathways of lipid metabolism that occur in MASLD provides mechanistic insights that could be exploited in the context of therapeutic interventions.

3.2.2. Oxidative Stress and Mitochondrial Dysfunction

Excess lipid buildup in hepatocytes enhances mitochondrial lipolysis and β-oxidation, leading to increased ROS production within the respiratory chain. The resulting increase in ROS levels disrupts mitochondrial integrity by increasing membrane permeability and impairing mitochondrial antioxidative defense mechanisms [138]. The ensuing ROS-mediated mitochondrial injury initiates a self-perpetuating cycle of ROS production. In palmitic acid-mediated lipotoxicity, the mitochondrial protein Sab interacts with JNK, causing electron transport chain (ETC) dysfunction, amplified ROS production, and eventually initiation of apoptosis [139]. Accumulated ROS activates the mitochondrial apoptosis pathway by opening the mitochondrial membrane permeability transition pore (MPTP). Subsequently, the uncoupling of the electron transport chain occurs, and ATP production is disrupted. The release of cytochrome c, which combines with apoptosis activator factor-1 (Apaf-1), subsequently activates caspase-9 and caspase-3, thereby inducing cell death [140]. The voltage-dependent anion channel (VDAC) plays a key role in sensing lipotoxicity by altering outer mitochondrial membrane permeability. Reduced GSK3-mediated phosphorylation of VDAC promotes calcium and water influx, leading cytochrome c release and apoptosis. In addition, oxidative stress overwhelms the body's antioxidant defense system leading to peroxidation of membrane lipids by polyunsaturated fatty acids. This increases the production of ROS and reactive nitrogen species (RNS), which contribute to further tissue damage as they diffuse into the surrounding extracellular space [141,142].

In both mice and humans, mitochondrial respiration is initially augmented in hepatic steatosis. For instance, patients with MASH display a higher degree of mitochondrial uncoupling, proton leakage, structural alterations, and diminished mitochondrial function, leading to disproportionate hepatic oxidative stress [143,144]. Noteworthy, mitochondrial autophagy (mitophagy) ensures the maintenance of metabolic and energy homeostasis by selectively eliminating mitochondria that generate excessive amounts of ROS [145]. This can hold important implications in treating MASLD. Moreover, cAMP-response element-binding protein H (CREBH), a key regulator of hepatic lipid metabolism has emerged as a promising therapeutic target as it enhances mitochondrial resistance to oxidative stress and inflammation in MASH [146].

Damage-associated molecular patterns (DAMPs), such as high mobility group box-1 protein (HMGB), released as a consequence of ROS-induced tissue injury, bind to TLR4 on Kupffer cells (KCs) [147]. This triggers NF-κB signaling, leading to proinflammatory cytokine release, thereby amplifying the inflammatory response. Moreover, DAMPs can also bind to TLR9 on KCs, amplifying TLR9-dependent ROS synthesis, further perpetuating a pro-inflammatory vicious cycle [148]. These findings underscore the contribution of ROS-induced hepatic injury and mitochondrial dysfunction in the metabolic and pathophysiologic impairments observed in patients with MASLD.

3.2.3. Hepatic Inflammation and Immune Response

Lipid accumulation in the liver causes lipotoxicity that in turn fosters a proinflammatory environment and steatohepatitis. The inflammatory response in MASH involves both the activation of liver immune cells and the recruitment of bone-marrow-derived myeloid cells [149]. ER stress can be propagated to neighboring hepatocytes via Connexin 43 channels as demonstrated in mice fed a high-fat diet [150,151]. Other players involved in sensing and controlling this metabolic and inflammatory process include inositol-requiring enzyme 1 alpha (IRE1α) and c-Jun N-terminal kinase (JNK) [152]. ER stress has been shown to drive the inflammatory response through the secretion of ceramide-enriched vesicles in a IRE1α-dependent mechanism [153].

Intracellular pattern-recognition receptors (PPRs), such as the NOD-like receptor protein-3 (NLRP3), play an important role in cytokine production in hepatocytes and immune cells. These receptors are primarily activated by microbial signals and DAMPs [e.g., adenosine triphosphate (ATP)]. Saturated fatty acids also activate the NLRP3 inflammasome, inducing the release of major proinflammatory cytokines, including IL-1β and IL-18 [154]. Inhibition of NLRP3 with sulforaphane improves high-fat diet-induced steatosis in mice, highlighting the role of this pathway in steatosis [155]. In addition, NOD-like receptor protein-6 (NLRP6), caspase activation and recruitment domain (CARD), and TLR signaling are also implicated in this process [156,157]. Moreover, B cells play an important role in the adaptive immune response that mediates hepatic inflammation by secreting profibrotic cytokines such as TNF-α and IL-6 and contributing to the formation of effector memory $CD4^+$ and $CD8^+$ T-cells in the liver [158,159]. Activation of these inflammatory pathways accelerates steatohepatitis progression, mediated by TNF-α, IL-1, IL-6, and IL-11, as supported by the amelioration of steatohepatitis in mice by inhibiting IL-6 and IL-1 [160–162].

Activated liver-resident Kupffer cells aggravate the inflammatory reactions [163]. In response to Kupffer cell-derived TNF-α and chemokine (C–C motif) ligand 2 (CCL2), innate immune cells such as macrophages and neutrophils migrate into the liver [164–166] to produce factors that promote steatohepatitis [e.g., neutrophil extracellular trap (NET)] [167], or to protect against it (e.g., macrophage-derived osteopontin) [168]. Antigen presenting cells are tightly associated with the ensuing inflammatory response in MASH, as evidenced by the abundance of dendritic cells and monocytes in hepatocytes of patients with MASH [166,169]. Type 1 conventional dendritic cells (cDC1) are responsible for inflammatory T-cell polarization [170]. The number of XCR1+ conventional type-1 dendritic cells increases in the liver and blood of mice and patients with MASH, and their genetic ablation curtails disease progression in mice [157]. Recent findings indicate that CXCR6+ cytotoxic T cells, activated by IL-15 rather than traditional antigen presentation, become more sensitive to metabolic triggers like acetate and extracellular ATP, thereby aggravating steatohepatitis in mice [171]. In MASLD, diverse metabolic changes lead to the conversion of regulatory T cells into T helper (TH) 17 cells [172]. This process is associated with elevated levels of IL-17, which correlates with specific inflammatory markers, particularly eotaxin, produced by smooth muscle cells and indicative of early atherosclerosis [173]. Conversely, the absence of cytotoxic T cells in mice has been shown to protect against diet-induced steatohepatitis [174]. This body of findings establishes the pathological involvement of innate immune cells and TH17 cells in mediating the inflammatory injury to hepatocytes in MASLD. Targeting these implicated mediators could be judicious in the context of MASLD prevention and treatment.

3.2.4. Fibrosis and Progression to Cirrhosis

Unresolved inflammatory responses and the activation of adaptive immune cells in the liver drive fibrosis, tissue dysfunction, and tumorigenesis. Hepatic stellate cells (HSCs), located in the subendothelial space of Disse, play a major role in maintaining liver integrity and vitamin A storage and secretion [175]. Activation of HSCs and their transformation into fibrogenic contractile myofibroblasts lead to scar tissue formation [176]. Excessive levels of fibrotic scar tissues lead to irreversible liver injury. Delineating the pathways governing HSC-mediated fibrinogenesis promises significant therapeutic applications [177]. Transforming growth factor-beta (TGF-β) is a potent pro-fibrogenic cytokine produced by hepatic macrophages. In patients, hepatocytes produce bone morphogenic proteins (BMPs), such as BMP8B and BMP9, which are members of the TGF-β superfamily. A key study demonstrated that exogenous BMP9 administration ameliorates liver disease in a CCl4-induced mouse model of hepatotoxicity, while BMP8B deficiency resulted in a significant reduction in liver fibrosis [178,179]. These findings highlight the importance of these proteins as potential therapeutic targets in liver disease management.

The activation of HSCs is mediated by various immune-dependent signals, including activation (phosphorylation) of the TGF-β/SMAD signaling pathways [180–182]. The depletion of retinol coupled with the accumulation of free cholesterol sensitizes HSCs to TGF-β signaling [183]. Moreover, PDGF, IL-1β, IL-6, and TNF-α, secreted by macrophages and T-cells, play a prominent profibrotic role [184–186]. Initially, IL-17A was thought to directly activate HSCs based on in vitro stimulation assays. However, more recent findings suggest that IL-17A instead prompts the proliferation of fibrogenic CD9+TREM2+ macrophages, driving hepatic fibrosis [187–190]. In addition, adipokines, like leptin and adiponectin, are also involved in the pathogenesis of hepatic fibrosis. While adiponectin exhibits robust antifibrotic properties, leptin is chiefly profibrogenic. Conversely, nuclear receptors, such as liver X receptor (LXR), farnesoid X receptor (FXR), and peroxisome proliferator-activated receptors (PPARγ and PPARδ), inhibit the activation of HSCs and fibrosis. Persistent inflammation eventually progresses to irreversible chronic inflammation, impairing liver repair and leading to extensive extracellular matrix deposition and fibrosis. Therefore, targeting these pathways may be an effective approach to slow the pro-fibrotic progression of liver injury.

3.3. *Risk Factors and Their Impact on MASH Progression*

Metabolic dysfunction is a central hallmark of MASLD pathogenesis, which is often regarded as the hepatic manifestation of metabolic syndrome [191]. The growing global obesity pandemic is paralleled by a remarkable increase in the incidence of MASLD. The concurrent surge in these metabolic diseases is largely attributed to overnutrition and to a sedentary lifestyle [192]. Notably, more than 70% of patients with T2D develop MASLD. Reciprocally, more than 20% of patients with MASLD present with T2DM, suggesting shared pathophysiological mechanisms [193,194]. The establishment of the role of insulin resistance in the pathogenesis of MASLD was originally proposed by Marchesini et al. [195]. Elevated serum insulin levels are strongly associated with hepatic ballooning and lobular inflammation [196]. Insulin resistance and chronic hyperinsulinemia induce intrahepatic fat accumulation by promoting de novo lipogenesis, partly through transcriptional upregulation of lipogenic genes expression by activating SREBP-1c. In addition, insulin resistance increases fatty acid mobilization from adipocytes eventually reaching the hepatocytes through the portal circulation [122]. Other inflammatory pathways are also critical in the development of hepatic insulin resistance. Interestingly, constitutive activation of nuclear factor kappa-B kinase subunit beta (IKK-β) in mice leads to hepatic insulin resistance, whereas hepatocyte-specific IKK-β knockout mice do not develop hepatic insulin resistance in response to sustained high-fat intake [197,198]. IKK-β activation is driven by oxidative stress and proinflammatory cytokines, particularly TNF-α, both of which are remarkably elevated in patients with MASLD. In addition, the activation of both protein kinase C epsilon (PKC-ε) and c-Jun N-terminal kinase 1 (JNK1) inhibit the phosphorylation of insulin receptor substrates (IRS-1 and IRS-2), blunting insulin signaling. Dyslipidemia is another important risk factor for MALSD, affecting ~70% of patients with MASLD and MASH. Dyslipidemia is characterized by a state of elevated triglyceride (TG) levels and decreased high-density lipoprotein cholesterol (HDL-C) [199]. Interestingly, the extent of visceral adipose tissue (VAT) is significantly associated with hepatic steatosis in patients with MASLD [200]. Chronic dyslipidemia upregulates the expression and activity of SREBP-1c, leading to hepatic lipid accumulation [201]. Moreover, insulin resistance in patients with T2D impairs lipid metabolism, dyslipidemia, oxidative stress, and membrane lipid peroxidation, accelerating the progression of MASLD to advanced stages of liver disease. The apolipoprotein B/apolipoprotein AI (ApoB/AI) ratio has also emerged as a valuable predictor for cardiovascular disease risk and is associated with MASLD prevalence [201,202]. Diet, weight gain, and sedentary lifestyle are well-established risk factors for MASLD. High fructose intake, from sweetened beverages and processed foods, is closely associated with MASLD development and progression [203]. In fact, one of the major dietary constituents involved in liver disease progression from MASLD to MASH is fructose as it promotes hepatic fat deposition and fibrosis [204,205]. This stems from its lipogenic role in serving as a substrate that fuels de novo lipogenesis in part by stimulating lipogenic enzymes transcription via SREBP1c and ChREBP [206,207]. The release of non-esterified fatty acids (NEFA) from VAT is a major contributor to hepatic steatosis. Accordingly, obesity is another important risk factor for MALSD and metabolic diseases. In obesity, elevated levels of circulating FFAs from VAT and subcutaneous adipose tissue (SAT) alter hepatic lipid metabolism to contribute to insulin resistance in hepatocytes and skeletal muscle cells and promote dyslipidemia. This highlights the importance of lifestyle modifications (i.e., dietary changes and increased physical activity) as essential components of MASLD therapy [208]. Other non-modifiable risk factors include advanced age (>60 years), which is associated with a more severe disease phenotype, characterized by a higher incidence of fibrosis. Moreover, single-nucleotide polymorphisms (SNPs) in the PNPLA3 gene, which regulate triacylglycerol breakdown in adipocytes, are closely linked to MASLD susceptibility [6,209].

Patients with MASLD exhibit an increased risk of CVD, as supported by two independent findings. First, metabolic manifestations in MASLD including T2D, dyslipidemia, hypertension, and obesity, all of which are independently linked to increased CVD. Remarkably, patients with MASLD with concurrent T2D are likely to exhibit the worst prognosis, although some studies rule out this association [210]. Other cross-sectional studies demonstrated an existing correlation between MASLD and atherosclerosis independent of T2D [211]. A recent study examining the link between atherosclerotic cardiovascular disease (ASCVD) risk scores and overall and cardiac-specific mortality rates in MASLD patients indicates that ASCVD is associated with a higher risk of both overall and cardiac-specific mortality [212]. Other studies suggest that the heightened risk and mortality rates from CVD may be due to advanced fibrosis (Stage 3 or 4) and T2D, independent of MASLD [213–216]. On the other hand, individuals with MASLD with viral hepatitis or who consume alcohol moderately exhibit a higher 10-year CVD risk compared to those with MASLD alone. This suggests that the impact of MASLD on CVD risk may be influenced by additional factors related to hepatic injury. Understanding the shared pathophysiological mechanisms between these diseases is crucial, as targeting one disease pathway could provide collateral benefits for treating the other comorbidities. Several interconnected pathophysiological pathways may link MASLD and T2D to an increased CVD risk, including a proatherogenic lipid phenotype, increased prothrombotic factors, insulin resistance, endothelial dysfunction, increased oxidative stress, low-grade inflammation, and intestinal dysbiosis [8,217–220]. ROS generation, secondary to hepatic inflammation, also plays a key role in the development of atherosclerotic lesions and disease progression. ROS induce endothelial cell dysfunction and vascular smooth muscle cell proliferation [221,222]. Moreover, insulin resistance and chronic hyperglycemia trigger aberrant ROS production, impairing vascular endothelial cells and accelerating smooth muscle cell proliferation, thereby fueling atherogenesis [223]. In addition to the role of inflammation in endothelial dysfunction, it is also responsible for decreased vascular tone and vascular plaque development. The prevalence of lean MASLD is approximately 8.4% of total MASLD reported cases. This diagnosis requires both evidence of hepatic steatosis and the occurrence of metabolic dysregulation, defined by the presence of at least two risk factors (i.e., increased waist circumference, hypertension, low serum HDL levels, high cholesterol levels, hypertriglyceridemia, hyperglycemia, insulin resistance, and chronic subclinical inflammation) [224–226]. A noteworthy study evaluated the importance of anthropometric measurements, including height, weight, body mass index (BMI), and circumference of various body parts (e.g., waist and hips), in predicting long-term outcomes of patients with MASLD. Stratifying MASLD patients by BMI and waist circumference has proven to be a more accurate prognostic biomarker. Notably, MASLD patients with lean BMI but obese waist-to-hip ratio have a significantly higher risk of mortality due to hypertension, hyperlipidemia, T2D, and insulin resistance. In addition, CVD mortality risk is nearly three times higher in individuals with lean BMI and obese waist circumference compared to those with overweight BMI and normal waist circumference. These findings reinforce the link between CVD-associated MASLD mortality and highlight the need for personalized therapeutic management based on individual body composition. Moreover, assessment of waist circumference should be incorporated in clinical practice [7].

4. Common Risk Factors and Pathways

Mounting evidence indicates a pathophysiological link between MASLD and atherosclerosis, although the shared mechanism(s) underlying concurrent disease progression is (are) yet to be elucidated. However, several overlapping etiologies have been identified. A strong association between MASLD and endothelial dysfunction, the chief hallmark of atherosclerosis, has been established [227]. Fetuin-A, an insulin signaling inhibitor that serves as a metabolic syndrome diagnostic biomarker, was found to be positively correlated with endothelial dysfunction and carotid artery atherosclerosis in a study involving 115 MASLD patients [228]. A separate report showed a significant decrease in brachial artery flow medial dilatation (FMD) in a sample of 52 patients with MASLD [229]. Moreover, a direct association between reduced NO in endothelial cells, impaired vasodilation, increased oxidative stress, increased inflammation, and endothelial dysfunction was demonstrated in MASLD. At the level of the endothelium, inducible nitric oxide synthase (iNOS) and endothelial nitric oxide synthase (eNOS) are responsible for nitric oxide production, a major regulator of vascular tone. In a stressful physiological milieu, NO is produced via eNOS and iNOS [230]. Evidence suggests that iNOS activation is more common in inflammatory conditions and can exacerbate insulin resistance and hyperglycemia, increase oxidative stress, and downregulate eNOS, all of which can lead to endothelial dysfunction. Abnormal eNOS activity was reported in insulin resistance, leading to low NO production [231,232]. Endothelial dysfunction in hepatic sinusoids triggers hepatic stellate and Kupffer cell activation [233,234]. Upon their activation, stellate and Kupffer cells produce several prothrombotic factors and recruit neutrophils and platelets, all of which partake in sinusoidal microthrombus development and parenchymal extinction, hence accelerating the evolution of fibrosis [235,236]. Therefore, endothelial dysfunction is not only a principal contributor to atherosclerosis, but also a key indicator of MASLD severity. In fact, a recent study documented increased levels of VCAM-1, NOX2 activity, endothelial progenitor cells, fetuin-A, and carotid artery intima media thickness (CIMT) in patients with MASLD [237]. In early-stage MASLD, inflammation acts as a critical bridge between liver fibrosis and atherosclerosis. Through oxidative stress and inflammation, neutrophils accelerate atherosclerosis and contribute to plaque instability. Epicardial adipose tissue produces pro-inflammatory molecules, including IL-1β, IL-6, MCP-1, and TNF-α, which contribute to myocardial inflammation in the early stages and to atherosclerosis in the later stages [238]. In a similar manner, disrupting insulin intracellular signaling of inflammatory pathways, mainly IKK/NF-κB and JNK/AP1 pathways, plays a key role in MASLD progression [239]. These pathways induce the production of hepatic CRP that stimulates NF-κB which further disrupts insulin signaling. Moreover, it was found that hepatic lipid accumulation leads to inflammation and activation of NF-κB. The latter induces the transcription of proinflammatory genes and cytokine production to lead to insulin resistance and MASLD [227]. Furthermore, inflammation leads to ROS production that, in turn, mediate the oxidation of polyunsaturated fatty acids to 4-hydroxy-nonenal (HNE), malonyl-aldehyde (MDA), and 4-oxy-2-nonenal (ONE). These markers are not only found in patients with MASLD but are also associated with vascular damage [240]. Caimi et al. investigated the link between metabolic syndrome and oxidative stress by assessing lipid peroxidation, measured as thiobarbituric acid-reactive substances (TBARS), nitric oxide metabolites (nitrite + nitrate) expressed as NOx, and their ratio TBARS/NOx in 106 patients with metabolic syndrome. In comparison to controls, the results revealed higher TRABS and NOx levels as well as lower TRABS/NOx ratio. This implies that redox and inflammatory status are important contributors, as there is a correlation between lipid peroxidation and inflammation in this group of patients [241]. When pro-inflammatory transcription factors like NF-κB and activator protein-1 (AP-1) are activated in adipocytes of obese individuals, inflammatory cytokines like TNF-α, IL-1β, and IL-6 are released. This creates a vicious cycle because the release of these cytokines increases ROS production [242,243].

Many studies focused on uncovering the mechanism by which central obesity causes oxidative stress. Obesity is marked by nutritional excess, adipocyte hypertrophy, and release of inflammatory molecules related to PKC and polyol pathways, which induce NADPH oxidase (NOXs), nitric oxide synthase, uncoupled endothelial NOS (eNOS), and myeloperoxidase activation. The resulting alteration in adipocyte's function affects the transcription of inflammatory factors, leading to oxidative stress and inflammation that subsequently halt antioxidant defense mechanisms. The product of this functional change is metabolic dysfunction [244].

Insulin resistance is associated with both MASLD and atherosclerosis. Under homeosteatic conditions, insulin binds to its receptor on endothelial cells and maintains vascular tone for proper tissue perfusion by promoting NO-dependent vasodilation and Endothelin-1-dependent vasoconstriction via PI3K and MAPK pathways, respectively. In the insulin-resistance state, insulin favors the MAPK/ET-1 pathway over the PI3K/NO pathway, tipping the balance towards more vasoconstriction with decreased endothelial vasodilation and endothelial dysfunction [11,245]. Likewise, the p38MAPK pathway is implicated in the development and progression of atherosclerosis. Smooth muscle cell proliferation, macrophage activation, and monocyte chemotaxis are among the processes that are activated by p38MAPK in several cell types typically found in atherosclerotic plaques. This pathway contributes to the spread of plaques in atherosclerotic disease [246]. Supporting data to this association was presented by the finding that metformin, an antidiabetic medication used to enhance insulin sensitivity in the liver of patients with insulin resistance, decreases ET-1 and increases NO blood levels. It was also shown that metformin therapy for 3 years reduces major cardiovascular complications significantly in patients with T2D [247]. Furthermore, insulin resistance downregulates lipoprotein lipase (LPL) and hepatic lipase (HL), leading to lipid profile disturbances and culminating in atherogenic dyslipidemia. As previously mentioned, insulin halts the activity of both lipases. These enzymes function in the catabolism of triglyceride rich lipoproteins [248]. This malfunction causes an increase in triglyceride and LDL and a decrease in HDL level, which is often reported in MASLD. Patients with MASLD exhibit a dose-dependent rise in fasting blood triglycerides and a fall of serum HDL, indicating a distinct pathophysiologic relationship between insulin resistance, dyslipidemia, and MASLD [227]. A recent study was carried out on a population of newly diagnosed insulin-sensitive patients with familial combined hyperlipidemia. The prevalence of hepatic steatosis in the study sample was 75%, and a markedly increased risk of atherosclerotic disease was observed in cases presenting with liver fibrosis [199]. Patients with MASLD exhibit high levels of triglycerides and LDL in addition to low HDL levels [249,250]. This lipid profile is associated with increased CETP activity, an enzyme that transfers cholesterol esters from HDL to VLDL and LDL in exchange for triglycerides. In MASLD, the activity of CETP is enhanced, leading to hypertriglyceridemia and the consequent production of larger VLDL particles. These particles are metabolized into atherogenic particles, small dense LDL and small HDL. Due to their small size, they have the capacity to pass through the endothelial layer more easily, initiating plaque formation in arteries [251]. Moreover, TGF-β, a key profibrogenic molecule, is a primary driver of hepatic fibrosis. In fact, it has a direct influence on hepatic stellate cell activation, transforming them into collagen-secreting myofibroblasts, promoting fibrogenesis. TGF-β also has a fibrotic role in the myocardium; when fibrosis develops in the heart, the injured myocardium releases pro-fibrotic substances such as angiotensin II, TGF-β1, and IL-1β, which combined perpetuate the inflammatory cycle [251]. Moreover, patients with atherosclerosis exhibit elevated levels of TGF-β1 and the long non-coding RNA-ATB (lncRNA-ATB), suggesting that these markers could be a useful diagnostic marker for atherosclerosis [252]. Thus, TGF-β1 emerges as a critical pathophysiological link, tethering hepatic fibrosis to atherosclerosis.

5. Loss of CEACAM1 Links Hepatic Fibrosis to Atherosclerosis

5.1. MASLD and Atherosclerosis: Twin Diseases

MASLD and atherosclerosis are often interconnected, representing different manifestations of the same underlying disease. MASLD involves fat buildup in the liver, while atherosclerosis is marked by fat accumulation in blood vessels. Hepatic inflammation, especially in MASH, is strongly linked to increased atherosclerosis compared to simple hepatic steatosis [253–255]. MASLD, a liver-related feature of metabolic syndrome [9,256–258], includes conditions like abdominal obesity, dyslipidemia, hypertension, insulin resistance, and glucose intolerance [259,260]. About 90% of MASLD patients exhibit one or more of these metabolic abnormalities, and 33% meet the full criteria for MetS [261,262]. This raises death risk, primarily due to CVD or liver complications [263,264]. The strong connection between MASH and atherosclerosis highlights the role of the liver in cardiovascular health, but the cause–effect relationship between these two health conditions remains elusive [265,266]. Identifying the mechanisms linking these diseases is key to developing better therapeutic strategies. Factors like insulin resistance, inflammation, lipid disorders, oxidative stress, and systemic release of oxidized LDL cholesterol may contribute to both conditions [256,267]. In insulin resistance, the liver and adipose tissue become targets and contributors to systemic inflammation, with increased lipolysis-derived NEFA and pro-inflammatory cytokines such as IL-6 and TNF-α [260]. Due to the heightened cardiovascular risk in MASLD patients, a multidisciplinary approach is critical to manage these interconnected cardiometabolic disorders effectively.

5.2. CEACAM1—Its Loss Links Reduced Insulin Clearance to MASH

In the liver, CEACAM1, a plasma membrane glycoprotein, belongs to a family of proteins containing four immunoglobulin-like (Ig) structures in its extracellular domain. It is ubiquitously expressed in many cell types, most predominantly in hepatocytes, followed by renal proximal tubule cells, the main sites of insulin clearance.

In hepatocytes, CEACAM1 is mainly expressed as two alternative spliced isoforms that differ by the length of their cytoplasmic tail (72–74 vs. 10–12 amino acids depending on species) and in their subcellular localization. In contrast to the short isoform (CEACAM1-4S), the long (CEACAM1-4L) contains two tyrosine sites (Y493 and Y520 in humans) within the well-conserved immunoreceptor tyrosine-based inhibitory motifs (ITIMs). While the expression of the short isoform is restricted to the bile canalicular domain of hepatocytes, CEACAM1-4L is mainly expressed in the sinusoidal domain in the space of Disse [268,269]. This localization of CEACAM1-4L positions it to undergo phosphorylation on Y493 (Y488 in rodents) by the insulin receptor tyrosine kinase upon its activation by insulin that is passively transported through the fenestrae of the capillaries lining the sinusoid [10,17]. CEACAM1-4L phosphorylation causes it to partake in the insulin–receptor complex to increase the rate of insulin targeting to its lysosomal degradation process in hepatocytes. This promotes insulin clearance, which, together with insulin secretion, serves to maintain the physiologic levels of insulin that reach peripheral target tissues and ensure proper insulin action (Figure 1).

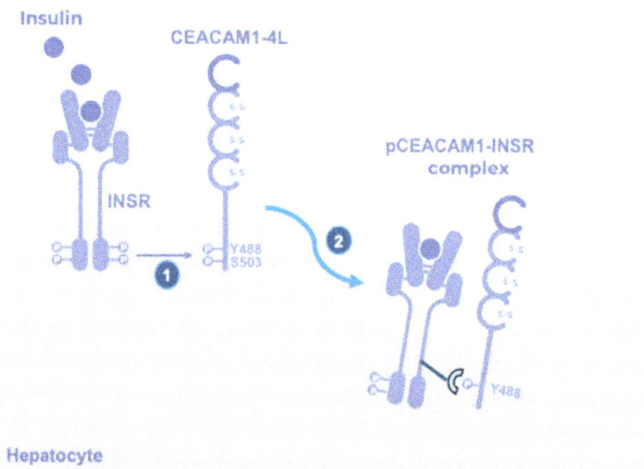

Figure 1. Upon its phosphorylation (*-p*) on tyrosine 488 (Y488) by insulin-activated insulin receptor tyrosine kinase (INSR) (1), CEACAM1 partakes in the insulin-INSR internalization complex (2). This stabilizes the complex and increases the rate of cellular uptake of insulin and its targeting to the lysosomal degradation process to be cleared.

The role of CEACAM1-4L in insulin clearance is tightly associated with its role in mediating a suppressive effect on FASN activity by acutely secreted insulin [270]. Following its endocytosis, phosphorylated CEACAM1-4L binds to cytoplasmic FASN, an event that detaches it from the insulin–receptor complex to allow insulin's dissociation from its receptor to undergo lysosomal degradation in late endosomes, as the receptor is recycled back to the plasma membrane. Binding of CEACAM1-4L to FASN causes suppression of its enzymatic activity, demonstrating that acutely, insulin exerts an anti-lipogenic effect in hepatocytes, as opposed to the well-accepted lipogenic effect of chronic hyperinsulinemia [270,271].

It is commonly believed that reduced insulin clearance plays a compensatory mechanism alongside insulin hypersecretion to prolong the function of pancreatic β-cells. Conversely, reduced insulin clearance has emerged in recent years as a risk factor for MetS and MASLD, particularly among Native Americans, African Americans, and Hispanic individuals of Mexican descent [272,273]. This is based on the notion that reduced insulin clearance drives chronic hyperinsulinemia, which in turn causes hepatic insulin resistance (by downregulating the insulin receptor) and promotes de novo lipogenesis and, subsequently, hepatic steatosis.

Bril et al. [274] and Watada et al. [275] have demonstrated that in patients with MASLD, hyperinsulinemia is mainly due to impaired insulin clearance, rather than aberrant insulin secretion. In a cohort of 1019 subjects from the second Portuguese prevalence study of type 2 diabetes (PREVADIAB2), we recently reported that circulating CEACAM1 levels decreases in parallel with reduced insulin clearance as the disease progresses from normoglycemia to hyperglycemia, concomitant with an increase in fatty liver index [276]. Consistent with a critical role for CEACAM1 in insulin and lipid metabolism, hepatic CEACAM1 levels are lower in obese individuals with insulin resistance and hepatic steatosis than age-matched insulin sensitive subjects, with the extent of fat accumulation being directly correlating with the degree of CEACAM1 reduction [18,19]. Furthermore, CEACAM1 protein levels are significantly lower in primary hepatocytes of obese individuals with steatotic livers compared to age-matched lean controls, indicating an inherent loss of hepatic CEACAM1 in obesity [18]. Hepatic CEACAM1 expression is significantly downregulated in patients with MASH and further declines in hepatocytes and liver sinusoidal endothelial cells as hepatic fibrosis advances [277]. Moreover, hepatic CEACAM1 levels are notably reduced in liver biopsies of obese South Korean subjects presenting with insulin resistance and microvesicular steatosis, even in the absence of T2D [19]. These findings underscore the need to delineate the mechanistic involvement of CEACAM1 in the pathogenesis of insulin resistance driven by impaired insulin clearance and associated comorbidities [278]. Notably, patients with T2D are more likely to present with concomitant hepatic steatosis and reduced insulin clearance compared to their non-diabetic counterparts [279]. Insulin clearance in these patients is rescued via PPARγ agonists, possibly through a CEACAM1-dependent mechanism, given the established role of PPARγ as a transcriptional inducer of CEACAM1 expression in hepatocytes and HSCs [280–282]. It is intriguing that the insulin sensitizers PPARγ agonists or secretagogues (GLP-1 receptor agonists) activate CEACAM1 transcription [281,283], thus suggesting that inducing CEACAM1 expression could constitute an effective targeted therapy.

Additionally, recent findings have underscored the interplay between elevated plasma NEFA, hepatic CEACAM1 expression, and impaired insulin clearance in the etiology of metabolic disease [271]. For instance, short-term exposure to a Western-style diet rapidly impaired insulin clearance and induced early hepatic insulin resistance in healthy South Asian men but not in their Caucasian counterparts, highlighting population-specific metabolic response to diet and predisposition to metabolic disease [284]. This reduction in insulin clearance was associated with increased NEFA levels, emphasizing the role of lipolysis-derived NEFA release in mediating CEACAM1 downregulation [271]. Mechanistically, NEFA likely suppress CEACAM1 expression via a PPARα-dependent pathway, initiating a vicious cycle wherein impaired insulin clearance causes hyperinsulinemia, further exacerbating insulin resistance and hepatic steatosis [285].

5.3. *Repositioning CEACAM1 as a Critical Immunometabolic Regulator*

In addition to its established regulatory role in insulin and lipid metabolism, CEACAM1 is also implicated in inflammation, particularly under states of nutritional excess. The homeostatic immuno-metabolic network, coupling hepatic lipid accumulation with inflammatory signaling, is orchestrated by the CEACAM1—CD36 axis [286]. This sophisticated molecular bridge governs fatty acid and lipopolysaccharide uptake, thereby influencing lipid droplet formation and modulating inflammatory responses in the liver.

CEACAM1 serves as a crucial immunological signaling mediator. It orchestrates immune and non-immune processes through both homophilic and heterophilic interactions. When CEACAM1-4L undergoes tyrosine phosphorylation by SRC-family kinases, ITIMs recruit SH2 domain-containing phosphatases, transducing inhibitory signaling cascades in

T-cells [287]. Conversely, the short isoform (CEACAM1-4S) lacks ITIMs and is therefore associated with non-inhibitory responses to exert a pro-inflammatory response. CEACAM1-4L has been implicated in immunosuppression and cancer immune evasion via interaction with TIM-3, partaking in checkpoint-mediated immune inhibition. Additionally, pathogen–CEACAM1 interaction facilitates microbial host invasion and immune bypass [287]. This corroborates CEACAM1's function as a key immunoregulatory molecule and a potential therapeutic target in inflammatory diseases [288].

Moreover, CEACAM1-4L expression in neutrophils modulates ischemia-reperfusion injury (IRI) during orthotopic liver transplantation. Specifically, elevated neutrophil CEACAM1-4L expression is associated with reduced NETosis, improved graft function, and lower rates of allograft rejection. Therefore, targeting CEACAM1-related pathways hold promises of mitigating aberrant inflammatory responses in the context of IRI, potentially improving organ transplant outcomes [289]. Aberrant alternative splicing of CEACAM1 disrupts the equilibrium between its L and S isoforms, driving aberrant inflammatory responses, immune evasion, and tumor progression. Antisense oligonucleotides represent a promising strategy to therapeutically tip the splicing balance towards the immunoregulatory CEACAM1-4L isoform [290–292].

In the vasculature, CEACAM1 is involved in maintaining endothelial barrier integrity, facilitating nitric oxide signaling, and promoting angiogenesis. The proinflammatory cytokine TNF-α significantly upregulates CEACAM1 in endothelial cells via NF-κB and β-catenin signaling, contributing to endothelial dysfunction and aging-associated inflammation [293]. CEACAM1 emerges therefore as a promising therapeutic target in the context of age-related cardiovascular disease.

In sum, CEACAM1 serves as a critical immune-metabolic regulator, integrating lipid trafficking, endothelial function, and inflammatory response. This underscores the potential contribution of CEACAM1 expression to multiple human disease processes.

5.4. *CEACAM1—Its Loss Links MASH to Atherosclerosis*

Patients with MASLD/MASH are at higher risk for cardiovascular diseases, such as atherosclerosis [294–297]. Furthermore, CEACAM1 levels are lower in hepatocytes (and liver sinusoidal endothelial cells) of patients with MASH and as hepatic fibrosis stage advances, in inverse relationship with plasma Endothelin-1 levels [298]. Similarly, rats selectively bred with low aerobic capacity exhibit all of the cardiometabolic features of MetS relative to those with high-aerobic capacity, including MASH [299] and atherosclerosis [300], in parallel to their lower hepatic CEACAM1 expression [299,300]. Moreover, the phenotype of cell-specific and global $Cc1^{-/-}$ models closely recapitulate the phenotypic presentation and pathophysiologic processes that occur in human MetS.

These observations have led to efforts to uncover potential CEACAM1-dependent common molecular pathways that link these cardiometabolic conditions. Accordingly, global ($Cc1^{-/-}$ mice) and liver-specific deletion (i.e., *AlbCre+Cc1$^{fl/fl}$* mice) of the Ceacam1 gene cause chronic hyperinsulinemia, mainly due to decreased insulin clearance. This is followed by hepatic insulin resistance, steatohepatitis, visceral obesity, and eventually systemic insulin resistance [20,21]. Additionally, these mutations cause human MASH-characteristic liver histology, including hepatic inflammation and fibrosis even when mice are fed a regular chow diet [191,301]. They also lead to cardiovascular abnormalities such as hypertension and endothelial and cardiac dysfunction [22,23]. Conversely, liver-specific reconstitution of CEACAM1 reverses insulin resistance with other features of metabolic dysfunction and hepatic fibrosis in $Cc1^{-/-}$ nulls, even when they are fed with a high-fat diet [302]. It also reverses hypertension and cardiac and endothelial dysfunction, at least in part resulting from curbing the hyperinsulinemia-driven release of Endothelin-1 in $Cc1^{-/-}$

nulls [23]. This underscores the role of the loss of hepatic CEACAM1 in linking metabolic to cardiovascular dysregulation [23,303].

AlbCre+Cc1$^{fl/fl}$ mice bred on *Ldlr$^{-/-}$* background and fed with an atherogenic diet developed chronic hyperinsulinemia due to impaired insulin clearance, high cholesterol levels, a proinflammatory state, and increased oxidative stress [15]. They also developed MASH (steatohepatitis, apoptosis, and fibrosis) and atherosclerotic plaque lesions. Mechanistically, reduced hepatic insulin clearance caused by the loss of CEACAM1 in hepatocytes led to hyperinsulinemia, which in turn drove the downregulation of the insulin receptor and systemic insulin resistance including in the aorta. This was followed by impaired Akt/eNOS and Shc/MAPK NF-kB pathways downstream of the insulin receptor, the former suppressing NO production, and the latter stimulating that of Endothelin-1 to shift the balance towards vasoconstriction, followed by portal hypertension and oxidative stress [15], key mechanisms underlying hepatic fibrosis. This mouse model provides an in vivo demonstration of how insulin resistance caused by hyperinsulinemia links MASH to atherosclerosis when coupled with hypercholesterolemia (Figure 2). Thus, insulin resistance, caused by impaired CEACAM1-dependent hepatic insulin clearance pathways, plays a key role in linking MASLD/MASH to atherosclerosis.

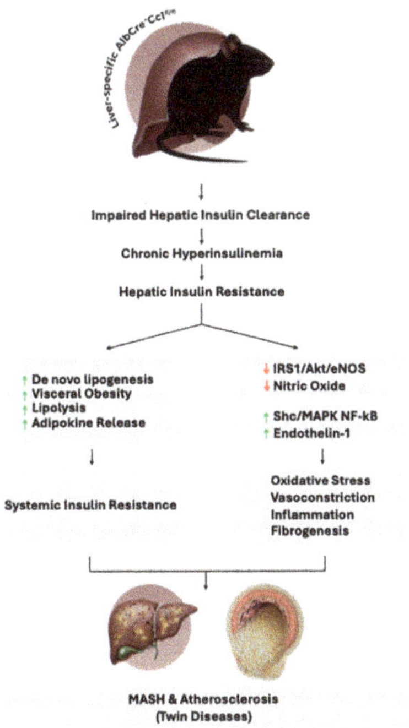

Figure 2. Hepatocyte-specific deletion of CEACAM1 links MASH to atherosclerosis. *AlbCre+Cc1$^{fl/fl}$* mutant mice with conditional deletion of the *Ceacam1* gene in hepatocytes were propagated on the *Ldlr$^{-/-}$* background. Beginning at 4 months of age, mice were fed ad libitum a high-cholesterol atherogenic diet for 2 months before they underwent metabolic phenotyping. Following sacrifice, tissues were removed for histological and cell signaling analysis. It was determined that the mice manifested concomitant presentation of MASH and atherosclerotic plaque lesions. An upward green arrow indicates an increase, while a downward red arrow indicates a decrease.

However, the role of insulin resistance, independent of dyslipidemia, remains unclear. Mice with endothelial-specific deletion of *Ceacam1* bred on *Ldlr$^{-/-}$* background and fed with an atherogenic diet developed hypercholesterolemia without insulin resistance. This led to vascular inflammation and hepatic and aortic fibrosis without an increase in atheroma formation [304]. Mechanistically, this was marked by decreased NO bioavailability and increased oxidative stress, caused by an impaired Akt/eNOS pathway downstream of the VEGF receptor. In addition, endothelial loss of CEACAM1 led to the hyperactivation of Shc/MAPK NF-kB signaling, followed by stimulating pro-inflammatory and pro-fibrogenic events (including excessive production and Endothelin-1 secretion) that led to endothelial dysfunction and aortic and hepatic fibrosis [304]. Nonetheless, these mice did not develop hyperinsulinemia, insulin resistance, aortic steatosis, liver steatosis, or atheroma [304,305]. This highlights the pivotal role of hyperinsulinemia-driven insulin resistance in the development of overt atherosclerosis and tissue steatosis. Collectively, these studies emphasize that inflammation can drive fibrosis, but hyperinsulinemia and insulin resistance are central to atherosclerosis progression and steatosis. This validates the use of insulin sensitizers to prevent atherosclerosis progression in patients with insulin resistance and MASLD/MASH. We posit that the efficacy of these drugs could be partly mediated by inducing CEACAM1 transcription [281,283].

6. Conclusions

This review presents CEACAM1 as a master immuno-metabolic regulator, coordinating hepatic insulin and lipid metabolism, immune cell-response, and endothelial/vascular physiology. The impairment of CEACAM1-related pathways contributes to the development of insulin resistance, MASLD/MASH, hepatic and aortic fibrosis, and cardiovascular disease. More specifically, impaired CEACAM1-dependent insulin clearance in hepatocytes promotes hyperinsulinemia, causing insulin resistance and precipitating hepatic steatosis, inflammation, and fibrosis, while also prompting endothelial dysfunction and vascular plaque formation. Although these findings are yet to lead to tangible clinical application, they lay a robust foundation for future interventions designed to target the immuno-metabolic dysregulation characteristic of metabolic liver diseases and atherosclerosis [286]. We posit that research directed toward developing strategies targeting CEACAM1 to mitigate cardiometabolic disease burden will disrupt the vicious cycle of hyperinsulinemia-induced hepatic and endothelial injury.

Author Contributions: Conceptualization, S.M.N. and H.E.G.; writing—original draft preparation, S.E.K., S.N.A.H., T.Y., C.E.R., N.G.H., N.M.D. and K.A.; writing—review and editing, S.E.K., S.N.A.H., T.Y., C.E.R., N.G.H., N.M.D., K.A., S.A., S.M.N. and H.E.G.; visualization, S.N.A.H., S.M.N. and H.E.G.; supervision, S.M.N. and H.E.G.; project administration, S.M.N. and H.E.G.; funding acquisition, S.M.N. All authors have read and agreed to the published version of the manuscript.

Funding: This research was funded by NIH R01-DK054254, R01DK124126, R01-MD012579, and R01-DK129877 to S.M.N.

Institutional Review Board Statement: Not applicable.

Informed Consent Statement: Not applicable.

Data Availability Statement: No new data were created or analyzed in this study. Data sharing is not applicable to this article.

Acknowledgments: All authors have reviewed and edited the output and take full responsibility for the content of this publication.

Conflicts of Interest: The authors declare no conflicts of interest.

References

1. Bergheanu, S.C.; Bodde, M.C.; Jukema, J.W. Pathophysiology and treatment of atherosclerosis: Current view and future perspective on lipoprotein modification treatment. *Neth. Heart J.* **2017**, *25*, 231–242. [CrossRef]

2. Timmis, A.; Kazakiewicz, D.; Townsend, N.; Huculeci, R.; Aboyans, V.; Vardas, P. Global epidemiology of acute coronary syndromes. *Nat. Rev. Cardiol.* **2023**, *20*, 778–788. [CrossRef] [PubMed]
3. Younossi, Z.M.; Golabi, P.; Paik, J.M.; Henry, A.; Van Dongen, C.; Henry, L. The global epidemiology of nonalcoholic fatty liver disease (NAFLD) and nonalcoholic steatohepatitis (NASH): A systematic review. *Hepatology* **2023**, *77*, 1335–1347. [CrossRef]
4. Riazi, K.; Azhari, H.; Charette, J.H.; Underwood, F.E.; King, J.A.; Afshar, E.E.; Swain, M.G.; Congly, S.E.; Kaplan, G.G.; Shaheen, A.A. The prevalence and incidence of NAFLD worldwide: A systematic review and meta-analysis. *Lancet Gastroenterol. Hepatol.* **2022**, *7*, 851–861. [CrossRef] [PubMed]
5. Tabas, I.; García-Cardeña, G.; Owens, G.K. Recent insights into the cellular biology of atherosclerosis. *J. Cell Biol.* **2015**, *209*, 13–22. [CrossRef]
6. Eslam, M.; George, J. Genetic contributions to NAFLD: Leveraging shared genetics to uncover systems biology. *Nat. Rev. Gastroenterol. Hepatol.* **2020**, *17*, 40–52. [CrossRef]
7. Golabi, P.; Paik, J.M.; Arshad, T.; Younossi, Y.; Mishra, A.; Younossi, Z.M. Mortality of NAFLD According to the Body Composition and Presence of Metabolic Abnormalities. *Hepatol. Commun.* **2020**, *4*, 1136–1148. [CrossRef]
8. Mantovani, A.; Csermely, A.; Petracca, G.; Beatrice, G.; Corey, K.E.; Simon, T.G.; Byrne, C.D.; Targher, G. Non-alcoholic fatty liver disease and risk of fatal and non-fatal cardiovascular events: An updated systematic review and meta-analysis. *Lancet Gastroenterol. Hepatol.* **2021**, *6*, 903–913. [CrossRef]
9. Targher, G.; Day, C.P.; Bonora, E. Risk of cardiovascular disease in patients with nonalcoholic fatty liver disease. *N. Engl. J. Med.* **2010**, *363*, 1341–1350. [CrossRef] [PubMed]
10. Najjar, S.M.; Perdomo, G. Hepatic Insulin Clearance: Mechanism and Physiology. *Physiology* **2019**, *34*, 198–215. [CrossRef]
11. Kim, J.A.; Montagnani, M.; Koh, K.K.; Quon, M.J. Reciprocal relationships between insulin resistance and endothelial dysfunction: Molecular and pathophysiological mechanisms. *Circulation* **2006**, *113*, 1888–1904. [CrossRef]
12. Ipsen, D.H.; Lykkesfeldt, J.; Tveden-Nyborg, P. Molecular mechanisms of hepatic lipid accumulation in non-alcoholic fatty liver disease. *Cell Mol. Life Sci.* **2018**, *75*, 3313–3327. [CrossRef] [PubMed]
13. Förstermann, U.; Xia, N.; Li, H. Roles of Vascular Oxidative Stress and Nitric Oxide in the Pathogenesis of Atherosclerosis. *Circ. Res.* **2017**, *120*, 713–735. [CrossRef] [PubMed]
14. Gimbrone, M.A., Jr.; García-Cardeña, G. Endothelial Cell Dysfunction and the Pathobiology of Atherosclerosis. *Circ. Res.* **2016**, *118*, 620–636. [CrossRef] [PubMed]
15. Ghadieh, H.E.; Abu Helal, R.; Muturi, H.T.; Issa, D.D.; Russo, L.; Abdallah, S.L.; Najjar, J.A.; Benencia, F.; Vazquez, G.; Li, W.; et al. Loss of Hepatic Carcinoembryonic Antigen-Related Cell Adhesion Molecule 1 Links Nonalcoholic Steatohepatitis to Atherosclerosis. *Hepatol. Commun.* **2020**, *4*, 1591–1609. [CrossRef]
16. Najjar, S.M.; Ledford, K.J.; Abdallah, S.L.; Paus, A.; Russo, L.; Kaw, M.K.; Ramakrishnan, S.K.; Muturi, H.T.; Raphael, C.K.; Lester, S.G.; et al. Ceacam1 deletion causes vascular alterations in large vessels. *Am. J. Physiol. Endocrinol. Metab.* **2013**, *305*, E519–E529. [CrossRef]
17. Najjar, S.M.; Caprio, S.; Gastaldelli, A. Insulin Clearance in Health and Disease. *Annu. Rev. Physiol.* **2023**, *85*, 363–381. [CrossRef]
18. Heinrich, G.; Muturi, H.T.; Rezaei, K.; Al-Share, Q.Y.; DeAngelis, A.M.; Bowman, T.A.; Ghadieh, H.E.; Ghanem, S.S.; Zhang, D.; Garofalo, R.S.; et al. Reduced Hepatic Carcinoembryonic Antigen-Related Cell Adhesion Molecule 1 Level in Obesity. *Front. Endocrinol.* **2017**, *8*, 54. [CrossRef]
19. Lee, W. The CEACAM1 expression is decreased in the liver of severely obese patients with or without diabetes. *Diagn. Pathol.* **2011**, *6*, 40. [CrossRef]
20. DeAngelis, A.M.; Heinrich, G.; Dai, T.; Bowman, T.A.; Patel, P.R.; Lee, S.J.; Hong, E.G.; Jung, D.Y.; Assmann, A.; Kulkarni, R.N.; et al. Carcinoembryonic antigen-related cell adhesion molecule 1: A link between insulin and lipid metabolism. *Diabetes* **2008**, *57*, 2296–2303. [CrossRef]
21. Ghadieh, H.E.; Russo, L.; Muturi, H.T.; Ghanem, S.S.; Manaserh, I.H.; Noh, H.L.; Suk, S.; Kim, J.K.; Hill, J.W.; Najjar, S.M. Hyperinsulinemia drives hepatic insulin resistance in male mice with liver-specific Ceacam1 deletion independently of lipolysis. *Metabolism* **2019**, *93*, 33–43. [CrossRef]
22. Huang, J.; Ledford, K.J.; Pitkin, W.B.; Russo, L.; Najjar, S.M.; Siragy, H.M. Targeted deletion of murine CEACAM 1 activates PI3K-Akt signaling and contributes to the expression of (Pro)renin receptor via CREB family and NF-kappaB transcription factors. *Hypertension* **2013**, *62*, 317–323. [CrossRef]
23. Russo, L.; Muturi, H.T.; Ghadieh, H.E.; Wisniewski, A.M.; Morgan, E.E.; Quadri, S.S.; Landesberg, G.P.; Siragy, H.M.; Vazquez, G.; Scalia, R.; et al. Liver-specific rescuing of CEACAM1 reverses endothelial and cardiovascular abnormalities in male mice with null deletion of Ceacam1 gene. *Mol. Metab.* **2018**, *9*, 98–113. [CrossRef] [PubMed]
24. Imakita, M.; Yutani, C.; Strong, J.P.; Sakurai, I.; Sumiyoshi, A.; Watanabe, T.; Mitsumata, M.; Kusumi, Y.; Katayama, S.; Mano, M.; et al. Second nation-wide study of atherosclerosis in infants, children and young adults in Japan. *Atherosclerosis* **2001**, *155*, 487–497. [CrossRef]

25. Takei, H.; Strong, J.P.; Yutani, C.; Malcom, G.T. Comparison of coronary and aortic atherosclerosis in youth from Japan and the USA. *Atherosclerosis* **2005**, *180*, 171–179. [CrossRef]
26. Hanke, H.; Lenz, C.; Finking, G. The discovery of the pathophysiological aspects of atherosclerosis—A review. *Acta Chir. Belg.* **2001**, *101*, 162–169. [CrossRef]
27. Konstantinov, I.E.; Mejevoi, N.; Anichkov, N.M.; Nikolai, N. Anichkov and his theory of atherosclerosis. *Tex. Heart Inst. J.* **2006**, *33*, 417–423. [PubMed]
28. Lusis, A.J. Atherosclerosis. *Nature* **2000**, *407*, 233–241. [CrossRef]
29. Reitsma, S.; Slaaf, D.W.; Vink, H.; van Zandvoort, M.A.; oude Egbrink, M.G. The endothelial glycocalyx: Composition, functions, and visualization. *Pflugers Arch.* **2007**, *454*, 345–359. [CrossRef] [PubMed]
30. Anderson, T.J. Assessment and treatment of endothelial dysfunction in humans. *J. Am. Coll. Cardiol.* **1999**, *34*, 631–638. [CrossRef]
31. Davignon, J.; Ganz, P. Role of endothelial dysfunction in atherosclerosis. *Circulation* **2004**, *109* (Suppl. S1), III27–III32. [CrossRef] [PubMed]
32. Berenji Ardestani, S.; Eftedal, I.; Pedersen, M.; Jeppesen, P.B.; Nørregaard, R.; Matchkov, V.V. Endothelial dysfunction in small arteries and early signs of atherosclerosis in ApoE knockout rats. *Sci. Rep.* **2020**, *10*, 15296. [CrossRef]
33. Mudau, M.; Genis, A.; Lochner, A.; Strijdom, H. Endothelial dysfunction: The early predictor of atherosclerosis. *Cardiovasc. J. Afr.* **2012**, *23*, 222–231. [CrossRef]
34. VanderLaan, P.A.; Reardon, C.A.; Getz, G.S. Site specificity of atherosclerosis: Site-selective responses to atherosclerotic modulators. *Arterioscler. Thromb. Vasc. Biol.* **2004**, *24*, 12–22. [CrossRef]
35. Chistiakov, D.A.; Orekhov, A.N.; Bobryshev, Y.V. Effects of shear stress on endothelial cells: Go with the flow. *Acta Physiol.* **2017**, *219*, 382–408. [CrossRef]
36. Kang, H.; Cancel, L.M.; Tarbell, J.M. Effect of shear stress on water and LDL transport through cultured endothelial cell monolayers. *Atherosclerosis* **2014**, *233*, 682–690. [CrossRef] [PubMed]
37. Nigro, P.; Abe, J.; Berk, B.C. Flow shear stress and atherosclerosis: A matter of site specificity. *Antioxid. Redox Signal* **2011**, *15*, 1405–1414. [CrossRef]
38. Zhou, J.; Li, Y.S.; Chien, S. Shear stress-initiated signaling and its regulation of endothelial function. *Arterioscler. Thromb. Vasc. Biol.* **2014**, *34*, 2191–2198. [CrossRef]
39. Souilhol, C.; Serbanovic-Canic, J.; Fragiadaki, M.; Chico, T.J.; Ridger, V.; Roddie, H.; Evans, P.C. Endothelial responses to shear stress in atherosclerosis: A novel role for developmental genes. *Nat. Rev. Cardiol.* **2020**, *17*, 52–63. [CrossRef]
40. Chien, S.; Shyy, J.Y. Effects of hemodynamic forces on gene expression and signal transduction in endothelial cells. *Biol. Bull.* **1998**, *194*, 390–391; discussion 392–393. [CrossRef] [PubMed]
41. Chiu, J.J.; Usami, S.; Chien, S. Vascular endothelial responses to altered shear stress: Pathologic implications for atherosclerosis. *Ann. Med.* **2009**, *41*, 19–28. [CrossRef]
42. Shyy, J.Y.; Lin, M.C.; Han, J.; Lu, Y.; Petrime, M.; Chien, S. The cis-acting phorbol ester "12-O-tetradecanoylphorbol 13-acetate"-responsive element is involved in shear stress-induced monocyte chemotactic protein 1 gene expression. *Proc. Natl. Acad. Sci. USA* **1995**, *92*, 8069–8073. [CrossRef]
43. Hsiai, T.K.; Cho, S.K.; Wong, P.K.; Ing, M.; Salazar, A.; Sevanian, A.; Navab, M.; Demer, L.L.; Ho, C.M. Monocyte recruitment to endothelial cells in response to oscillatory shear stress. *FASEB J.* **2003**, *17*, 1648–1657. [CrossRef]
44. Kraiss, L.W.; Geary, R.L.; Mattsson, E.J.; Vergel, S.; Au, Y.P.; Clowes, A.W. Acute reductions in blood flow and shear stress induce platelet-derived growth factor-A expression in baboon prosthetic grafts. *Circ. Res.* **1996**, *79*, 45–53. [CrossRef] [PubMed]
45. Wilcox, J.N.; Smith, K.M.; Williams, L.T.; Schwartz, S.M.; Gordon, D. Platelet-derived growth factor mRNA detection in human atherosclerotic plaques by in situ hybridization. *J. Clin. Investig.* **1988**, *82*, 1134–1143. [CrossRef] [PubMed]
46. Landmesser, U.; Hornig, B.; Drexler, H. Endothelial dysfunction in hypercholesterolemia: Mechanisms, pathophysiological importance, and therapeutic interventions. *Semin. Thromb. Hemost.* **2000**, *26*, 529–537. [CrossRef]
47. Chen, J.Y.; Ye, Z.X.; Wang, X.F.; Chang, J.; Yang, M.W.; Zhong, H.H.; Hong, F.F.; Yang, S.L. Nitric oxide bioavailability dysfunction involves in atherosclerosis. *Biomed. Pharmacother.* **2018**, *97*, 423–428. [CrossRef]
48. Carlström, M. Nitric oxide signalling in kidney regulation and cardiometabolic health. *Nat. Rev. Nephrol.* **2021**, *17*, 575–590. [CrossRef]
49. Casino, P.R.; Kilcoyne, C.M.; Quyyumi, A.A.; Hoeg, J.M.; Panza, J.A. The role of nitric oxide in endothelium-dependent vasodilation of hypercholesterolemic patients. *Circulation* **1993**, *88*, 2541–2547. [CrossRef]
50. Panza, J.A.; Casino, P.R.; Kilcoyne, C.M.; Quyyumi, A.A. Role of endothelium-derived nitric oxide in the abnormal endothelium-dependent vascular relaxation of patients with essential hypertension. *Circulation* **1993**, *87*, 1468–1474. [CrossRef] [PubMed]
51. Esper, R.J.; Nordaby, R.A.; Vilariño, J.O.; Paragano, A.; Cacharrón, J.L.; Machado, R.A. Endothelial dysfunction: A comprehensive appraisal. *Cardiovasc. Diabetol.* **2006**, *5*, 4. [CrossRef] [PubMed]

52. Lee, K.S.; Kim, J.; Kwak, S.N.; Lee, K.S.; Lee, D.K.; Ha, K.S.; Won, M.H.; Jeoung, D.; Lee, H.; Kwon, Y.G.; et al. Functional role of NF-kappaB in expression of human endothelial nitric oxide synthase. *Biochem. Biophys. Res. Commun.* **2014**, *448*, 101–107. [CrossRef]
53. Schulz, E.; Gori, T.; Münzel, T. Oxidative stress and endothelial dysfunction in hypertension. *Hypertens. Res.* **2011**, *34*, 665–673. [CrossRef]
54. Alexander, R.W.; Dzau, V.J. Vascular biology: The past 50 years. *Circulation* **2000**, *102* (Suppl. S4), IV112–IV116. [CrossRef]
55. Chroni, A.; Leondaritis, G.; Karlsson, H. Lipids and lipoproteins in atherosclerosis. *J. Lipids* **2011**, *2011*, 160104. [CrossRef]
56. Goldstein, J.L.; Brown, M.S. The LDL receptor. *Arterioscler. Thromb. Vasc. Biol.* **2009**, *29*, 431–438. [CrossRef]
57. Babitt, J.; Trigatti, B.; Rigotti, A.; Smart, E.J.; Anderson, R.G.; Xu, S.; Krieger, M. Murine SR-BI, a high density lipoprotein receptor that mediates selective lipid uptake, is N-glycosylated and fatty acylated and colocalizes with plasma membrane caveolae. *J. Biol. Chem.* **1997**, *272*, 13242–13249. [CrossRef] [PubMed]
58. Santibanez, J.F.; Blanco, F.J.; Garrido-Martin, E.M.; Sanz-Rodriguez, F.; del Pozo, M.A.; Bernabeu, C. Caveolin-1 interacts and cooperates with the transforming growth factor-beta type I receptor ALK1 in endothelial caveolae. *Cardiovasc. Res.* **2008**, *77*, 791–799. [CrossRef]
59. Wang, D.X.; Pan, Y.Q.; Liu, B.; Dai, L. Cav-1 promotes atherosclerosis by activating JNK-associated signaling. *Biochem. Biophys. Res. Commun.* **2018**, *503*, 513–520. [CrossRef]
60. Takahashi, Y.; Zhu, H.; Yoshimoto, T. Essential roles of lipoxygenases in LDL oxidation and development of atherosclerosis. *Antioxid. Redox Signal* **2005**, *7*, 425–431. [CrossRef] [PubMed]
61. Yu, X.H.; Zheng, X.L.; Tang, C.K. Nuclear Factor-κB Activation as a Pathological Mechanism of Lipid Metabolism and Atherosclerosis. *Adv. Clin. Chem.* **2015**, *70*, 1–30. [CrossRef]
62. Teh, Y.C.; Ding, J.L.; Ng, L.G.; Chong, S.Z. Capturing the Fantastic Voyage of Monocytes Through Time and Space. *Front. Immunol.* **2019**, *10*, 834. [CrossRef]
63. Ley, K.; Laudanna, C.; Cybulsky, M.I.; Nourshargh, S. Getting to the site of inflammation: The leukocyte adhesion cascade updated. *Nat. Rev. Immunol.* **2007**, *7*, 678–689. [CrossRef] [PubMed]
64. Gerhardt, T.; Ley, K. Monocyte trafficking across the vessel wall. *Cardiovasc. Res.* **2015**, *107*, 321–330. [CrossRef]
65. Lin, J.; Kakkar, V.; Lu, X. Impact of MCP-1 in atherosclerosis. *Curr. Pharm. Des.* **2014**, *20*, 4580–4588. [CrossRef]
66. Italiani, P.; Boraschi, D. From Monocytes to M1/M2 Macrophages: Phenotypical vs. Functional Differentiation. *Front. Immunol.* **2014**, *5*, 514. [CrossRef]
67. Shapouri-Moghaddam, A.; Mohammadian, S.; Vazini, H.; Taghadosi, M.; Esmaeili, S.A.; Mardani, F.; Seifi, B.; Mohammadi, A.; Afshari, J.T.; Sahebkar, A. Macrophage plasticity, polarization, and function in health and disease. *J. Cell Physiol.* **2018**, *233*, 6425–6440. [CrossRef]
68. De Paoli, F.; Staels, B.; Chinetti-Gbaguidi, G. Macrophage phenotypes and their modulation in atherosclerosis. *Circ. J.* **2014**, *78*, 1775–1781. [CrossRef] [PubMed]
69. Chistiakov, D.A.; Bobryshev, Y.V.; Orekhov, A.N. Macrophage-mediated cholesterol handling in atherosclerosis. *J. Cell Mol. Med.* **2016**, *20*, 17–28. [CrossRef] [PubMed]
70. Younis, N.; Sharma, R.; Soran, H.; Charlton-Menys, V.; Elseweidy, M.; Durrington, P.N. Glycation as an atherogenic modification of LDL. *Curr. Opin. Lipidol.* **2008**, *19*, 378–384. [CrossRef]
71. Weber, C.; Noels, H. Atherosclerosis: Current pathogenesis and therapeutic options. *Nat. Med.* **2011**, *17*, 1410–1422. [CrossRef]
72. Libby, P. Vascular biology of atherosclerosis: Overview and state of the art. *Am. J. Cardiol.* **2003**, *91*, 3–6. [CrossRef]
73. Sheedy, F.J.; Grebe, A.; Rayner, K.J.; Kalantari, P.; Ramkhelawon, B.; Carpenter, S.B.; Becker, C.E.; Ediriweera, H.N.; Mullick, A.E.; Golenbock, D.T.; et al. CD36 coordinates NLRP3 inflammasome activation by facilitating intracellular nucleation of soluble ligands into particulate ligands in sterile inflammation. *Nat. Immunol.* **2013**, *14*, 812–820. [CrossRef] [PubMed]
74. Choi, H.Y.; Rahmani, M.; Wong, B.W.; Allahverdian, S.; McManus, B.M.; Pickering, J.G.; Chan, T.; Francis, G.A. ATP-binding cassette transporter A1 expression and apolipoprotein A-I binding are impaired in intima-type arterial smooth muscle cells. *Circulation* **2009**, *119*, 3223–3231. [CrossRef] [PubMed]
75. Watson, M.G.; Byrne, H.M.; Macaskill, C.; Myerscough, M.R. A two-phase model of early fibrous cap formation in atherosclerosis. *J. Theor. Biol.* **2018**, *456*, 123–136. [CrossRef] [PubMed]
76. Sharif, H.; Akash, M.S.H.; Rehman, K.; Irshad, K.; Imran, I. Pathophysiology of atherosclerosis: Association of risk factors and treatment strategies using plant-based bioactive compounds. *J. Food Biochem.* **2020**, *44*, e13449. [CrossRef] [PubMed]
77. Cheezum, M.K.; Kim, A.; Bittencourt, M.S.; Kassop, D.; Nissen, A.; Thomas, D.M.; Nguyen, B.; Glynn, R.J.; Shah, N.R.; Villines, T.C. Association of tobacco use and cessation with coronary atherosclerosis. *Atherosclerosis* **2017**, *257*, 201–207. [CrossRef]
78. Elagizi, A.; Kachur, S.; Lavie, C.J.; Carbone, S.; Pandey, A.; Ortega, F.B.; Milani, R.V. An Overview and Update on Obesity and the Obesity Paradox in Cardiovascular Diseases. *Prog. Cardiovasc. Dis.* **2018**, *61*, 142–150. [CrossRef]
79. Kinlen, D.; Cody, D.; O'Shea, D. Complications of obesity. *QJM* **2018**, *111*, 437–443. [CrossRef]
80. Endo, A. A gift from nature: The birth of the statins. *Nat. Med.* **2008**, *14*, 1050–1052. [CrossRef]

81. Fan, J.; Watanabe, T. Atherosclerosis: Known and unknown. *Pathol. Int.* **2022**, *72*, 151–160. [CrossRef]
82. Singh, M.; Kapoor, A.; Bhatnagar, A. Physiological and Pathological Roles of Aldose Reductase. *Metabolites* **2021**, *11*, 655. [CrossRef]
83. Turer, A.T.; Hill, J.A.; Elmquist, J.K.; Scherer, P.E. Adipose tissue biology and cardiomyopathy: Translational implications. *Circ. Res.* **2012**, *111*, 1565–1577. [CrossRef]
84. Liu, J.; Pan, S.; Wang, X.; Liu, Z.; Zhang, Y. Role of advanced glycation end products in diabetic vascular injury: Molecular mechanisms and therapeutic perspectives. *Eur. J. Med. Res.* **2023**, *28*, 553. [CrossRef]
85. Singh, S.; Siva, B.V.; Ravichandiran, V. Advanced Glycation End Products: Key player of the pathogenesis of atherosclerosis. *Glycoconj. J.* **2022**, *39*, 547–563. [CrossRef]
86. D'Souza, A.; Hussain, M.; Howarth, F.C.; Woods, N.M.; Bidasee, K.; Singh, J. Pathogenesis and pathophysiology of accelerated atherosclerosis in the diabetic heart. *Mol. Cell Biochem.* **2009**, *331*, 89–116. [CrossRef] [PubMed]
87. Alpert, M.A.; Omran, J.; Bostick, B.P. Effects of Obesity on Cardiovascular Hemodynamics, Cardiac Morphology, and Ventricular Function. *Curr. Obes. Rep.* **2016**, *5*, 424–434. [CrossRef] [PubMed]
88. Wong, C.; Marwick, T.H. Obesity cardiomyopathy: Pathogenesis and pathophysiology. *Nat. Clin. Pract. Cardiovasc. Med.* **2007**, *4*, 436–443. [CrossRef]
89. Nakamura, M.; Sadoshima, J. Cardiomyopathy in obesity, insulin resistance and diabetes. *J. Physiol.* **2020**, *598*, 2977–2993. [CrossRef] [PubMed]
90. Alí, A.; Boutjdir, M.; Aromolaran, A.S. Cardiolipotoxicity, Inflammation, and Arrhythmias: Role for Interleukin-6 Molecular Mechanisms. *Front. Physiol.* **2018**, *9*, 1866. [CrossRef]
91. Cheng, W.; Cui, C.; Liu, G.; Ye, C.; Shao, F.; Bagchi, A.K.; Mehta, J.L.; Wang, X. NF-κB, A Potential Therapeutic Target in Cardiovascular Diseases. *Cardiovasc. Drugs Ther.* **2023**, *37*, 571–584. [CrossRef]
92. Nagueh, S.F.; Smiseth, O.A.; Appleton, C.P.; Byrd, B.F., 3rd; Dokainish, H.; Edvardsen, T.; Flachskampf, F.A.; Gillebert, T.C.; Klein, A.L.; Lancellotti, P.; et al. Recommendations for the Evaluation of Left Ventricular Diastolic Function by Echocardiography: An Update from the American Society of Echocardiography and the European Association of Cardiovascular Imaging. *J. Am. Soc. Echocardiogr.* **2016**, *29*, 277–314. [CrossRef]
93. Groenewegen, A.; Rutten, F.H.; Mosterd, A.; Hoes, A.W. Epidemiology of heart failure. *Eur. J. Heart Fail.* **2020**, *22*, 1342–1356. [CrossRef]
94. Lang, R.M.; Badano, L.P.; Mor-Avi, V.; Afilalo, J.; Armstrong, A.; Ernande, L.; Flachskampf, F.A.; Foster, E.; Goldstein, S.A.; Kuznetsova, T.; et al. Recommendations for cardiac chamber quantification by echocardiography in adults: An update from the American Society of Echocardiography and the European Association of Cardiovascular Imaging. *J. Am. Soc. Echocardiogr.* **2015**, *28*, 1–39.e14. [CrossRef] [PubMed]
95. Park, J.H.; Lee, J.H.; Lee, S.Y.; Choi, J.O.; Shin, M.S.; Kim, M.J.; Jung, H.O.; Park, J.R.; Sohn, I.S.; Kim, H.; et al. Normal 2-Dimensional Strain Values of the Left Ventricle: A Substudy of the Normal Echocardiographic Measurements in Korean Population Study. *J. Cardiovasc. Ultrasound* **2016**, *24*, 285–293. [CrossRef]
96. Taylor, R.J.; Moody, W.E.; Umar, F.; Edwards, N.C.; Taylor, T.J.; Stegemann, B.; Townend, J.N.; Hor, K.N.; Steeds, R.P.; Mazur, W.; et al. Myocardial strain measurement with feature-tracking cardiovascular magnetic resonance: Normal values. *Eur. Heart J. Cardiovasc. Imaging* **2015**, *16*, 871–881. [CrossRef]
97. Lieb, W.; Xanthakis, V.; Sullivan, L.M.; Aragam, J.; Pencina, M.J.; Larson, M.G.; Benjamin, E.J.; Vasan, R.S. Longitudinal tracking of left ventricular mass over the adult life course: Clinical correlates of short- and long-term change in the framingham offspring study. *Circulation* **2009**, *119*, 3085–3092. [CrossRef] [PubMed]
98. McDonagh, T.A.; Metra, M.; Adamo, M.; Gardner, R.S.; Baumbach, A.; Böhm, M.; Burri, H.; Butler, J.; Čelutkienė, J.; Chioncel, O.; et al. 2023 Focused update of the 2021 ESC Guidelines for the diagnosis and treatment of acute and chronic heart failure. *G. Ital. Cardiol.* **2024**, *25*, 202–213. [CrossRef] [PubMed]
99. van der Ende, M.Y.; Juarez-Orozco, L.E.; Waardenburg, I.; Lipsic, E.; Schurer, R.A.J.; van der Werf, H.W.; Benjamin, E.J.; van Veldhuisen, D.J.; Snieder, H.; van der Harst, P. Sex-Based Differences in Unrecognized Myocardial Infarction. *J. Am. Heart Assoc.* **2020**, *9*, e015519. [CrossRef] [PubMed]
100. Boonman-de Winter, L.J.; Rutten, F.H.; Cramer, M.J.; Landman, M.J.; Zuithoff, N.P.; Liem, A.H.; Hoes, A.W. Efficiently screening heart failure in patients with type 2 diabetes. *Eur. J. Heart Fail.* **2015**, *17*, 187–195. [CrossRef]
101. Garawi, F.; Devries, K.; Thorogood, N.; Uauy, R. Global differences between women and men in the prevalence of obesity: Is there an association with gender inequality? *Eur. J. Clin. Nutr.* **2014**, *68*, 1101–1106. [CrossRef]
102. Abel, E.D. Insulin signaling in the heart. *Am. J. Physiol. Endocrinol. Metab.* **2021**, *321*, E130–E145. [CrossRef] [PubMed]
103. Cai, W.; Sakaguchi, M.; Kleinridders, A.; Gonzalez-Del Pino, G.; Dreyfuss, J.M.; O'Neill, B.T.; Ramirez, A.K.; Pan, H.; Winnay, J.N.; Boucher, J.; et al. Domain-dependent effects of insulin and IGF-1 receptors on signalling and gene expression. *Nat. Commun.* **2017**, *8*, 14892. [CrossRef]
104. Petersen, M.C.; Shulman, G.I. Mechanisms of Insulin Action and Insulin Resistance. *Physiol. Rev.* **2018**, *98*, 2133–2223. [CrossRef]

105. Chopra, I.; Li, H.F.; Wang, H.; Webster, K.A. Phosphorylation of the insulin receptor by AMP-activated protein kinase (AMPK) promotes ligand-independent activation of the insulin signalling pathway in rodent muscle. *Diabetologia* **2012**, *55*, 783–794. [CrossRef]
106. Fazio, S.; Mercurio, V.; Fazio, V.; Ruvolo, A.; Affuso, F. Insulin Resistance/Hyperinsulinemia, Neglected Risk Factor for the Development and Worsening of Heart Failure with Preserved Ejection Fraction. *Biomedicines* **2024**, *12*, 806. [CrossRef]
107. Younossi, Z.M.; Koenig, A.B.; Abdelatif, D.; Fazel, Y.; Henry, L.; Wymer, M. Global epidemiology of nonalcoholic fatty liver disease-Meta-analytic assessment of prevalence, incidence, and outcomes. *Hepatology* **2016**, *64*, 73–84. [CrossRef] [PubMed]
108. Goldberg, D.; Ditah, I.C.; Saeian, K.; Lalehzari, M.; Aronsohn, A.; Gorospe, E.C.; Charlton, M. Changes in the Prevalence of Hepatitis C Virus Infection, Nonalcoholic Steatohepatitis, and Alcoholic Liver Disease Among Patients With Cirrhosis or Liver Failure on the Waitlist for Liver Transplantation. *Gastroenterology* **2017**, *152*, 1090–1099.e1. [CrossRef] [PubMed]
109. Zafrani, E.S. Non-alcoholic fatty liver disease: An emerging pathological spectrum. *Virchows Arch.* **2004**, *444*, 3–12. [CrossRef]
110. Younossi, Z.; Anstee, Q.M.; Marietti, M.; Hardy, T.; Henry, L.; Eslam, M.; George, J.; Bugianesi, E. Global burden of NAFLD and NASH: Trends, predictions, risk factors and prevention. *Nat. Rev. Gastroenterol. Hepatol.* **2018**, *15*, 11–20. [CrossRef]
111. Eslam, M.; Sanyal, A.J.; George, J. Toward More Accurate Nomenclature for Fatty Liver Diseases. *Gastroenterology* **2019**, *157*, 590–593. [CrossRef] [PubMed]
112. Sarin, S.K.; Kumar, M.; Eslam, M.; George, J.; Al Mahtab, M.; Akbar, S.M.F.; Jia, J.; Tian, Q.; Aggarwal, R.; Muljono, D.H.; et al. Liver diseases in the Asia-Pacific region: A Lancet Gastroenterology & Hepatology Commission. *Lancet Gastroenterol. Hepatol.* **2020**, *5*, 167–228. [CrossRef] [PubMed]
113. Paik, J.M.; Henry, L.; De Avila, L.; Younossi, E.; Racila, A.; Younossi, Z.M. Mortality Related to Nonalcoholic Fatty Liver Disease Is Increasing in the United States. *Hepatol. Commun.* **2019**, *3*, 1459–1471. [CrossRef]
114. Sayiner, M.; Stepanova, M.; Pham, H.; Noor, B.; Walters, M.; Younossi, Z.M. Assessment of health utilities and quality of life in patients with non-alcoholic fatty liver disease. *BMJ Open Gastroenterol.* **2016**, *3*, e000106. [CrossRef]
115. Lu, Y.C.; Chang, C.C.; Wang, C.P.; Hung, W.C.; Tsai, I.T.; Tang, W.H.; Wu, C.C.; Wei, C.T.; Chung, F.M.; Lee, Y.J.; et al. Circulating fatty acid-binding protein 1 (FABP1) and nonalcoholic fatty liver disease in patients with type 2 diabetes mellitus. *Int. J. Med. Sci.* **2020**, *17*, 182–190. [CrossRef]
116. Wang, G.; Bonkovsky, H.L.; de Lemos, A.; Burczynski, F.J. Recent insights into the biological functions of liver fatty acid binding protein 1. *J. Lipid Res.* **2015**, *56*, 2238–2247. [CrossRef]
117. Koonen, D.P.; Jacobs, R.L.; Febbraio, M.; Young, M.E.; Soltys, C.L.; Ong, H.; Vance, D.E.; Dyck, J.R. Increased hepatic CD36 expression contributes to dyslipidemia associated with diet-induced obesity. *Diabetes* **2007**, *56*, 2863–2871. [CrossRef]
118. Buttet, M.; Poirier, H.; Traynard, V.; Gaire, K.; Tran, T.T.; Sundaresan, S.; Besnard, P.; Abumrad, N.A.; Niot, I. Deregulated Lipid Sensing by Intestinal CD36 in Diet-Induced Hyperinsulinemic Obese Mouse Model. *PLoS ONE* **2016**, *11*, e0145626. [CrossRef]
119. Auinger, A.; Valenti, L.; Pfeuffer, M.; Helwig, U.; Herrmann, J.; Fracanzani, A.L.; Dongiovanni, P.; Fargion, S.; Schrezenmeir, J.; Rubin, D. A promoter polymorphism in the liver-specific fatty acid transport protein 5 is associated with features of the metabolic syndrome and steatosis. *Horm. Metab. Res.* **2010**, *42*, 854–859. [CrossRef]
120. Donnelly, K.L.; Smith, C.I.; Schwarzenberg, S.J.; Jessurun, J.; Boldt, M.D.; Parks, E.J. Sources of fatty acids stored in liver and secreted via lipoproteins in patients with nonalcoholic fatty liver disease. *J. Clin. Investig.* **2005**, *115*, 1343–1351. [CrossRef] [PubMed]
121. Hong, S.; Gordon, D.; Stec, D.E.; Hinds, T.D. Bilirubin: A Ligand of the PPARα Nuclear Receptor. In *Nuclear Receptors: The Art and Science of Modulator Design and Discovery*; Badr, M.Z., Ed.; Springer International Publishing: Cham, Switzerland, 2021; pp. 463–482.
122. Eberlé, D.; Hegarty, B.; Bossard, P.; Ferré, P.; Foufelle, F. SREBP transcription factors: Master regulators of lipid homeostasis. *Biochimie* **2004**, *86*, 839–848. [CrossRef] [PubMed]
123. Knebel, B.; Haas, J.; Hartwig, S.; Jacob, S.; Kollmer, C.; Nitzgen, U.; Muller-Wieland, D.; Kotzka, J. Liver-specific expression of transcriptionally active SREBP-1c is associated with fatty liver and increased visceral fat mass. *PLoS ONE* **2012**, *7*, e31812. [CrossRef] [PubMed]
124. Iizuka, K.; Takao, K.; Yabe, D. ChREBP-Mediated Regulation of Lipid Metabolism: Involvement of the Gut Microbiota, Liver, and Adipose Tissue. *Front. Endocrinol.* **2020**, *11*, 587189. [CrossRef]
125. Iizuka, K.; Bruick, R.K.; Liang, G.; Horton, J.D.; Uyeda, K. Deficiency of carbohydrate response element-binding protein (ChREBP) reduces lipogenesis as well as glycolysis. *Proc. Natl. Acad. Sci. USA* **2004**, *101*, 7281–7286. [CrossRef]
126. Hinds, T.D., Jr.; Hosick, P.A.; Chen, S.; Tukey, R.H.; Hankins, M.W.; Nestor-Kalinoski, A.; Stec, D.E. Mice with hyperbilirubinemia due to Gilbert's syndrome polymorphism are resistant to hepatic steatosis by decreased serine 73 phosphorylation of PPARalpha. *Am. J. Physiol. Endocrinol. Metab.* **2017**, *312*, E244–E252. [CrossRef]
127. Stec, D.E.; John, K.; Trabbic, C.J.; Luniwal, A.; Hankins, M.W.; Baum, J.; Hinds, T.D., Jr. Bilirubin Binding to PPARalpha Inhibits Lipid Accumulation. *PLoS ONE* **2016**, *11*, e0153427. [CrossRef]

128. Hinds, T.D., Jr.; Adeosun, S.O.; Alamodi, A.A.; Stec, D.E. Does bilirubin prevent hepatic steatosis through activation of the PPARalpha nuclear receptor? *Med. Hypotheses* **2016**, *95*, 54–57. [CrossRef]
129. Hinds, T.D., Jr.; Burns, K.A.; Hosick, P.A.; McBeth, L.; Nestor-Kalinoski, A.; Drummond, H.A.; AlAmodi, A.A.; Hankins, M.W.; Vanden Heuvel, J.P.; Stec, D.E. Biliverdin Reductase A Attenuates Hepatic Steatosis by Inhibition of Glycogen Synthase Kinase (GSK) 3beta Phosphorylation of Serine 73 of Peroxisome Proliferator-activated Receptor (PPAR) alpha. *J. Biol. Chem.* **2016**, *291*, 25179–25191. [CrossRef]
130. Francque, S.; Verrijken, A.; Caron, S.; Prawitt, J.; Paumelle, R.; Derudas, B.; Lefebvre, P.; Taskinen, M.R.; Van Hul, W.; Mertens, I.; et al. PPARalpha gene expression correlates with severity and histological treatment response in patients with non-alcoholic steatohepatitis. *J. Hepatol.* **2015**, *63*, 164–173. [CrossRef] [PubMed]
131. Wang, Y.; Nakajima, T.; Gonzalez, F.J.; Tanaka, N. PPARs as Metabolic Regulators in the Liver: Lessons from Liver-Specific PPAR-Null Mice. *Int. J. Mol. Sci.* **2020**, *21*, 2061. [CrossRef]
132. Hu, X.; Tanaka, N.; Guo, R.; Lu, Y.; Nakajima, T.; Gonzalez, F.J.; Aoyama, T. PPARalpha protects against trans-fatty-acid-containing diet-induced steatohepatitis. *J. Nutr. Biochem.* **2017**, *39*, 77–85. [CrossRef]
133. Ota, T.; Gayet, C.; Ginsberg, H.N. Inhibition of apolipoprotein B100 secretion by lipid-induced hepatic endoplasmic reticulum stress in rodents. *J. Clin. Investig.* **2008**, *118*, 316–332. [CrossRef] [PubMed]
134. Charlton, M.; Sreekumar, R.; Rasmussen, D.; Lindor, K.; Nair, K.S. Apolipoprotein synthesis in nonalcoholic steatohepatitis. *Hepatology* **2002**, *35*, 898–904. [CrossRef] [PubMed]
135. Neuschwander-Tetri, B.A. Hepatic lipotoxicity and the pathogenesis of nonalcoholic steatohepatitis: The central role of non-triglyceride fatty acid metabolites. *Hepatology* **2010**, *52*, 774–788. [CrossRef] [PubMed]
136. Fuchs, M.; Sanyal, A.J. Lipotoxicity in NASH. *J. Hepatol.* **2012**, *56*, 291–293. [CrossRef]
137. Sinha, R.A. Autophagy: A Cellular Guardian against Hepatic Lipotoxicity. *Genes* **2023**, *14*, 553. [CrossRef]
138. Rector, R.S.; Thyfault, J.P.; Uptergrove, G.M.; Morris, E.M.; Naples, S.P.; Borengasser, S.J.; Mikus, C.R.; Laye, M.J.; Laughlin, M.H.; Booth, F.W.; et al. Mitochondrial dysfunction precedes insulin resistance and hepatic steatosis and contributes to the natural history of non-alcoholic fatty liver disease in an obese rodent model. *J. Hepatol.* **2010**, *52*, 727–736. [CrossRef]
139. Win, S.; Than, T.A.; Le, B.H.; García-Ruiz, C.; Fernandez-Checa, J.C.; Kaplowitz, N. Sab (Sh3bp5) dependence of JNK mediated inhibition of mitochondrial respiration in palmitic acid induced hepatocyte lipotoxicity. *J. Hepatol.* **2015**, *62*, 1367–1374. [CrossRef]
140. Tang, S.P.; Mao, X.L.; Chen, Y.H.; Yan, L.L.; Ye, L.P.; Li, S.W. Reactive Oxygen Species Induce Fatty Liver and Ischemia-Reperfusion Injury by Promoting Inflammation and Cell Death. *Front. Immunol.* **2022**, *13*, 870239. [CrossRef] [PubMed]
141. Delli Bovi, A.P.; Marciano, F.; Mandato, C.; Siano, M.A.; Savoia, M.; Vajro, P. Oxidative Stress in Non-alcoholic Fatty Liver Disease. An Updated Mini Review. *Front. Med.* **2021**, *8*, 595371. [CrossRef]
142. Grohmann, M.; Wiede, F.; Dodd, G.T.; Gurzov, E.N.; Ooi, G.J.; Butt, T.; Rasmiena, A.A.; Kaur, S.; Gulati, T.; Goh, P.K.; et al. Obesity Drives STAT-1-Dependent NASH and STAT-3-Dependent HCC. *Cell* **2018**, *175*, 1289–1306.e20. [CrossRef]
143. Koliaki, C.; Szendroedi, J.; Kaul, K.; Jelenik, T.; Nowotny, P.; Jankowiak, F.; Herder, C.; Carstensen, M.; Krausch, M.; Knoefel, W.T.; et al. Adaptation of hepatic mitochondrial function in humans with non-alcoholic fatty liver is lost in steatohepatitis. *Cell Metab.* **2015**, *21*, 739–746. [CrossRef]
144. Greatorex, S.; Kaur, S.; Xirouchaki, C.E.; Goh, P.K.; Wiede, F.; Genders, A.J.; Tran, M.; Jia, Y.; Raajendiran, A.; Brown, W.A.; et al. Mitochondria- and NOX4-dependent antioxidant defense mitigates progression to nonalcoholic steatohepatitis in obesity. *J. Clin. Investig.* **2023**, *134*, e162533. [CrossRef] [PubMed]
145. Zhu, L.; Wu, X.; Liao, R. Mechanism and regulation of mitophagy in nonalcoholic fatty liver disease (NAFLD): A mini-review. *Life Sci.* **2023**, *312*, 121162. [CrossRef] [PubMed]
146. Zhang, J.; Zhao, Y.; Wang, S.; Li, G.; Xu, K. CREBH alleviates mitochondrial oxidative stress through SIRT3 mediating deacetylation of MnSOD and suppression of Nlrp3 inflammasome in NASH. *Free Radic. Biol. Med.* **2022**, *190*, 28–41. [CrossRef]
147. Tsung, A.; Klune, J.R.; Zhang, X.; Jeyabalan, G.; Cao, Z.; Peng, X.; Stolz, D.B.; Geller, D.A.; Rosengart, M.R.; Billiar, T.R. HMGB1 release induced by liver ischemia involves Toll-like receptor 4 dependent reactive oxygen species production and calcium-mediated signaling. *J. Exp. Med.* **2007**, *204*, 2913–2923. [CrossRef] [PubMed]
148. Xu, L.; Ge, F.; Hu, Y.; Yu, Y.; Guo, K.; Miao, C. Sevoflurane Postconditioning Attenuates Hepatic Ischemia-Reperfusion Injury by Limiting HMGB1/TLR4/NF-kappaB Pathway via Modulating microRNA-142 in vivo and in vitro. *Front. Pharmacol.* **2021**, *12*, 646307. [CrossRef]
149. Schwarzler, J.; Grabherr, F.; Grander, C.; Adolph, T.E.; Tilg, H. The pathophysiology of MASLD: An immunometabolic perspective. *Expert. Rev. Clin. Immunol.* **2024**, *20*, 375–386. [CrossRef]
150. Lebeaupin, C.; Vallee, D.; Hazari, Y.; Hetz, C.; Chevet, E.; Bailly-Maitre, B. Endoplasmic reticulum stress signalling and the pathogenesis of non-alcoholic fatty liver disease. *J. Hepatol.* **2018**, *69*, 927–947. [CrossRef]
151. Tirosh, A.; Tuncman, G.; Calay, E.S.; Rathaus, M.; Ron, I.; Tirosh, A.; Yalcin, A.; Lee, Y.G.; Livne, R.; Ron, S.; et al. Intercellular Transmission of Hepatic ER Stress in Obesity Disrupts Systemic Metabolism. *Cell Metab.* **2021**, *33*, 319–333.e6. [CrossRef]

152. Urano, F.; Wang, X.; Bertolotti, A.; Zhang, Y.; Chung, P.; Harding, H.P.; Ron, D. Coupling of stress in the ER to activation of JNK protein kinases by transmembrane protein kinase IRE1. *Science* **2000**, *287*, 664–666. [CrossRef]
153. Kakazu, E.; Mauer, A.S.; Yin, M.; Malhi, H. Hepatocytes release ceramide-enriched pro-inflammatory extracellular vesicles in an IRE1alpha-dependent manner. *J. Lipid Res.* **2016**, *57*, 233–245. [CrossRef]
154. Wen, H.; Gris, D.; Lei, Y.; Jha, S.; Zhang, L.; Huang, M.T.; Brickey, W.J.; Ting, J.P. Fatty acid-induced NLRP3-ASC inflammasome activation interferes with insulin signaling. *Nat. Immunol.* **2011**, *12*, 408–415. [CrossRef]
155. Yang, G.; Lee, H.E.; Lee, J.Y. A pharmacological inhibitor of NLRP3 inflammasome prevents non-alcoholic fatty liver disease in a mouse model induced by high fat diet. *Sci. Rep.* **2016**, *6*, 24399. [CrossRef]
156. Chen, Y.; Ma, K. NLRC4 inflammasome activation regulated by TNF-alpha promotes inflammatory responses in nonalcoholic fatty liver disease. *Biochem. Biophys. Res. Commun.* **2019**, *511*, 524–530. [CrossRef] [PubMed]
157. Arroyo, V.; Angeli, P.; Moreau, R.; Jalan, R.; Claria, J.; Trebicka, J.; Fernandez, J.; Gustot, T.; Caraceni, P.; Bernardi, M.; et al. The systemic inflammation hypothesis: Towards a new paradigm of acute decompensation and multiorgan failure in cirrhosis. *J. Hepatol.* **2021**, *74*, 670–685. [CrossRef] [PubMed]
158. Barrow, F.; Khan, S.; Fredrickson, G.; Wang, H.; Dietsche, K.; Parthiban, P.; Robert, S.; Kaiser, T.; Winer, S.; Herman, A.; et al. Microbiota-Driven Activation of Intrahepatic B Cells Aggravates NASH Through Innate and Adaptive Signaling. *Hepatology* **2021**, *74*, 704–722. [CrossRef]
159. Zhang, F.; Jiang, W.W.; Li, X.; Qiu, X.Y.; Wu, Z.; Chi, Y.J.; Cong, X.; Liu, Y.L. Role of intrahepatic B cells in non-alcoholic fatty liver disease by secreting pro-inflammatory cytokines and regulating intrahepatic T cells. *J. Dig. Dis.* **2016**, *17*, 464–474. [CrossRef] [PubMed]
160. Crespo, J.; Cayon, A.; Fernandez-Gil, P.; Hernandez-Guerra, M.; Mayorga, M.; Dominguez-Diez, A.; Fernandez-Escalante, J.C.; Pons-Romero, F. Gene expression of tumor necrosis factor alpha and TNF-receptors, p55 and p75, in nonalcoholic steatohepatitis patients. *Hepatology* **2001**, *34*, 1158–1163. [CrossRef]
161. Hotamisligil, G.S.; Shargill, N.S.; Spiegelman, B.M. Adipose expression of tumor necrosis factor-alpha: Direct role in obesity-linked insulin resistance. *Science* **1993**, *259*, 87–91. [CrossRef]
162. Kamari, Y.; Shaish, A.; Vax, E.; Shemesh, S.; Kandel-Kfir, M.; Arbel, Y.; Olteanu, S.; Barshack, I.; Dotan, S.; Voronov, E.; et al. Lack of interleukin-1alpha or interleukin-1beta inhibits transformation of steatosis to steatohepatitis and liver fibrosis in hypercholesterolemic mice. *J. Hepatol.* **2011**, *55*, 1086–1094. [CrossRef]
163. Huby, T.; Gautier, E.L. Immune cell-mediated features of non-alcoholic steatohepatitis. *Nat. Rev. Immunol.* **2022**, *22*, 429–443. [CrossRef]
164. Tosello-Trampont, A.C.; Landes, S.G.; Nguyen, V.; Novobrantseva, T.I.; Hahn, Y.S. Kuppfer cells trigger nonalcoholic steatohepatitis development in diet-induced mouse model through tumor necrosis factor-alpha production. *J. Biol. Chem.* **2012**, *287*, 40161–40172. [CrossRef]
165. Pan, J.; Ou, Z.; Cai, C.; Li, P.; Gong, J.; Ruan, X.Z.; He, K. Fatty acid activates NLRP3 inflammasomes in mouse Kupffer cells through mitochondrial DNA release. *Cell Immunol.* **2018**, *332*, 111–120. [CrossRef]
166. Baeck, C.; Wehr, A.; Karlmark, K.R.; Heymann, F.; Vucur, M.; Gassler, N.; Huss, S.; Klussmann, S.; Eulberg, D.; Luedde, T.; et al. Pharmacological inhibition of the chemokine CCL2 (MCP-1) diminishes liver macrophage infiltration and steatohepatitis in chronic hepatic injury. *Gut* **2012**, *61*, 416–426. [CrossRef]
167. van der Windt, D.J.; Sud, V.; Zhang, H.; Varley, P.R.; Goswami, J.; Yazdani, H.O.; Tohme, S.; Loughran, P.; O'Doherty, R.M.; Minervini, M.I.; et al. Neutrophil extracellular traps promote inflammation and development of hepatocellular carcinoma in nonalcoholic steatohepatitis. *Hepatology* **2018**, *68*, 1347–1360. [CrossRef]
168. Han, H.; Ge, X.; Komakula, S.S.B.; Desert, R.; Das, S.; Song, Z.; Chen, W.; Athavale, D.; Gaskell, H.; Lantvit, D.; et al. Macrophage-derived Osteopontin (SPP1) Protects From Nonalcoholic Steatohepatitis. *Gastroenterology* **2023**, *165*, 201–217. [CrossRef] [PubMed]
169. Henning, J.R.; Graffeo, C.S.; Rehman, A.; Fallon, N.C.; Zambirinis, C.P.; Ochi, A.; Barilla, R.; Jamal, M.; Deutsch, M.; Greco, S.; et al. Dendritic cells limit fibroinflammatory injury in nonalcoholic steatohepatitis in mice. *Hepatology* **2013**, *58*, 589–602. [CrossRef]
170. Deczkowska, A.; David, E.; Ramadori, P.; Pfister, D.; Safran, M.; Li, B.; Giladi, A.; Jaitin, D.A.; Barboy, O.; Cohen, M.; et al. XCR1(+) type 1 conventional dendritic cells drive liver pathology in non-alcoholic steatohepatitis. *Nat. Med.* **2021**, *27*, 1043–1054. [CrossRef] [PubMed]
171. Dudek, M.; Pfister, D.; Donakonda, S.; Filpe, P.; Schneider, A.; Laschinger, M.; Hartmann, D.; Huser, N.; Meiser, P.; Bayerl, F.; et al. Auto-aggressive CXCR6(+) CD8 T cells cause liver immune pathology in NASH. *Nature* **2021**, *592*, 444–449. [CrossRef]
172. Hang, S.; Paik, D.; Yao, L.; Kim, E.; Trinath, J.; Lu, J.; Ha, S.; Nelson, B.N.; Kelly, S.P.; Wu, L.; et al. Bile acid metabolites control T(H)17 and T(reg) cell differentiation. *Nature* **2019**, *576*, 143–148. [CrossRef] [PubMed]
173. Tarantino, G.; Costantini, S.; Finelli, C.; Capone, F.; Guerriero, E.; La Sala, N.; Gioia, S.; Castello, G. Is serum Interleukin-17 associated with early atherosclerosis in obese patients? *J. Transl. Med.* **2014**, *12*, 214. [CrossRef]

174. Wolf, M.J.; Adili, A.; Piotrowitz, K.; Abdullah, Z.; Boege, Y.; Stemmer, K.; Ringelhan, M.; Simonavicius, N.; Egger, M.; Wohlleber, D.; et al. Metabolic activation of intrahepatic CD8+ T cells and NKT cells causes nonalcoholic steatohepatitis and liver cancer via cross-talk with hepatocytes. *Cancer Cell* **2014**, *26*, 549–564. [CrossRef]
175. Senoo, H.; Yoshikawa, K.; Morii, M.; Miura, M.; Imai, K.; Mezaki, Y. Hepatic stellate cell (vitamin A-storing cell) and its relative—Past, present and future. *Cell Biol. Int.* **2010**, *34*, 1247–1272. [CrossRef]
176. Kamm, D.R.; McCommis, K.S. Hepatic stellate cells in physiology and pathology. *J. Physiol.* **2022**, *600*, 1825–1837. [CrossRef]
177. Tsuchida, T.; Friedman, S.L. Mechanisms of hepatic stellate cell activation. *Nat. Rev. Gastroenterol. Hepatol.* **2017**, *14*, 397–411. [CrossRef] [PubMed]
178. Breitkopf-Heinlein, K.; Meyer, C.; Konig, C.; Gaitantzi, H.; Addante, A.; Thomas, M.; Wiercinska, E.; Cai, C.; Li, Q.; Wan, F.; et al. BMP-9 interferes with liver regeneration and promotes liver fibrosis. *Gut* **2017**, *66*, 939–954. [CrossRef] [PubMed]
179. Vacca, M.; Leslie, J.; Virtue, S.; Lam, B.Y.H.; Govaere, O.; Tiniakos, D.; Snow, S.; Davies, S.; Petkevicius, K.; Tong, Z.; et al. Bone morphogenetic protein 8B promotes the progression of non-alcoholic steatohepatitis. *Nat. Metab.* **2020**, *2*, 514–531. [CrossRef]
180. Xu, F.; Liu, C.; Zhou, D.; Zhang, L. TGF-beta/SMAD Pathway and Its Regulation in Hepatic Fibrosis. *J. Histochem. Cytochem.* **2016**, *64*, 157–167. [CrossRef]
181. Hellerbrand, C.; Stefanovic, B.; Giordano, F.; Burchardt, E.R.; Brenner, D.A. The role of TGFbeta1 in initiating hepatic stellate cell activation in vivo. *J. Hepatol.* **1999**, *30*, 77–87. [CrossRef]
182. Cai, B.; Dongiovanni, P.; Corey, K.E.; Wang, X.; Shmarakov, I.O.; Zheng, Z.; Kasikara, C.; Davra, V.; Meroni, M.; Chung, R.T.; et al. Macrophage MerTK Promotes Liver Fibrosis in Nonalcoholic Steatohepatitis. *Cell Metab.* **2020**, *31*, 406–421.e7. [CrossRef]
183. Tomita, K.; Teratani, T.; Suzuki, T.; Shimizu, M.; Sato, H.; Narimatsu, K.; Okada, Y.; Kurihara, C.; Irie, R.; Yokoyama, H.; et al. Free cholesterol accumulation in hepatic stellate cells: Mechanism of liver fibrosis aggravation in nonalcoholic steatohepatitis in mice. *Hepatology* **2014**, *59*, 154–169. [CrossRef]
184. Kagan, P.; Sultan, M.; Tachlytski, I.; Safran, M.; Ben-Ari, Z. Both MAPK and STAT3 signal transduction pathways are necessary for IL-6-dependent hepatic stellate cells activation. *PLoS ONE* **2017**, *12*, e0176173. [CrossRef]
185. Ying, H.Z.; Chen, Q.; Zhang, W.Y.; Zhang, H.H.; Ma, Y.; Zhang, S.Z.; Fang, J.; Yu, C.H. PDGF signaling pathway in hepatic fibrosis pathogenesis and therapeutics (Review). *Mol. Med. Rep.* **2017**, *16*, 7879–7889. [CrossRef] [PubMed]
186. Gieling, R.G.; Wallace, K.; Han, Y.P. Interleukin-1 participates in the progression from liver injury to fibrosis. *Am. J. Physiol. Gastrointest. Liver Physiol.* **2009**, *296*, G1324–G1331. [CrossRef]
187. Li, F.; Hao, X.; Chen, Y.; Bai, L.; Gao, X.; Lian, Z.; Wei, H.; Sun, R.; Tian, Z. The microbiota maintain homeostasis of liver-resident gammadeltaT-17 cells in a lipid antigen/CD1d-dependent manner. *Nat. Commun.* **2017**, *7*, 13839. [CrossRef]
188. Fabre, T.; Barron, A.M.S.; Christensen, S.M.; Asano, S.; Bound, K.; Lech, M.P.; Wadsworth, M.H., 2nd; Chen, X.; Wang, C.; Wang, J.; et al. Identification of a broadly fibrogenic macrophage subset induced by type 3 inflammation. *Sci. Immunol.* **2023**, *8*, eadd8945. [CrossRef] [PubMed]
189. Marinovic, S.; Lenartic, M.; Mladenic, K.; Sestan, M.; Kavazovic, I.; Benic, A.; Krapic, M.; Rindlisbacher, L.; Cokaric Brdovcak, M.; Sparano, C.; et al. NKG2D-mediated detection of metabolically stressed hepatocytes by innate-like T cells is essential for initiation of NASH and fibrosis. *Sci. Immunol.* **2023**, *8*, eadd1599. [CrossRef]
190. Ma, H.Y.; Yamamoto, G.; Xu, J.; Liu, X.; Karin, D.; Kim, J.Y.; Alexandrov, L.B.; Koyama, Y.; Nishio, T.; Benner, C.; et al. IL-17 signaling in steatotic hepatocytes and macrophages promotes hepatocellular carcinoma in alcohol-related liver disease. *J. Hepatol.* **2020**, *72*, 946–959. [CrossRef]
191. Najjar, S.M.; Russo, L. CEACAM1 loss links inflammation to insulin resistance in obesity and non-alcoholic steatohepatitis (NASH). *Semin. Immunopathol.* **2014**, *36*, 55–71. [CrossRef] [PubMed]
192. Diehl, A.M.; Farpour-Lambert, N.J.; Zhao, L.; Tilg, H. Why we need to curb the emerging worldwide epidemic of nonalcoholic fatty liver disease. *Nat. Metab.* **2019**, *1*, 1027–1029. [CrossRef] [PubMed]
193. Tilg, H.; Moschen, A.R.; Roden, M. NAFLD and diabetes mellitus. *Nat. Rev. Gastroenterol. Hepatol.* **2017**, *14*, 32–42. [CrossRef]
194. Roden, M.; Shulman, G.I. The integrative biology of type 2 diabetes. *Nature* **2019**, *576*, 51–60. [CrossRef]
195. Marchesini, G.; Brizi, M.; Morselli-Labate, A.M.; Bianchi, G.; Bugianesi, E.; McCullough, A.J.; Forlani, G.; Melchionda, N. Association of nonalcoholic fatty liver disease with insulin resistance. *Am. J. Med.* **1999**, *107*, 450–455. [CrossRef]
196. Enooku, K.; Kondo, M.; Fujiwara, N.; Sasako, T.; Shibahara, J.; Kado, A.; Okushin, K.; Fujinaga, H.; Tsutsumi, T.; Nakagomi, R.; et al. Hepatic IRS1 and ss-catenin expression is associated with histological progression and overt diabetes emergence in NAFLD patients. *J. Gastroenterol.* **2018**, *53*, 1261–1275. [CrossRef]
197. Cai, D.; Yuan, M.; Frantz, D.F.; Melendez, P.A.; Hansen, L.; Lee, J.; Shoelson, S.E. Local and systemic insulin resistance resulting from hepatic activation of IKK-beta and NF-kappaB. *Nat. Med.* **2005**, *11*, 183–190. [CrossRef] [PubMed]
198. Arkan, M.C.; Hevener, A.L.; Greten, F.R.; Maeda, S.; Li, Z.W.; Long, J.M.; Wynshaw-Boris, A.; Poli, G.; Olefsky, J.; Karin, M. IKK-beta links inflammation to obesity-induced insulin resistance. *Nat. Med.* **2005**, *11*, 191–198. [CrossRef]

199. Mandraffino, G.; Morace, C.; Franzè, M.S.; Nassisi, V.; Sinicropi, D.; Cinquegrani, M.; Saitta, C.; Scoglio, R.; Marino, S.; Belvedere, A.; et al. Fatty Liver as Potential Biomarker of Atherosclerotic Damage in Familial Combined Hyperlipidemia. *Biomedicines* **2022**, *10*, 1770. [CrossRef]
200. Jacobs, K.; Brouha, S.; Bettencourt, R.; Barrett-Connor, E.; Sirlin, C.; Loomba, R. Association of Nonalcoholic Fatty Liver Disease With Visceral Adiposity but Not Coronary Artery Calcification in the Elderly. *Clin. Gastroenterol. Hepatol.* **2016**, *14*, 1337–1344.e3. [CrossRef]
201. Soto, A.; Spongberg, C.; Martinino, A.; Giovinazzo, F. Exploring the Multifaceted Landscape of MASLD: A Comprehensive Synthesis of Recent Studies, from Pathophysiology to Organoids and Beyond. *Biomedicines* **2024**, *12*, 397. [CrossRef] [PubMed]
202. Zhang, Q.Q.; Lu, L.G. Nonalcoholic Fatty Liver Disease: Dyslipidemia, Risk for Cardiovascular Complications, and Treatment Strategy. *J. Clin. Transl. Hepatol.* **2015**, *3*, 78–84. [CrossRef]
203. Vos, M.B.; Lavine, J.E. Dietary fructose in nonalcoholic fatty liver disease. *Hepatology* **2013**, *57*, 2525–2531. [CrossRef] [PubMed]
204. Lee, D.; Chiavaroli, L.; Ayoub-Charette, S.; Khan, T.A.; Zurbau, A.; Au-Yeung, F.; Cheung, A.; Liu, Q.; Qi, X.; Ahmed, A.; et al. Important Food Sources of Fructose-Containing Sugars and Non-Alcoholic Fatty Liver Disease: A Systematic Review and Meta-Analysis of Controlled Trials. *Nutrients* **2022**, *14*, 2846. [CrossRef]
205. Abdelmalek, M.F.; Suzuki, A.; Guy, C.; Unalp-Arida, A.; Colvin, R.; Johnson, R.J.; Diehl, A.M.; Nonalcoholic Steatohepatitis Clinical Research Network. Increased fructose consumption is associated with fibrosis severity in patients with nonalcoholic fatty liver disease. *Hepatology* **2010**, *51*, 1961–1971. [CrossRef]
206. Andres-Hernando, A.; Orlicky, D.J.; Kuwabara, M.; Ishimoto, T.; Nakagawa, T.; Johnson, R.J.; Lanaspa, M.A. Deletion of Fructokinase in the Liver or in the Intestine Reveals Differential Effects on Sugar-Induced Metabolic Dysfunction. *Cell Metab.* **2020**, *32*, 117–127.e3. [CrossRef]
207. Herman, M.A.; Samuel, V.T. The Sweet Path to Metabolic Demise: Fructose and Lipid Synthesis. *Trends Endocrinol. Metab.* **2016**, *27*, 719–730. [CrossRef] [PubMed]
208. Younossi, Z.M.; Zelber-Sagi, S.; Henry, L.; Gerber, L.H. Lifestyle interventions in nonalcoholic fatty liver disease. *Nat. Rev. Gastroenterol. Hepatol.* **2023**, *20*, 708–722. [CrossRef]
209. Romeo, S.; Kozlitina, J.; Xing, C.; Pertsemlidis, A.; Cox, D.; Pennacchio, L.A.; Boerwinkle, E.; Cohen, J.C.; Hobbs, H.H. Genetic variation in PNPLA3 confers susceptibility to nonalcoholic fatty liver disease. *Nat. Genet.* **2008**, *40*, 1461–1465. [CrossRef]
210. Davis, T.M.E. Diabetes and metabolic dysfunction-associated fatty liver disease. *Metabolism* **2021**, *123*, 154868. [CrossRef] [PubMed]
211. Ismaiel, A.; Dumitrascu, D.L. Cardiovascular Risk in Fatty Liver Disease: The Liver-Heart Axis-Literature Review. *Front. Med.* **2019**, *6*, 202. [CrossRef]
212. Golabi, P.; Fukui, N.; Paik, J.; Sayiner, M.; Mishra, A.; Younossi, Z.M. Mortality Risk Detected by Atherosclerotic Cardiovascular Disease Score in Patients With Nonalcoholic Fatty Liver Disease. *Hepatol. Commun.* **2019**, *3*, 1050–1060. [CrossRef]
213. Kasper, P.; Martin, A.; Lang, S.; Kutting, F.; Goeser, T.; Demir, M.; Steffen, H.M. NAFLD and cardiovascular diseases: A clinical review. *Clin. Res. Cardiol.* **2021**, *110*, 921–937. [CrossRef]
214. Kim, D.; Kim, W.R.; Kim, H.J.; Therneau, T.M. Association between noninvasive fibrosis markers and mortality among adults with nonalcoholic fatty liver disease in the United States. *Hepatology* **2013**, *57*, 1357–1365. [CrossRef]
215. Tana, C.; Ballestri, S.; Ricci, F.; Di Vincenzo, A.; Ticinesi, A.; Gallina, S.; Giamberardino, M.A.; Cipollone, F.; Sutton, R.; Vettor, R.; et al. Cardiovascular Risk in Non-Alcoholic Fatty Liver Disease: Mechanisms and Therapeutic Implications. *Int. J. Environ. Res. Public Health* **2019**, *16*, 3104. [CrossRef]
216. Haring, R.; Wallaschofski, H.; Nauck, M.; Dorr, M.; Baumeister, S.E.; Volzke, H. Ultrasonographic hepatic steatosis increases prediction of mortality risk from elevated serum gamma-glutamyl transpeptidase levels. *Hepatology* **2009**, *50*, 1403–1411. [CrossRef]
217. Adams, L.A.; Anstee, Q.M.; Tilg, H.; Targher, G. Non-alcoholic fatty liver disease and its relationship with cardiovascular disease and other extrahepatic diseases. *Gut* **2017**, *66*, 1138–1153. [CrossRef] [PubMed]
218. Han, E.; Lee, Y.H.; Kim, Y.D.; Kim, B.K.; Park, J.Y.; Kim, D.Y.; Ahn, S.H.; Lee, B.W.; Kang, E.S.; Cha, B.S.; et al. Nonalcoholic Fatty Liver Disease and Sarcopenia Are Independently Associated With Cardiovascular Risk. *Am. J. Gastroenterol.* **2020**, *115*, 584–595. [CrossRef]
219. Yki-Jarvinen, H. Non-alcoholic fatty liver disease as a cause and a consequence of metabolic syndrome. *Lancet Diabetes Endocrinol.* **2014**, *2*, 901–910. [CrossRef]
220. Ballestri, S.; Lonardo, A.; Bonapace, S.; Byrne, C.D.; Loria, P.; Targher, G. Risk of cardiovascular, cardiac and arrhythmic complications in patients with non-alcoholic fatty liver disease. *World J. Gastroenterol.* **2014**, *20*, 1724–1745. [CrossRef] [PubMed]
221. Incalza, M.A.; D'Oria, R.; Natalicchio, A.; Perrini, S.; Laviola, L.; Giorgino, F. Oxidative stress and reactive oxygen species in endothelial dysfunction associated with cardiovascular and metabolic diseases. *Vasc. Pharmacol.* **2018**, *100*, 1–19. [CrossRef] [PubMed]

222. Stahl, E.P.; Dhindsa, D.S.; Lee, S.K.; Sandesara, P.B.; Chalasani, N.P.; Sperling, L.S. Nonalcoholic Fatty Liver Disease and the Heart: JACC State-of-the-Art Review. *J. Am. Coll. Cardiol.* **2019**, *73*, 948–963. [CrossRef]
223. Pasterkamp, G. Methods of accelerated atherosclerosis in diabetic patients. *Heart* **2013**, *99*, 743–749. [CrossRef]
224. Eslam, M.; Sanyal, A.J.; George, J.; International Consensus Panel. MAFLD: A Consensus-Driven Proposed Nomenclature for Metabolic Associated Fatty Liver Disease. *Gastroenterology* **2020**, *158*, 1999–2014.e1. [CrossRef] [PubMed]
225. Eslam, M.; Sarin, S.K.; Wong, V.W.; Fan, J.G.; Kawaguchi, T.; Ahn, S.H.; Zheng, M.H.; Shiha, G.; Yilmaz, Y.; Gani, R.; et al. The Asian Pacific Association for the Study of the Liver clinical practice guidelines for the diagnosis and management of metabolic associated fatty liver disease. *Hepatol. Int.* **2020**, *14*, 889–919. [CrossRef] [PubMed]
226. Eslam, M.; Newsome, P.N.; Sarin, S.K.; Anstee, Q.M.; Targher, G.; Romero-Gomez, M.; Zelber-Sagi, S.; Wai-Sun Wong, V.; Dufour, J.F.; Schattenberg, J.M.; et al. A new definition for metabolic dysfunction-associated fatty liver disease: An international expert consensus statement. *J. Hepatol.* **2020**, *73*, 202–209. [CrossRef] [PubMed]
227. Fargion, S.; Porzio, M.; Fracanzani, A.L. Nonalcoholic fatty liver disease and vascular disease: State-of-the-art. *World J. Gastroenterol.* **2014**, *20*, 13306–13324. [CrossRef] [PubMed]
228. Dogru, T.; Genc, H.; Tapan, S.; Aslan, F.; Ercin, C.N.; Ors, F.; Kara, M.; Sertoglu, E.; Karslioglu, Y.; Bagci, S.; et al. Plasma fetuin-A is associated with endothelial dysfunction and subclinical atherosclerosis in subjects with nonalcoholic fatty liver disease. *Clin. Endocrinol.* **2013**, *78*, 712–717. [CrossRef]
229. Villanova, N.; Moscatiello, S.; Ramilli, S.; Bugianesi, E.; Magalotti, D.; Vanni, E.; Zoli, M.; Marchesini, G. Endothelial dysfunction and cardiovascular risk profile in nonalcoholic fatty liver disease. *Hepatology* **2005**, *42*, 473–480. [CrossRef]
230. Wilcox, J.N.; Subramanian, R.R.; Sundell, C.L.; Tracey, W.R.; Pollock, J.S.; Harrison, D.G.; Marsden, P.A. Expression of multiple isoforms of nitric oxide synthase in normal and atherosclerotic vessels. *Arterioscler. Thromb. Vasc. Biol.* **1997**, *17*, 2479–2488. [CrossRef]
231. Fujimoto, M.; Shimizu, N.; Kunii, K.; Martyn, J.A.; Ueki, K.; Kaneki, M. A role for iNOS in fasting hyperglycemia and impaired insulin signaling in the liver of obese diabetic mice. *Diabetes* **2005**, *54*, 1340–1348. [CrossRef]
232. Chauhan, S.D.; Seggara, G.; Vo, P.A.; Macallister, R.J.; Hobbs, A.J.; Ahluwalia, A. Protection against lipopolysaccharide-induced endothelial dysfunction in resistance and conduit vasculature of iNOS knockout mice. *FASEB J.* **2003**, *17*, 773–775. [CrossRef]
233. Francque, S.; Laleman, W.; Verbeke, L.; Van Steenkiste, C.; Casteleyn, C.; Kwanten, W.; Van Dyck, C.; D'Hondt, M.; Ramon, A.; Vermeulen, W.; et al. Increased intrahepatic resistance in severe steatosis: Endothelial dysfunction, vasoconstrictor overproduction and altered microvascular architecture. *Lab. Investig.* **2012**, *92*, 1428–1439. [CrossRef]
234. Miyao, M.; Kotani, H.; Ishida, T.; Kawai, C.; Manabe, S.; Abiru, H.; Tamaki, K. Pivotal role of liver sinusoidal endothelial cells in NAFLD/NASH progression. *Lab. Investig.* **2015**, *95*, 1130–1144. [CrossRef] [PubMed]
235. Lafoz, E.; Ruart, M.; Anton, A.; Oncins, A.; Hernández-Gea, V. The Endothelium as a Driver of Liver Fibrosis and Regeneration. *Cells* **2020**, *9*, 929. [CrossRef]
236. Hilscher, M.B.; Sehrawat, T.; Arab, J.P.; Zeng, Z.; Gao, J.; Liu, M.; Kostallari, E.; Gao, Y.; Simonetto, D.A.; Yaqoob, U.; et al. Mechanical Stretch Increases Expression of CXCL1 in Liver Sinusoidal Endothelial Cells to Recruit Neutrophils, Generate Sinusoidal Microthombi, and Promote Portal Hypertension. *Gastroenterology* **2019**, *157*, 193–209.e9. [CrossRef]
237. Ogresta, D.; Mrzljak, A.; Cigrovski Berkovic, M.; Bilic-Curcic, I.; Stojsavljevic-Shapeski, S.; Virovic-Jukic, L. Coagulation and Endothelial Dysfunction Associated with NAFLD: Current Status and Therapeutic Implications. *J. Clin. Transl. Hepatol.* **2022**, *10*, 339–355. [CrossRef]
238. Mazurek, T.; Zhang, L.; Zalewski, A.; Mannion, J.D.; Diehl, J.T.; Arafat, H.; Sarov-Blat, L.; O'Brien, S.; Keiper, E.A.; Johnson, A.G.; et al. Human epicardial adipose tissue is a source of inflammatory mediators. *Circulation* **2003**, *108*, 2460–2466. [CrossRef] [PubMed]
239. Duan, Y.; Pan, X.; Luo, J.; Xiao, X.; Li, J.; Bestman, P.L.; Luo, M. Association of Inflammatory Cytokines With Non-Alcoholic Fatty Liver Disease. *Front. Immunol.* **2022**, *13*, 880298. [CrossRef]
240. Kathirvel, E.; Chen, P.; Morgan, K.; French, S.W.; Morgan, T.R. Oxidative stress and regulation of anti-oxidant enzymes in cytochrome P4502E1 transgenic mouse model of non-alcoholic fatty liver. *J. Gastroenterol. Hepatol.* **2010**, *25*, 1136–1143. [CrossRef] [PubMed]
241. Caimi, G.; Lo Presti, R.; Montana, M.; Noto, D.; Canino, B.; Averna, M.R.; Hopps, E. Lipid peroxidation, nitric oxide metabolites, and their ratio in a group of subjects with metabolic syndrome. *Oxid. Med. Cell Longev.* **2014**, *2014*, 824756. [CrossRef]
242. Fernández-Sánchez, A.; Madrigal-Santillán, E.; Bautista, M.; Esquivel-Soto, J.; Morales-González, A.; Esquivel-Chirino, C.; Durante-Montiel, I.; Sánchez-Rivera, G.; Valadez-Vega, C.; Morales-González, J.A. Inflammation, oxidative stress, and obesity. *Int. J. Mol. Sci.* **2011**, *12*, 3117–3132. [CrossRef]
243. Huang, C.J.; McAllister, M.J.; Slusher, A.L.; Webb, H.E.; Mock, J.T.; Acevedo, E.O. Obesity-Related Oxidative Stress: The Impact of Physical Activity and Diet Manipulation. *Sports Med. Open* **2015**, *1*, 32. [CrossRef]
244. Masenga, S.K.; Kabwe, L.S.; Chakulya, M.; Kirabo, A. Mechanisms of Oxidative Stress in Metabolic Syndrome. *Int. J. Mol. Sci.* **2023**, *24*, 7898. [CrossRef]

245. Potenza, M.A.; Marasciulo, F.L.; Chieppa, D.M.; Brigiani, G.S.; Formoso, G.; Quon, M.J.; Montagnani, M. Insulin resistance in spontaneously hypertensive rats is associated with endothelial dysfunction characterized by imbalance between NO and ET-1 production. *Am. J. Physiol. Heart Circ. Physiol.* **2005**, *289*, H813–H822. [CrossRef]
246. Reustle, A.; Torzewski, M. Role of p38 MAPK in Atherosclerosis and Aortic Valve Sclerosis. *Int. J. Mol. Sci.* **2018**, *19*, 3761. [CrossRef]
247. Hong, J.; Zhang, Y.; Lai, S.; Lv, A.; Su, Q.; Dong, Y.; Zhou, Z.; Tang, W.; Zhao, J.; Cui, L.; et al. Effects of metformin versus glipizide on cardiovascular outcomes in patients with type 2 diabetes and coronary artery disease. *Diabetes Care* **2013**, *36*, 1304–1311. [CrossRef]
248. Yanai, H.; Adachi, H.; Hakoshima, M.; Iida, S.; Katsuyama, H. Metabolic-Dysfunction-Associated Steatotic Liver Disease-Its Pathophysiology, Association with Atherosclerosis and Cardiovascular Disease, and Treatments. *Int. J. Mol. Sci.* **2023**, *24*, 5473. [CrossRef] [PubMed]
249. Amor, A.J.; Pinyol, M.; Solà, E.; Catalan, M.; Cofán, M.; Herreras, Z.; Amigó, N.; Gilabert, R.; Sala-Vila, A.; Ros, E.; et al. Relationship between noninvasive scores of nonalcoholic fatty liver disease and nuclear magnetic resonance lipoprotein abnormalities: A focus on atherogenic dyslipidemia. *J. Clin. Lipidol.* **2017**, *11*, 551–561.e7. [CrossRef]
250. DeFilippis, A.P.; Blaha, M.J.; Martin, S.S.; Reed, R.M.; Jones, S.R.; Nasir, K.; Blumenthal, R.S.; Budoff, M.J. Nonalcoholic fatty liver disease and serum lipoproteins: The Multi-Ethnic Study of Atherosclerosis. *Atherosclerosis* **2013**, *227*, 429–436. [CrossRef] [PubMed]
251. Heeren, J.; Scheja, L. Metabolic-associated fatty liver disease and lipoprotein metabolism. *Mol. Metab.* **2021**, *50*, 101238. [CrossRef] [PubMed]
252. Yu, H.; Ma, S.; Sun, L.; Gao, J.; Zhao, C. TGF-β1 upregulates the expression of lncRNA-ATB to promote atherosclerosis. *Mol. Med. Rep.* **2019**, *19*, 4222–4228. [CrossRef] [PubMed]
253. Ekstedt, M.; Franzen, L.E.; Mathiesen, U.L.; Thorelius, L.; Holmqvist, M.; Bodemar, G.; Kechagias, S. Long-term follow-up of patients with NAFLD and elevated liver enzymes. *Hepatology* **2006**, *44*, 865–873. [CrossRef] [PubMed]
254. Xu, X.; Lu, L.; Dong, Q.; Li, X.; Zhang, N.; Xin, Y.; Xuan, S. Research advances in the relationship between nonalcoholic fatty liver disease and atherosclerosis. *Lipids Health Dis.* **2015**, *14*, 158. [CrossRef] [PubMed]
255. Duell, P.B.; Welty, F.K.; Miller, M.; Chait, A.; Hammond, G.; Ahmad, Z.; Cohen, D.E.; Horton, J.D.; Pressman, G.S.; Toth, P.P.; et al. Nonalcoholic Fatty Liver Disease and Cardiovascular Risk: A Scientific Statement From the American Heart Association. *Arterioscler. Thromb. Vasc. Biol.* **2022**, *42*, e168–e185. [CrossRef]
256. Bieghs, V.; Rensen, P.C.; Hofker, M.H.; Shiri-Sverdlov, R. NASH and atherosclerosis are two aspects of a shared disease: Central role for macrophages. *Atherosclerosis* **2012**, *220*, 287–293. [CrossRef]
257. Sookoian, S.; Gianotti, T.F.; Rosselli, M.S.; Burgueno, A.L.; Castano, G.O.; Pirola, C.J. Liver transcriptional profile of atherosclerosis-related genes in human nonalcoholic fatty liver disease. *Atherosclerosis* **2011**, *218*, 378–385. [CrossRef]
258. Abdallah, L.R.; de Matos, R.C.; YPDM, E.S.; Vieira-Soares, D.; Muller-Machado, G.; Pollo-Flores, P. Non-alcoholic Fatty Liver Disease and Its Links with Inflammation and Atherosclerosis. *Curr. Atheroscler. Rep.* **2020**, *22*, 7. [CrossRef]
259. Gaggini, M.; Morelli, M.; Buzzigoli, E.; DeFronzo, R.A.; Bugianesi, E.; Gastaldelli, A. Non-alcoholic fatty liver disease (NAFLD) and its connection with insulin resistance, dyslipidemia, atherosclerosis and coronary heart disease. *Nutrients* **2013**, *5*, 1544–1560. [CrossRef]
260. Zhu, B.; Wu, H.; Li, K.S.; Eisa-Beygi, S.; Singh, B.; Bielenberg, D.R.; Huang, W.; Chen, H. Two sides of the same coin: Non-alcoholic fatty liver disease and atherosclerosis. *Vasc. Pharmacol.* **2024**, *154*, 107249. [CrossRef]
261. Abd El-Kader, S.M.; El-Den Ashmawy, E.M. Non-alcoholic fatty liver disease: The diagnosis and management. *World J. Hepatol.* **2015**, *7*, 846–858. [CrossRef]
262. Pacifico, L.; Nobili, V.; Anania, C.; Verdecchia, P.; Chiesa, C. Pediatric nonalcoholic fatty liver disease, metabolic syndrome and cardiovascular risk. *World J. Gastroenterol.* **2011**, *17*, 3082–3091. [CrossRef]
263. Muzurovic, E.; Peng, C.C.; Belanger, M.J.; Sanoudou, D.; Mikhailidis, D.P.; Mantzoros, C.S. Nonalcoholic Fatty Liver Disease and Cardiovascular Disease: A Review of Shared Cardiometabolic Risk Factors. *Hypertension* **2022**, *79*, 1319–1326. [CrossRef]
264. Hamaguchi, M.; Kojima, T.; Takeda, N.; Nagata, C.; Takeda, J.; Sarui, H.; Kawahito, Y.; Yoshida, N.; Suetsugu, A.; Kato, T.; et al. Nonalcoholic fatty liver disease is a novel predictor of cardiovascular disease. *World J. Gastroenterol.* **2007**, *13*, 1579–1584. [CrossRef]
265. Anstee, Q.M.; Targher, G.; Day, C.P. Progression of NAFLD to diabetes mellitus, cardiovascular disease or cirrhosis. *Nat. Rev. Gastroenterol. Hepatol.* **2013**, *10*, 330–344. [CrossRef]
266. Castillo-Nunez, Y.; Almeda-Valdes, P.; Gonzalez-Galvez, G.; Arechavaleta-Granell, M.D.R. Metabolic dysfunction-associated steatotic liver disease and atherosclerosis. *Curr. Diab. Rep.* **2024**, *24*, 158–166. [CrossRef]
267. Lonardo, A.; Nascimbeni, F.; Mantovani, A.; Targher, G. Hypertension, diabetes, atherosclerosis and NASH: Cause or consequence? *J. Hepatol.* **2018**, *68*, 335–352. [CrossRef] [PubMed]

268. Sundberg, U.; Beauchemin, N.; Obrink, B. The cytoplasmic domain of CEACAM1-L controls its lateral localization and the organization of desmosomes in polarized epithelial cells. *J. Cell Sci.* **2004**, *117 Pt 7*, 1091–1104. [CrossRef]
269. Sundberg, U.; Obrink, B. CEACAM1 isoforms with different cytoplasmic domains show different localization, organization and adhesive properties in polarized epithelial cells. *J. Cell Sci.* **2002**, *115 Pt 6*, 1273–1284. [CrossRef] [PubMed]
270. Najjar, S.M.; Yang, Y.; Fernstrom, M.A.; Lee, S.J.; Deangelis, A.M.; Rjaily, G.A.; Al-Share, Q.Y.; Dai, T.; Miller, T.A.; Ratnam, S.; et al. Insulin acutely decreases hepatic fatty acid synthase activity. *Cell Metab.* **2005**, *2*, 43–53. [CrossRef] [PubMed]
271. Najjar, S.M.; Abdolahipour, R.; Ghadieh, H.E.; Jahromi, M.S.; Najjar, J.A.; Abuamreh, B.A.M.; Zaidi, S.; Kumarasamy, S.; Muturi, H.T. Regulation of Insulin Clearance by Non-Esterified Fatty Acids. *Biomedicines* **2022**, *10*, 1899. [CrossRef]
272. Aldroubi, B.G.; Najjar, J.A.; Youssef, T.S.; Rizk, C.E.; Abuamreh, B.A.M.; Aramouni, K.; Ghadieh, H.E.; Najjar, S.M. Cell-specific regulation of insulin action and hepatic fibrosis by CEACAM1. *Metab. Target. Organ. Damage* **2024**, *4*, 34. [CrossRef]
273. Shaheen, M.; Pan, D.; Schrode, K.M.; Kermah, D.; Puri, V.; Zarrinpar, A.; Elisha, D.; Najjar, S.M.; Friedman, T.C. Reassessment of the Hispanic Disparity: Hepatic Steatosis Is More Prevalent in Mexican Americans Than Other Hispanics. *Hepatol. Commun.* **2021**, *5*, 2068–2079. [CrossRef]
274. Bril, F.; Lomonaco, R.; Orsak, B.; Ortiz-Lopez, C.; Webb, A.; Tio, F.; Hecht, J.; Cusi, K. Relationship between disease severity, hyperinsulinemia, and impaired insulin clearance in patients with nonalcoholic steatohepatitis. *Hepatology* **2014**, *59*, 2178–2187. [CrossRef] [PubMed]
275. Watada, H.; Tamura, Y. Impaired insulin clearance as a cause rather than a consequence of insulin resistance. *J. Diabetes Investig.* **2017**, *8*, 723–725. [CrossRef] [PubMed]
276. Patarrao, R.S.; Meneses, M.J.; Ghadieh, H.E.; Herrera, L.; Duarte, S.; Ribeiro, R.T.; Raposo, J.F.; Schmitt, V.; Singer, B.B.; Gastaldelli, A.; et al. Insights into circulating CEACAM1 in insulin clearance and disease progression: Evidence from the Portuguese PREVADIAB2 study. *Eur. J. Clin. Investig.* **2024**, *54* (Suppl. S2), e14344. [CrossRef] [PubMed]
277. Zaidi, S.; Asalla, S.; Muturi, H.T.; Russo, L.; Abdolahipour, R.; Belew, G.D.; Iglesias, M.B.; Feraudo, M.; Leon, L.; Kuo, E.; et al. Loss of CEACAM1 in hepatocytes causes hepatic fibrosis. *Eur. J. Clin. Investig.* **2024**, *54*, e14177. [CrossRef]
278. Ghadieh, H.E.; Gastaldelli, A.; Najjar, S.M. Role of Insulin Clearance in Insulin Action and Metabolic Diseases. *Int. J. Mol. Sci.* **2023**, *24*, 7156. [CrossRef]
279. Kotronen, A.; Juurinen, L.; Tiikkainen, M.; Vehkavaara, S.; Yki-Jarvinen, H. Increased liver fat, impaired insulin clearance, and hepatic and adipose tissue insulin resistance in type 2 diabetes. *Gastroenterology* **2008**, *135*, 122–130. [CrossRef]
280. Tiikkainen, M.; Hakkinen, A.M.; Korsheninnikova, E.; Nyman, T.; Makimattila, S.; Yki-Jarvinen, H. Effects of rosiglitazone and metformin on liver fat content, hepatic insulin resistance, insulin clearance, and gene expression in adipose tissue in patients with type 2 diabetes. *Diabetes* **2004**, *53*, 2169–2176. [CrossRef]
281. Ghadieh, H.E.; Muturi, H.T.; Russo, L.; Marino, C.C.; Ghanem, S.S.; Khuder, S.S.; Hanna, J.C.; Jash, S.; Puri, V.; Heinrich, G.; et al. Exenatide induces carcinoembryonic antigen-related cell adhesion molecule 1 expression to prevent hepatic steatosis. *Hepatol. Commun.* **2018**, *2*, 35–47. [CrossRef]
282. Muturi, H.T.; Ghadieh, H.E.; Asalla, S.; Lester, S.G.; Belew, G.D.; Zaidi, S.; Abdolahipour, R.; Shrestha, A.P.; Portuphy, A.O.; Stankus, H.L.; et al. Conditional deletion of CEACAM1 in hepatic stellate cells causes their activation. *Mol. Metab.* **2024**, *88*, 02010. [CrossRef]
283. Ghadieh, H.E.; Muturi, H.T.; Najjar, S.M. Exenatide Prevents Diet-induced Hepatocellular Injury in A CEACAM1-Dependent Mechanism. *J. Diabetes Treat.* **2017**, *2017*, 10-29011. [CrossRef]
284. Bakker, L.E.; van Schinkel, L.D.; Guigas, B.; Streefland, T.C.; Jonker, J.T.; van Klinken, J.B.; van der Zon, G.C.; Lamb, H.J.; Smit, J.W.; Pijl, H.; et al. A 5-day high-fat, high-calorie diet impairs insulin sensitivity in healthy, young South Asian men but not in Caucasian men. *Diabetes* **2014**, *63*, 248–258. [CrossRef]
285. Ramakrishnan, S.K.; Khuder, S.S.; Al-Share, Q.Y.; Russo, L.; Abdallah, S.L.; Patel, P.R.; Heinrich, G.; Muturi, H.T.; Mopidevi, B.R.; Oyarce, A.M.; et al. PPARalpha (Peroxisome Proliferator-activated Receptor alpha) Activation Reduces Hepatic CEACAM1 Protein Expression to Regulate Fatty Acid Oxidation during Fasting-refeeding Transition. *J. Biol. Chem.* **2016**, *291*, 8121–8129. [CrossRef]
286. Najjar, S.M.; Shively, J.E. Regulation of lipid storage and inflammation in the liver by CEACAM1. *Eur. J. Clin. Investig.* **2024**, *54* (Suppl. S2), e14338. [CrossRef]
287. Gandhi, A.K.; Huang, Y.H.; Sun, Z.J.; Kim, W.M.; Kondo, Y.; Hanley, T.; Beauchemin, N.; Blumberg, R.S. Structural aspects of CEACAM1 interactions. *Eur. J. Clin. Investig.* **2024**, *54* (Suppl. S2), e14357. [CrossRef]
288. Gotz, L.; Rueckschloss, U.; Najjar, S.M.; Ergun, S.; Kleefeldt, F. Carcinoembryonic antigen-related cell adhesion molecule 1 in cancer: Blessing or curse? *Eur. J. Clin. Investig.* **2024**, *54* (Suppl. S2), e14337. [CrossRef]
289. Dery, K.J.; Yao, S.; Cheng, B.; Kupiec-Weglinski, J.W. New therapeutic concepts against ischemia-reperfusion injury in organ transplantation. *Expert. Rev. Clin. Immunol.* **2023**, *19*, 1205–1224. [CrossRef]
290. Dery, K.J.; Najjar, S.M.; Beauchemin, N.; Shively, J.E.; Kupiec-Weglinski, J.W. Mechanism and function of CEACAM1 splice isoforms. *Eur. J. Clin. Investig.* **2024**, *54* (Suppl. S2), e14350. [CrossRef]

291. Kim, W.M.; Huang, Y.H.; Gandhi, A.; Blumberg, R.S. CEACAM1 structure and function in immunity and its therapeutic implications. *Semin. Immunol.* **2019**, *42*, 101296. [CrossRef]
292. Yao, S.; Kasargod, A.; Chiu, R.; Torgerson, T.R.; Kupiec-Weglinski, J.W.; Dery, K.J. The Coming Age of Antisense Oligos for the Treatment of Hepatic Ischemia/Reperfusion (IRI) and Other Liver Disorders: Role of Oxidative Stress and Potential Antioxidant Effect. *Antioxidants* **2024**, *13*, 678. [CrossRef]
293. Gotz, L.; Rueckschloss, U.; Ergun, S.; Kleefeldt, F. CEACAM1 in vascular homeostasis and inflammation. *Eur. J. Clin. Investig.* **2024**, *54* (Suppl. S2), e14345. [CrossRef]
294. Stefan, N.; Haring, H.U.; Cusi, K. Non-alcoholic fatty liver disease: Causes, diagnosis, cardiometabolic consequences, and treatment strategies. *Lancet Diabetes Endocrinol.* **2019**, *7*, 313–324. [CrossRef]
295. Alkhouri, N.; Carter-Kent, C.; Elias, M.; Feldstein, A.E. Atherogenic dyslipidemia and cardiovascular risk in children with nonalcoholic fatty liver disease. *Clin. Lipidol.* **2011**, *6*, 305–314. [CrossRef]
296. Di Pino, A.; DeFronzo, R.A. Insulin Resistance and Atherosclerosis: Implications for Insulin-Sensitizing Agents. *Endocr. Rev.* **2019**, *40*, 1447–1467. [CrossRef]
297. Lim, S.; Taskinen, M.R.; Boren, J. Crosstalk between nonalcoholic fatty liver disease and cardiometabolic syndrome. *Obes. Rev.* **2019**, *20*, 599–611. [CrossRef]
298. Muturi, H.T.; Ghadieh, H.E.; Abdolahipour, R.; Stankus, H.L.; Belew, G.D.; Liu, J.K.; Jahromi, M.S.; Lee, A.D.; Singer, B.B.; Angeli-Pahim, I.; et al. Loss of CEACAM1 in endothelial cells causes hepatic fibrosis. *Metabolism* **2023**, *144*, 155562. [CrossRef]
299. Bowman, T.A.; Ramakrishnan, S.K.; Kaw, M.; Lee, S.J.; Patel, P.R.; Golla, V.K.; Bourey, R.E.; Haram, P.M.; Koch, L.G.; Britton, S.L.; et al. Caloric restriction reverses hepatic insulin resistance and steatosis in rats with low aerobic capacity. *Endocrinology* **2010**, *151*, 5157–5164. [CrossRef]
300. Wisloff, U.; Najjar, S.M.; Ellingsen, O.; Haram, P.M.; Swoap, S.; Al-Share, Q.; Fernstrom, M.; Rezaei, K.; Lee, S.J.; Koch, L.G.; et al. Cardiovascular risk factors emerge after artificial selection for low aerobic capacity. *Science* **2005**, *307*, 418–420. [CrossRef]
301. Heinrich, G.; Ghadieh, H.E.; Ghanem, S.S.; Muturi, H.T.; Rezaei, K.; Al-Share, Q.Y.; Bowman, T.A.; Zhang, D.; Garofalo, R.S.; Yin, L.; et al. Loss of Hepatic CEACAM1: A Unifying Mechanism Linking Insulin Resistance to Obesity and Non-Alcoholic Fatty Liver Disease. *Front. Endocrinol.* **2017**, *8*, 8. [CrossRef]
302. Helal, R.A.; Russo, L.; Ghadieh, H.E.; Muturi, H.T.; Asalla, S.; Lee, A.D.; Gatto-Weis, C.; Najjar, S.M. Regulation of hepatic fibrosis by carcinoembryonic antigen-related cell adhesion molecule 1. *Metabolism* **2021**, *121*, 154801. [CrossRef] [PubMed]
303. Russo, L.; Muturi, H.T.; Ghadieh, H.E.; Ghanem, S.S.; Bowman, T.A.; Noh, H.L.; Dagdeviren, S.; Dogbey, G.Y.; Kim, J.K.; Heinrich, G.; et al. Liver-specific reconstitution of CEACAM1 reverses the metabolic abnormalities caused by its global deletion in male mice. *Diabetologia* **2017**, *60*, 2463–2474. [CrossRef]
304. Abu Helal, R.; Muturi, H.T.; Lee, A.D.; Li, W.; Ghadieh, H.E.; Najjar, S.M. Aortic Fibrosis in Insulin-Sensitive Mice with Endothelial Cell-Specific Deletion of Ceacam1 Gene. *Int. J. Mol. Sci.* **2022**, *23*, 4335. [CrossRef] [PubMed]
305. Muturi, H.T.; Khuder, S.S.; Ghadieh, H.E.; Esakov, E.L.; Noh, H.; Kang, H.; McInerney, M.F.; Kim, J.K.; Lee, A.D.; Najjar, S.M. Insulin Sensitivity Is Retained in Mice with Endothelial Loss of Carcinoembryonic Antigen Cell Adhesion Molecule 1. *Cells* **2021**, *10*, 2093. [CrossRef] [PubMed]

livers

MDPI

Review

The Pivotal Role of the Membrane-Bound O-Acyltransferase Domain Containing 7 in Non-Alcoholic Fatty Liver Disease

Preethi Chandrasekaran [1,*] and Ralf Weiskirchen [2,*]

[1] UT Southwestern Medical Center Dallas, 5323 Harry Hines Blvd. ND10.504, Dallas, TX 75390-9014, USA
[2] Institute of Molecular Pathobiochemistry, Experimental Gene Therapy and Clinical Chemistry (IFMPEGKC), Rheinisch-Westfälische Technische Hochschule (RWTH) University Hospital Aachen, D-52074 Aachen, Germany
* Correspondence: Preethi.Chandrasekaran@utsouthwestern.edu (P.C.); rweiskirchen@ukaachen.de (R.W.)

Abstract: Non-alcoholic fatty liver disease (NAFLD) is a common and prevalent disorder affecting 25 percent of the adults in the United States and 32 percent of adults globally. It is one of the common causes of chronic liver disease characterized by steatosis, which can lead to inflammation, fibrosis, and cirrhosis. NAFLD is strongly associated with obesity and insulin resistance. Multiple genetic variants have been consistently found to be associated with NAFLD; one of them is found in the TMC4-*MBOAT7* loci. One variant (rs641738 C>T) within *MBOAT7* encoding lysophosphatidyl inositol acyltransferase increases the risk for NAFLD development and triggers hepatic inflammation by regulating arachidonic acid levels. This review provides an overview of the *MBOAT7* gene, pathogenesis of NAFLD, understanding the regulation of *MBOAT7* and mechanistic link between *MBOAT7* and NAFLD. It further summarizes pathophysiologically relevant in vivo and in vitro studies on *MBOAT7* and challenges in treating complex NAFLD with recent progress made in the treatment of NAFLD. As such, this review provides useful information on *MBOAT7* and NAFLD interrelation, which has the potential of deciphering novel therapeutic targets rather than well-known genetic variants such as PNPLA3 and TM6SF2.

Keywords: non-alcoholic fatty liver disease; *MBOAT7*; lipid metabolism; hepatic steatosis; fibrosis; therapeutic targets; insulin resistance; pathogenesis

1. Introduction

NAFLD is a complex, multifactorial disease encompassing a broad spectrum of disorders including hepatic steatosis, fibrosis, cirrhosis, and progression to hepatocellular carcinoma and is strongly associated with metabolic syndrome including diabetes mellitus, insulin resistance and obesity. Noteworthy, the total number of populations with non-alcoholic fatty liver disease (NAFLD) exceeds the combined population with obesity and diabetes mellitus globally [1]. In addition, multiple studies have established a strong association between NAFLD and increased risk of cardiovascular diseases and its complications. More importantly, NAFLD is recognized as an independent risk factor in cardiovascular diseases [2]. These diseases share multiple pathophysiological features and are closely interrelated in their progression.

According to histology, NAFLD is defined by the presence of hepatic lipid accumulation in >5% of hepatocytes [2]. NAFLD has been predicted to be the most frequent indication for liver transplantation by 2030 [3]. It further contributes to extra-hepatic chronic complications and regulatory pathways [4]. The current gender-based prevalence of NAFLD is approximately 30–40% in men and 15–20% in women [5].

Recent studies have identified several genetic susceptibility variants comprising of single-nucleotide polymorphisms in *PNPLA3* (rs738409), *TM6SF2* (rs8542926), and *LXPLAL1* (rs12137855) [6]. The contributions of the *PNPLA3* polymorphism in NAFLD have been widely studied, while in contrast, the molecular biochemical mechanistic insights underlying the *MBOAT7* polymorphism are little understood [6]. Recently, the identification of genetic variant rs641738 near two genes encoding the *MBOAT7* gene and transmembrane channel-like 4 (TMC4) in determining the risk of NAFLD and its complications has gained utmost importance and still needs further exploration for a targeted drug design to treat complex NAFLD [7]. However, the available data presently suggest that TMC4 is not expressed abundantly in the human liver, and previous studies revealed that the CRISPR/Cas9-mediated TMC4 knockout in mice does not provoke hepatic steatosis [8]. More importantly, it has been reported that *MBOAT7* loss of function alone promotes liver disease progression via the accumulation of lysophosphatidylinositol lipids, thereby highlighting the unique role of *MBOAT7* in NAFLD pathogenesis [8].

MBOA7 is a lysophophosphatidylinositol (LPI) acyltransferase preferentially transferring polyunsaturated fatty acids (PUFAs) to LPI. Emerging genome-wide association studies reported that a genetic variant within the *MBOAT7* gene is closely related to non-alcoholic steatohepatitis (NASH), attributed to an increase in triglyceride synthesis through canonical and non-canonical pathways of de novo lipogenesis [9]. This review summarizes our knowledge of *MBOAT7* and NAFLD association, which potentially opens new avenues for drug design strategies to treat this multi-system disease. The selectivity of *MBOAT7* for long PUFAs such as arachidonic acids suggests that an abundance of specific phosphoinositols are regulated by *MBOAT7* without alterations in total phosphoinositol content [8].

2. *MBOAT7* Gene—An Overview

The *MBOAT7* gene, also known as lysophosphatidylinositol acyltransferase 1 (LPLAT1), is located on the long arm of human chromosome 19 (19q13.42) and encodes an enzyme with a size of 472 amino acids. The protein is highly expressed in liver, heart, testis, and adipose tissue, and has a molecular mass of 52,765 Da [10]. The *MBOAT7* protein is a highly conserved member of the membrane-bound O-acyltransferases family of integral membrane proteins composed of six transmembrane domains present on the endoplasmic reticulum, lipid droplets, and mitochondria-associated membranes (Figure 1) [10–12].

The encoded protein is a lysophosphatidylinositol acyltransferase having specificity for the arachidonoyl-CoA acyl donor, involved in reacylation of phospholipids (PLs) as a part of Land cycle (remodeling of PL) [9]. The lysophospholipid acyl transferase activity of *MBOAT7* preferentially incorporates arachidonic acid into PLs [9]. In the liver, *MBOAT7* participates in the regulation of triglyceride metabolism through the phosphatidylinositol acyl-chain remodeling regulation. *MBOAT7* plays a unique role in Land's cycle, in diversifying the fatty acid composition of membrane phosphatidylinositol (PI) species and not PLs with other head groups.

The two enzymatic reactions of the Land's cycle include diacylation of unsaturated PLs from the sn-2 position of PLs catalyzed by phospholipases and esterification of fatty acids to lysophospholipid catalyzed by acyltransferases resulting in the release of newly modeled PLs [11,12]. *MBOAT7* incorporates free PUFAs such as arachidonic acid into lysophospholipids and releases newly modeled PLs with a higher degree of unsaturation [11]. The *MBOAT7* mutations thus lead to the accumulation of intracellular free arachidonic acid, which is used as a substrate for the synthesis of inflammatory lipid mediators. In addition, the higher PI availability associated with weak *MBOAT7* enzymatic activity is used to synthesize diacylglycerols, which are the main precursors of triglycerides stored in lipid droplets [11].

In a cryo-EM structure model proposed by Wang and colleagues [12], the arachidonoyl-CoA substrate enters the enzyme tunnel from the cytoplasmic leaflet of the ER and lyso-PI enters the tunnel from a luminal leaflet with a side channel harboring its single acyl chain and positions the sn-2 hydroxyl group of the glycerol backbone near the His356 residue located in the catalytic domain [12].

```
Human      MSPEEWTYLVVLLISIPIGFLFKKAGPGLKRWGAAAVGLGLTLFTCGPHTLHSLVTILGT 60
Rat        MTPEEWTYLMVLLISIPVGFLFKKAGPGLKRWGAAAVGLGLTLFTCGPHSLHSLITILGT 60
Mouse      MTPEEWTYLMVLLISIPVGFLFKKAGPGLKRWGAAAVGLGLTLFTCGPHSLHSLITILGT 60
           *:*******:*******:*******************************:****:*****

Human      WALIQAQPCSCHALALAWTFSYLLFFRALSLLGLPTPTPFTNAVQLLLTLKLVSLASEVQ 120
Rat        WALIQAQPCSCHALALAWTFSYLLFFRALSLLGLPTPTPFTNAVQLLLTLKLVSLASEVQ 120
Mouse      WALIQAQPCSCHALALAWTFSYLLFFRALSLLGLPTPTPFTNAVQLLLTLKLVSLASEVQ 120
           ************************************************************

Human      DLHLAQRKEMASGFSKGPTLGLLPDVPSLMETLSYSYCYVGIMTGPFFRYRTYLDWLEQP 180
Rat        DLHLAQRKEMASGFSKEPTLGLLPDVPSLMETLSYSYCYVGIMTGPFFRYRTYLDWLEQP 180
Mouse      DLHLAQRKEIASGFHKEPTLGLLPEVPSLMETLSYSYCYVGIMTGPFFRYRTYLDWLEQP 180
           *********:**** * *******:***********************************

Human      FPGAVPSLRPLLRRAWPAPLFGLLFLLSSHLFPLEAVREDAFYARPLPARLFYMIPVFFA 240
Rat        FPEAVPSLRPLLRRAWPAPLFGLLFLLSSHLFPLEAVREDAFYARPLPTRLFYMIPVFFA 240
Mouse      FPEAVPSLRPLLRRAWPAPLFGLLFLLSSHLFPLEAVREDAFYARPLPTRLFYMIPVFFA 240
           ** *********************************************:***********

Human      FRMRFYVAWIAAECGCIAAGFGAYPVAAKARAGGGPTLQCPPPSSPEKAASLEYDYETIR 300
Rat        FRMRFYVAWIAAECGCIAAGFGAYPVAAKARAGGGPTLQCPPPSSPEIAASLEYDYEAIR 300
Mouse      FRMRFYVAWIAAECGCIAAGFGAYPVAAKARAGGGPTLQCPPPSSPEIAASLEYDYETIR 300
           *********************************************** *********:**

Human      NIDCYSTDFCVRVRDGMRYWNMTVQWWLAQYIYKSAPARSYVLRSAWTMLLSAYWHGLHP 360
Rat        NIDCYGTDFCVRVRDGMRYWNMTVQWWLAQYIYKSAPFRSYVLRSAWTMLLSAYWHGLHP 360
Mouse      NIDCYGTDFCVRVRDGMRYWNMTVQWWLAQYIYKSAPFRSYVLRSAWTMLLSAYWHGLHP 360
           *****.******************************* **********************

Human      GYYLSFLTIPLCLAAEGRLESALRGRLSPGGQKAWDWVHWFLKMRAYDYMCMGFVLLSLA 420
Rat        GYYLSFMTIPLCLAAEGYLESALRRHLSPGGQKAWDWFHWFLKMRAYDYMCMGFVLLSMG 420
Mouse      GYYLSFMTIPLCLAAEGYLESALRRHLSPGGQKAWDWVHWFLKMRAYDYMCMGFVLLSMA 420
           ******:********** ****** :***********.********************:.

Human      DTLRYWASIYFCIHFLALAALGLGLALGGGSPSRRKAASQPTS-LAPEKLREE        472
Rat        DTLRYWASIYFWVHFLALACLGLGLALGGGSPSKRKTPSQATTSQAKEKLREE        473
Mouse      DTLRYWASIYFWVHFLALACLGLGLVLGGGSPSKRKTPSQATSSQAKEKLREE        473
           *********** :******.*****.*******:**: ** *:  * ******
```

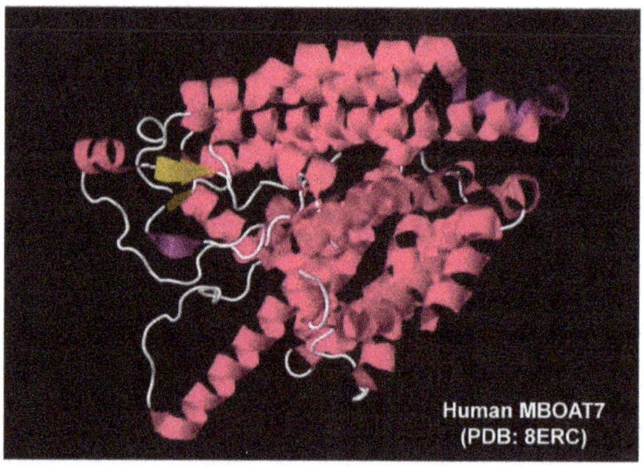

Figure 1. *MBOAT7*, a highly conserved O-acyltransferase. Sequence comparison of human, rat, and mouse *MBOAT7* proteins demonstrating the high degree of sequence similarity. Amino acid residues conserved in all three sequences are indicated by asterisks, while conserved amino acid residues with strongly similar properties are marked by colons, and amino acids with weakly similar properties are indicated by periods. The protein sequences were taken from protein sequences (human: NP_077274, rat: XP_038966897, mouse: NP_084210) deposited in the National Library of Medicine [13] and the alignment was performed using the EMBL-EBI Clustal Omega multiple sequence alignment tool [14]). Human *MBOAT7* is composed of 11 transmembrane helical segments that are connected by short intervening helices and loops. For more details about the structure of human *MBOAT7*, refer to [12]. The structure of human *MBOAT7* was generated with Jmol using the structure coordinates deposited in the RCSB Protein data base (access. no.: 8ERC).

3. Pathogenesis of NAFLD

NAFLD is defined by elevated hepatic lipid accumulation exceeding 5% of liver weight in the absence of heavy alcohol consumption. NAFLD entails a wide spectrum of conditions ranging from uncomplicated steatosis to NASH progressing to fibrosis and cirrhosis with few cases further progressing to hepatocellular carcinoma (HCC) [15]. The pathogenesis of NAFLD is closely related to obesity, glucose intolerance, and dyslipidemia [15]. Unhealthy dietary habits, highly fructose-enriched diets, excessive calorie intake, and lack of exercise along with genetic predisposition are the major contributors to this pathological condition [16]. The biological associations between fatty liver and inherited risk factors and their interplay with environmental factors are primary goals in the study of NAFLD pathophysiology.

In addition, multiple studies have established a strong correlation between NAFLD and increased risk of cardiovascular complications [17]. A recent retrospective study showed that NAFLD determined early atherosclerosis and progression, independently of traditional cardiovascular risk factors [18]. Few longitudinal and retrospective studies have demonstrated interesting findings on NAFLD association with hypertension, chronic kidney disease, and cardiometabolic comorbidities [19]. It is certainly evident that dysregulation of lipid and glucose metabolism and activation of the prothrombotic system are some of the mechanisms involved in NAFLD leading to cardiometabolic complications.

A 'Multi-hit' hypothesis has been proposed in previous studies to understand NAFLD pathogenesis [20]. Insulin resistance is the first hit responsible for hepatic steatosis either due to impaired insulin receptor activity or derangement of insulin response through downstream signaling cascade. Insulin resistance favors lipid storage dismissal, increasing the efflux of free fatty acids from adipose tissue to the liver where they are stored as triglycerides [21]. In addition, fat deposition is exacerbated by hyperinsulinemia by inducing de novo lipogenesis from glucose through sterol regulatory element binding protein 1 (SREBP1). Mitochondria dysfunctions and changes in PUFAs are also responsible for steatosis onset [22].

Under normal conditions, there is a balance and dynamic equilibrium between fatty acid storage and expenditure, in which the liver is the key organ involved in regulatory systemic lipid metabolism via coordinating lipid uptake, synthesis, oxidation, and export. Peripheral lipolysis, de novo lipogenesis, dietary-derived chylomicrons, and intermediate density lipoprotein particles are the main free fatty acid sources contributing to hepatic lipid accumulation [23]. Insulin resistance decreases the utilization of triglycerides in peripheral tissues and increased lipolysis in adipose tissue, leading to increased influx of free fatty acids to the liver. In addition, increased hepatic influx of chylomicrons and very-low-density lipoprotein (VLDL) can be caused by decreased lysophosphatidylinositol activity. These mechanisms mainly contribute to excess triglycerides and TC accumulation in the liver, which in turn enhances the assembly of VLDL particles, further worsening dyslipidemia [23].

There is much evidence illustrating the association between NAFLD pathogenesis and inflammatory responses [24]. In NAFLD, hepatic immune cell populations exhibit an immunogenic phenotype composed of Kupffer cells, monocyte-derived macrophages, and dendritic cells, whose transcriptional alterations were elucidated by single-cell RNA-seq technology determining NAFLD progression [24]. In line with this, an interesting finding illustrated a NASH-associated macrophage subset, with TREM2 expression linked to NASH severity. In particular, a specialized circulating monocyte-derived TREM2 $CD9^+$ macrophage subpopulation that promotes liver fibrosis seems to play an essential role in NASH-associated fibrogenesis [25].

Recent clinical studies have shed light on NAFLD severity being associated with inflammatory markers such as TNF, IL-1, IL-6, and high-sensitivity C-reactive protein. It is suggested that NAFLD may induce systemic inflammation, insulin resistance, and oxidative stress via these pro-inflammatory molecules [26].

NAFLD is a perfect example of ectopic fat accumulation, meaning that lipid accumulation occurs in another site other than adipose tissue. This in turn is associated with increased secretion of hepatokines, increased gluconeogenesis, and inhibition of insulin signaling [27]. Hepatic lipid accumulation causes insulin resistance and chronic inflammation, increasing the risk of fibrosis, cirrhosis, and HCC. Besides liver lipid metabolism, the other possibilities contributing to the pathogenesis of NAFLD include adipose tissue dysfunction/inflammation, dysbiosis of gut microbiota, and gut barrier function regulating several intrahepatic metabolic and inflammatory pathways (Figure 2) [28,29].

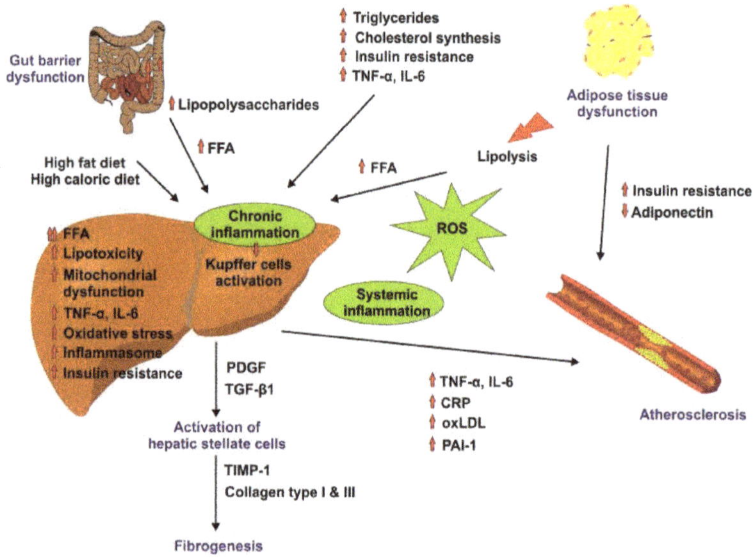

Figure 2. Factors driving pathogenesis of NAFLD and formation of atherosclerosis. Lipopolysaccharides that destroy the gut barrier function, high-caloric diets and elevated concentrations of free fatty acids (FFAs) lead to hepatic inflammation. This in turn leads to activation of hepatic stellate cells and production of cytokines (e.g., PDGF, TGF-β1) that drive fibrogenesis. Additionally, adipose tissue dysfunction and lipolysis leads to formation of insulin resistance and reactive oxygen species (ROS) that further drive the inflammatory process. Hepatic inflammation can result in systemic inflammation and factors (e.g., TNF-α, IL-6, CRP, oxLDL, PAI-1) that in concert with elevated concentrations of fat trigger atherosclerosis. Upward pointing arrows indicate increased concentrations/symptoms, while arrows pointing downwards lower concentrations/symptoms. This figure was redrawn in modified form from [29].

It is interesting to note that obesity is strongly associated with NAFLD but not an independent factor. Adipose tissue dysfunction is the key contributor to NAFLD in patients with lipodystrophy by increasing the hepatic/peripheral insulin resistance and promoting hepatic inflammation (Figure 3) [8,30].

In addition to these factors, the long chain fatty acids are esterified with glycerol-3-phosphate to mono-acylglycerols, diacylglycerols, and triacylglycerols in hepatocytes. The production of these intermediates is increased by lipid synthesis and lipid products like ceramides, which play crucial roles in causing resistance in the insulin signaling pathway, promoting hepatic inflammation and the progression of NAFLD [2,27].

Further, it is likely that the putative underlying mechanisms linking NAFLD, chronic kidney disease, and cardiovascular disease have their origin from inflamed visceral adipose tissue [4]. This in turn exacerbates atherogenic dyslipidemia, releasing a myriad of pro-inflammatory molecules, thrombogenic molecules, contributing to the pathophysiology of cardiovascular disease and chronic kidney disease. The co-existence of obesity further exerts additional effects, leading to functional derangements in the heart, kidneys, and vasculature [4].

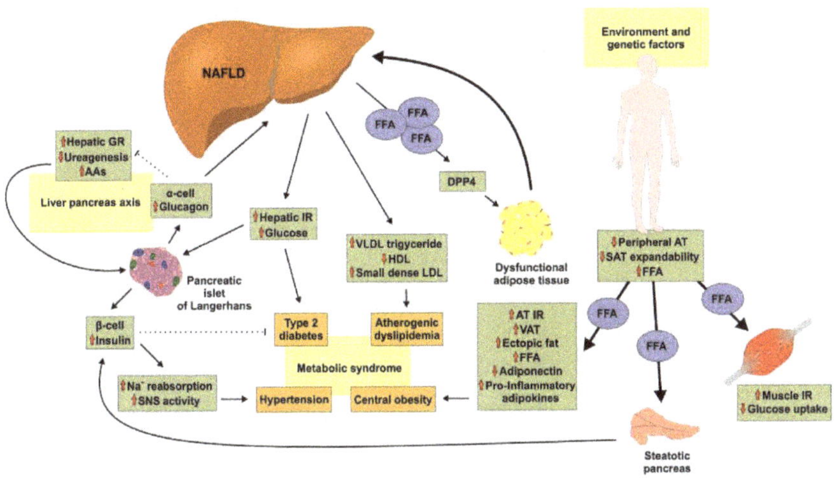

Figure 3. NAFLD as a result of obesity and metabolic syndrome. Increased free fatty acids (FFAs) result in dysfunction of peripheral adipose tissue (AT), expansion of subcutaneous adipose tissue SAT), central obesity, type 2 diabetes, insulin resistance (IR), and central obesity that form key features in the metabolic syndrome. These changes can be monitored by alterations in blood parameters (VLDL, triglyceride, small dense LDL, glucose). These changes are further associated with increased activity of sympathetic nervous system (SNS), glucagon increase, hepatic clearance of amino acids (AA), and increased ureagenesis. Epigenetic and genetic factors predispose to NAFLD pathogenesis. Upward pointing arrows indicate increased concentrations/symptoms, while arrows pointing downwards lower concentrations/symptoms. Solid arrows mark stimulatory effects, while dashed lines indicate inhibitory effects. For more information refer to the text. Abbreviations used are AA: arachidonic acid; GR: glucagon resistance; LDL: low-density lipoprotein(s). This figure was redrawn in modified form from [30].

4. Mechanistic Link between *MBOAT7* and NAFLD and Related In Vivo/In Vitro Studies

It is crucial to further understand the molecular mechanisms underlying the progression of liver disease from simple steatosis to more advanced fibrotic disease. *MBOAT7* association with NAFLD has emerged as a new lipid metabolic pathway as growing evidence suggests the pivotal role of *MBOAT7* as a driver of NAFLD development and progression. Few studies have provided vital clues into its broader role and mechanistic insights.

MBOAT7 preferentially esterifies lysophosphatidylinositol (LPI) lipids to arachidonoyl-CoA to form major phosphoinositol (PI) species (38:4) in the inner leaflet of cell membranes. Phospholipases, prominently phospholipase A2 (PLA2), cleave fatty acid from the sn2 position and *MBOAT7* selectively re-esterifies new PUFAs in that position, completing the remodeling cycle [31]. *MBOAT7* loss of function could alter cellular signal transduction, protein–lipid interactions, vesicular transport, and membrane fusion events, given the fact that *MBOAT7* generates the most abundant PI species (38:4) and key cellular phosphatidylinositol phosphates (PI 18:0/20:4) and PI ([18:0/20:4]-4,5P2). Another potential way by which *MBOAT7* loss of function could promote NASH is by abnormal accumulation of LPI substrates in liver, as evidenced by multiple mice studies. These LPI substrates serve as relevant lipid signals promoting pro-inflammatory and pro-fibrotic effects [31].

The liver-specific knockout of *MBOAT7* induces hepatic fat accumulation by increasing de novo lipogenesis driven by SREBP1, which is a key lipogenic transcription factor involved in fatty acid biosynthesis [22]. The non-canonical pathway, on the other hand, suggests that *MBOAT7* depletion causes a simultaneous increase in PI synthesis and PI degradation mediated by a protein with PLC activity resulting in diacylglycerol, a substrate of triglyceride synthesis [32].

Lee and coworkers unraveled the first evidence of *MBOAT7* enzymatic activity in *Caenorhabditis elegans* by RNA-interference-based genetic screening [33]. In *C. elegans*, eicosapentaenoic acid is the predominant PUFA, which is decreased by *MBOAT7* deletion. It also exhibited reduced PI species and PI3P-related events [33]. Similarly, it has been shown that obese people have low levels of *MBOAT7* in their livers and genetically modified obese mice with low *MBOAT7* levels developed more severe NAFLD [8]. Strikingly, excess fat accumulation was noticed in human liver cells with low levels of *MBOAT7*. New approaches to therapeutic strategies in treating NAFLD in patients with *MBOAT7* mutations can be developed with *MBOAT7* being a critical mediator of NAFLD.

Several studies revealed that the hepatic *MBOAT7* expression levels were suppressed in high-fat-diet mice and obese leptin-deficient mice and that *MBOAT7* levels in adipose tissue were negatively correlated with insulin sensitivity and impaired glucose tolerance (Figure 4) [21,34].

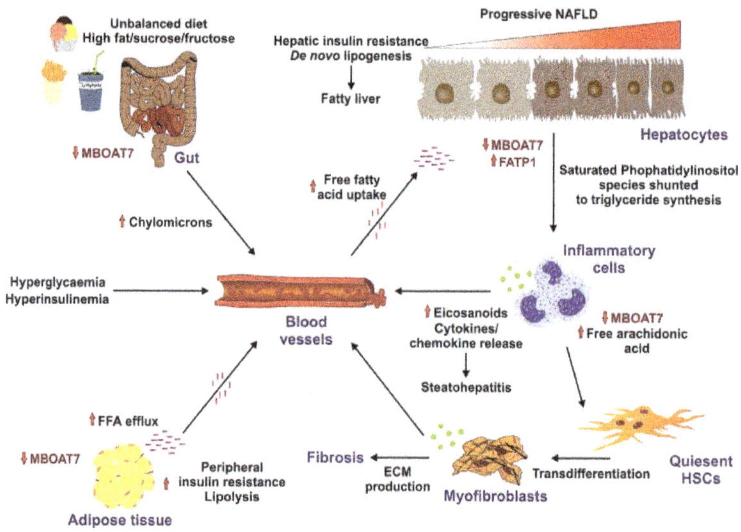

Figure 4. Factors promoting insulin resistance. High-caloric diets enriched in fat, sucrose, and fructose are risk factors for insulin resistance development. In the gut, the unbalanced diet results in downregulation of *MBOAT7* and formation of chylomicrons. Elevated concentrations of systemic free fatty acids are taken up by hepatocytes, resulting in increased de novo lipogenesis and fatty liver. This provokes the infiltration of the liver with inflammatory cells, which results in elevated concentrations of cytokines and chemokines, provoking steatohepatitis and transdifferentiation of quiescent hepatic stellate cells (HSCs) to extracellular-matrix-producing (ECM) myofibroblasts leading to hepatic fibrosis. Similarly, to the liver and the gut, *MBOAT7* is downregulated in the adipose, triggering peripheral insulin resistance. Solid arrows mark stimulatory effects. Small red lines indicate free fatty acids in the circulation, while small purple lines indicate tissue-bound free fatty acids. All these factors promote formation of hyperglycemia, hyperinsulinemia, and insulin resistance. This figure was redrawn in modified form from [34].

On a similar context, liver-specific deletion of *MBOAT7* increased liver fat content in chow-diet-fed mice under fasting-re-feeding conditions. This hepatic lipid accumulation is shown to be caused due to an increase in de novo lipogenesis driven by SREBP1, supported by normalization of hepatic fat content by liver-specific deletion of *MBOAT7* and SREBP cleavage-activating protein *Scap* [22].

In addition to the in vivo studies, Tanaka et al. investigated the impact of *MBOAT7* deletion on PI content and fat accumulation in cultured hepatocytes. This study suggested that depletion of *MBOAT7* in hepatocytes resulted in hepatic fat accumulation through increased triglyceride synthesis [32]. Here, it was proposed that hepatic lipid accumulation is due to a novel non-canonical pathway supplying substrates from PI to triglycerides through a futile cycle [32].

A wealth of recent data show that *MBOAT7* overexpression in mice had beneficial effects on NASH pathology by significantly decreasing hepatic triglyceride levels and normalizing liver injury markers such as alanine aminotransferase and aspartate aminotransferase [35]. Longo et al. showed that *MBOAT7* rs641738 and TM6SF2 E167k alters lipid droplet accumulation, mitochondrial morphology, and metabolic reprogramming towards HCC in vitro [36]. Strikingly, Krawczyk et al. confirmed the association of *MBOAT7* with a more severe stage of fibrosis increasing plasma triglycerides, cholesterol, LDL, and glucose levels [37].

An interesting study by Raja et al. shed light on *MBOAT7* rs641738 associations with NAFLD based on ethnicity [38]. It was shown that *MBOAT7* is a strong contributor to the progression of NAFLD in the Caucasian and Chinese population, while it is not significant in Afro-American and Hispanic populations [39]. Yet another unique finding by Massey et al. showed diet-induced metabolic disturbances, hyperinsulinemia, and systemic insulin resistance in mice with adipocyte-specific disruption of the *MBOAT7* gene [21].

Furthermore, liver-specific knockdown of *MBOAT7* by antisense oligonucleotides revealed large alterations in liver lipid storage characterized by the accumulation of triglycerides, free cholesterol, and cholesterol esters in high-fat-diet-fed mice [8]. In addition, *MBOAT7* knockdown was associated with liver injury as indicated by elevated aspartate aminotransferase and alanine aminotransferase in these animals. Aligned with these alterations, knockdown of *MBOAT7* in high-fat-diet-fed mice resulted in alterations in LPI and PI lipids in a tissue-specific manner such as selective reduction in 38:3 and 38:4 species of circulating PI lipids and significant accumulation of 16:0 and 18:1 LPI species in the liver, inducing an imbalance of local lipid mediators that originate from PI metabolism.

A recent meta-analysis of 42 studies including more than 1 million participants showed that the *MBOAT7* variation is firmly associated with the severity of NAFLD in European adults [40]. Another interesting study suggests that *MBOAT7* is a negative regulator of TLR signaling and highlights that *MBOAT7* modulation can be beneficial for suppressing inflammation associated with the dysregulation of Toll-like receptor signaling such as metabolic-associated fatty liver diseases (MAFLD) [24].

5. Challenges and Recent Progress in Treating Complex NAFLD

NAFLD represents a 'silent epidemic' as it is often asymptomatic in nature with increased prevalence among adults with obesity, type 2 diabetes, insulin resistance, and metabolic syndrome [41]. It represents a growing public health challenge owing to lack of approved therapies at present [42]. Individuals with NAFLD present at least one feature of metabolic syndrome, making it an even more challenging multi-systemic disease. In addition, the complexity is increased by the fact that many patients remain undiagnosed in early phases of the disease [43]. Variability in NAFLD-related risk factors, substantial mortality, and morbidity are a few other challenges in the management of this disease [43]. Therefore, it is important to adopt a holistic approach in managing this diversified condition.

At present, NAFLD is treated with lifestyle modifications such as weight loss and dietary changes as there is no approved therapy yet for this multi-factorial disease [42]. Multiple drug strategies are being developed and tested to treat advanced NAFLD and target inflammatory, fibrotic, and metabolic pathways. More recently, a structure and model were reported for the catalytic mechanism of human *MBOAT7*, which reveals a twisted tunnel from the cytosol and luminal side providing access for arachidonoyl-CoA and lyso-PI. This structure might be important in the identification of small molecule inhibitors for targeted drug therapy in treating NAFLD [12].

There is one other study, which elucidated that increased expression of *MBOAT7* is co-related with detrimental outcomes in HCC, emphasizing the role of *MBOAT7* inhibitors as useful therapeutic targets in treating HCC [44].

A profound study by Thangapandi et al. provided combined mice and human datasets and demonstrated that targeting PI signaling might be a potential therapeutic option for treating NAFLD and fibrosis. Their study unfolded a novel finding that *MBOAT7* deficiency in mice and humans points to an inflammation-independent pathway of liver fibrosis mediated by lipid signaling, opening new avenues for potential targets for NAFLD [45]. It was also shown via lipidomics that in addition to PI and LPI, phosphoglycerol, lysophophatidylglycerol, and phosphatidic acids were increased in *MBOAT7*-deficient livers.

For patients with biopsy-proven NASH, vitamin E and pioglitazone supplements are recommended, although there are concerns regarding side effects [46]. As previously mentioned, intestinal microbiota play an important role in NAFLD pathogenesis. Thus, probiotics, antibiotics, and prebiotics might play a therapeutic role via modulating gut microbiota [47].

Genetic screening for polymorphisms to identify the individuals at high risk for NAFLD will help in deeper understanding of specific therapeutic strategies. Modulators of bile acid signaling medications to improve insulin sensitivity are being tested in patients with NASH as a possible therapeutic approach [48].

Currently, there are several innovative pipeline drugs that are tested in clinical trials for the treatment of NAFLD/NASH (Figure 5).

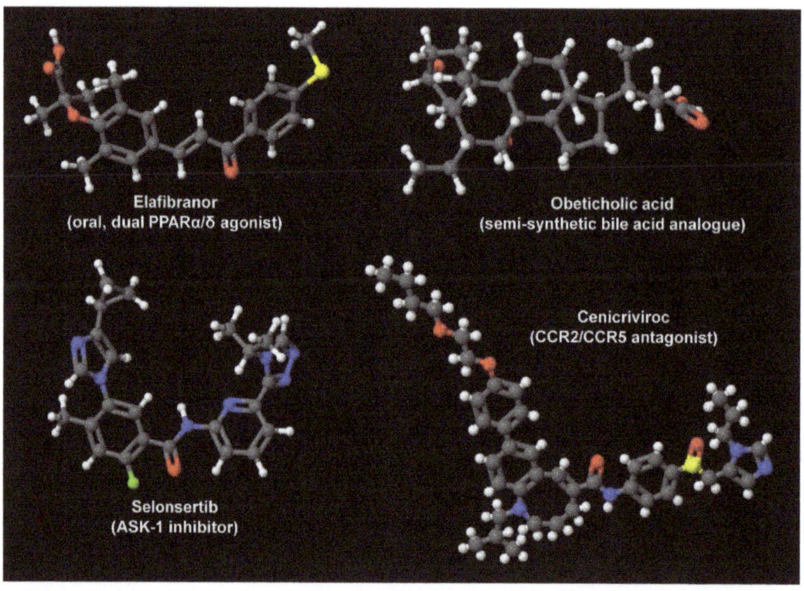

Figure 5. Drug candidates for treatment of NAFLD/NASH. Depicted are the oral, dual PPARα/δ agonist Elafibranor, the semi-synthetic bile acid analogue obeticholic acid, the ASK-1 inhibitor Selonsertib, and the CCR2/CCR5 antagonist Cenicriviroc. These are only some drugs that are tested in ongoing studies. In addition, there are several TLR4 antagonists and macrolide antibiotics that are tested in ongoing trials. Their variable mode of action demonstrates that there are many independent options to target the pathogenesis of NAFLD/NASH. All structures depicted were generated with the open-source molecule viewer Jmol, version 14.2.15_2015.07.09 [49] using information depicted in PubChem [50] for Elafibranor (PubChem CID: 9864881), obeticholic acid (PubChem CID: 447715), Selonsertib (PubChem CID: 71245288), and Cenicriviroc (PubChem CID: 11285792), respectively.

Elafibranor, which acts as a dual-peroxisome proliferation-activated receptor (PPAR) α/δ agonist, improves glucose metabolism and insulin sensitivity and decreases inflammation. In a phase 2b randomized control study (NCT0164849, GOLDEN-505), the effects of Elafibranor (120.80 mg/day) were studied for 52 weeks. NASH was resolved in 19% of patients compared to 9% in the placebo group. In addition, a phase 3 RCT (NCT02704403, RESOLVE-IT) is being evaluated on the effects of Elafibranor (120 mg/day for 72 weeks). Additional novel PPAR agonists such as Saroglitazar and Lanifibranor are also being tested [51].

Obeticholic acid, a semi-synthetic bile activator of Farnesoid X receptors, regulates lipid/glucose homeostasis, promotes insulin sensitivity, and modulates liver fibrosis. In a phase 2b RCT (NCT01264598, FLINT), obeticholic acid (25 mg/day) was tested for 72 weeks in patients with a NAFLD score greater than 4. Remarkably, 45% of the patients showed histological improvement compared with 21% in the placebo group [52]. This trial progressed to a phase 3 RCT (NCT02548351 REGENERATE), which is currently recruiting patients with biopsy-proven NASH to assess obeticholic acid's effects and to evaluate the long-term effects over a 7-year period [53].

The involvement of inflammatory cells and cascade of inflammatory events is well known in hepatocyte injury. Cenicriviroc (CVC) functions as a dual antagonist of CCR2 and CCR5 and demonstrated decreased fibrosis in preclinical models. A phase 2 RCT (NCT02217475, CENTAUR) with CVC 150 mg/day was evaluated in 289 patients with NASH, fibrosis, and diabetes mellitus. Although there was no significant improvement in NASH after 12 months, liver fibrosis improved in 20% patients as compared to 10% in the placebo group. A phase 3 RCT (NCT03028740 AURORA) was initiated to evaluate the effects of 150 mg/day CVC with long-term follow-up over a 5-year period [54].

TNF-α signaling plays an important role in hepatocyte injury and apoptosis, which in turn activates the apoptosis signal-regulating kinase 1 (ASK1) leading to hepatic inflammation, fibrosis, and hepatocyte apoptosis. Selonsertib, a selective inhibitor of ASK1, was tested for its effects on patients with NASH and fibrosis in a phase 2 RCT (NCT02466516). The patients showed fibrosis improvement after 24 weeks of treatment. Two phase 3 trials (NCT03053050 STELLAR3, NCT03053063 STELLAR 4) are being conducted currently to evaluate the effects of Selonsertib at week 48 and further monitor at 240 weeks [55].

In principle, there are also ways to directly target *MBOAT7* gene expression or activity. Since the suppression of *MBOAT7* was shown to drive hepatic fat accumulation and NAFLD development [8,56], the overexpression of *MBOAT7* or approaches leading to increased endogenous expression of *MBOAT7* should have beneficial effects on the outcome of NAFLD. Therapeutic gene therapy has been used in a plethora of diseases so far [57]. In particular, engineered hepatotropic adeno-associated viruses, retroviral vectors, or lentiviral delivery systems expressing *MBOAT7* under transcriptional control of liver-specific promoters could be used to increase the overall concentration of *MBOAT7* in the liver. Similarly, the transfer of nanoparticles, liposomes, polymers, virus-like particles, erythrocyte ghosts, and exosomes that are loaded with *MBOAT7* expression constructs, or special in vivo or ex vivo gene transfer techniques might be scalable alternatives to increase MBOAT quantities [57].

Similarly, strategies that enhance the translation and stability of endogenous or exogenous mRNA that were already used in other disease scenarios could be applied [58]. Finally, in the long term, there will be gene replacement techniques available (e.g., CRISPR/Cas9) that will allow for the replacement of *MBOAT7* mutations that are associated with increased accumulation of intracellular free fatty acids and hepatic steatosis. Nevertheless, although gene therapy is a promising therapeutic strategy that made remarkable advancements during the last decade, there are still many hurdles in the use of this promising therapy [59].

Nevertheless, a proof-of-concept study has recently shown that the overexpression of *MBOAT7* in mice fed either a choline-deficient high-fat diet or a Gubra Amylin NASH diet and subsequent infected with an adeno-associated virus expressing *MBOAT7* failed to improve in terms of NASH pathology [35]. However, in the mentioned study, the authors demonstrated that *MBOAT7* overexpression slightly improved liver weights, triglycerides, and plasma alanine and aspartate transaminases [35]. It is possible that *MBOAT7* needs additional factors to be therapeutically effective in NAFLD/NASH. This again highlights the complexity of the NAFLD/NASH pathogenesis that is driven by many genetic and epigenetic factors and pinpoints the fact that further studies are urgently needed to identify proper targeted therapies for NALFD/NASH.

6. Future Directions in Management of NAFLD

Collectively, NAFLD is a complex disease associated with increased adiposity, diabetes mellitus, and insulin resistance. Patients with mild NAFLD, which is relatively benign, are usually managed with lifestyle modifications through diet and exercise, whereas patients with NASH and fibrosis are usually managed with different classes of medications along with lifestyle modifications. The treatment of the final stages of disease progression, which are NASH-induced cirrhosis and HCC, is focused on preventing and treating the complications associated with it and liver transplant as a last resort [60]. Although lifestyle interventions are beneficial, the effects are short-lived. Additional research is needed to identify the most effective and customized treatment strategies for treating NASH in different patient populations.

7. Conclusions

NAFLD imposes a huge health burden globally due to its risk of progression to cirrhosis, fibrosis, and HCC and lack of well-defined approved therapies. NAFLD is the most common chronic liver disorder affecting more than one-third of the population worldwide and its pathogenesis is closely related to insulin resistance, dyslipidemia, obesity, and adipose tissue dysfunction. The pathogenesis of NAFLD is based on a 'Multihit' hypothesis with the main hit being hepatic triglyceride accumulation and susceptibility to liver injury by the increased influx of free fatty acids in insulin resistance and obesity. This is mediated by inflammatory cytokines, mitochondrial dysfunction, and oxidative stress leading to steatohepatitis and fibrosis. In the last few years, some robust studies elucidated the associations between genetic polymorphisms (e.g., in *PNPLA3, TM6SF2, GCKR, HSD17B13, PSD3, APOE*, and *MBOAT7*) and NAFLD. Single-nucleotide polymorphisms in *MBOAT7* are broadly associated with increased risk of initiation and progression of NAFLD to NASH and fibrosis and in a few cases to HCC. Multiple in vitro and in vivo studies have unraveled that *MBOAT7* deficiency in mice and humans alters the hepatic PL composition and LPI to promote hyperinsulinemia and hepatic insulin resistance. *MBOAT7* catalyzes the desaturation of the second acyl chain of PLs and transfers PUFAs, in the form of acyl-CoA to lyso-PLs, using arachidonic acid as a substrate, regulating the amount of free arachidonic acid, which is a potent trigger for hepatic inflammation and fibrosis and a precursor of multiple pro-inflammatory mediators such as eicosanoids. The treatment of this multi-spectrum disease is complex and challenging as there are plethora of factors involved in its pathogenesis and progression. Currently, there is no approved standard therapy for treating NAFLD. Multiple drugs are in phase 2 and phase 3 trials with the goal of developing potent and customized treatment strategies. An improved knowledge of pathophysiological links between NAFLD and *MBOAT7* will certainly help decrease the global burden of this complicated, wide-spectrum disease by opening new horizons in treatment strategies.

Author Contributions: Conceptualization, P.C.; resources, R.W.; data curation, P.C. and R.W.; writing—original draft preparation, P.C.; writing—review and editing, P.C. and R.W.; supervision, R.W.; funding acquisition, R.W. All authors have read and agreed to the published version of the manuscript.

Funding: RW is supported by the German Research Foundation (grants WE2554/13-1, WE2554/15-1, and WE 2554/17-1), the Deutsche Krebshilfe (grant 70115581), and the Interdisciplinary Centre for Clinical Research within the faculty of Medicine at the RWTH Aachen University (grant PTD 1-5). The funders had no role in the design of this article or in the decision to publish it.

Institutional Review Board Statement: Not applicable.

Informed Consent Statement: Not applicable.

Data Availability Statement: This review only presents data that were previously published. No new data were generated.

Acknowledgments: The authors are grateful to Sabine Weiskirchen (IFMPEGKC, RWTH University Hospital Aachen, Aachen, Germany) for drawing Figures 2–4 for this review.

Conflicts of Interest: The authors declare no conflict of interest.

References

1. Dowman, J.K.; Tomlinson, J.W.; Newsome, P.N. Pathogenesis of non-alcoholic fatty liver disease. *Qjm* **2010**, *103*, 71–83. [CrossRef]
2. Anstee, Q.M.; Targher, G.; Day, C.P. Progression of NAFLD to diabetes mellitus, cardiovascular disease or cirrhosis. *Nat. Rev. Gastroenterol. Hepatol.* **2013**, *10*, 330–344. [CrossRef]
3. Shaker, M.; Tabbaa, A.; Albeldawi, M.; Alkhouri, N. Liver transplantation for nonalcoholic fatty liver disease: New challenges and new opportunities. *World J. Gastroenterol.* **2014**, *20*, 5320–5330. [CrossRef]
4. Armstrong, M.J.; Adams, L.A.; Canbay, A.; Syn, W.K. Extrahepatic complications of nonalcoholic fatty liver disease. *Hepatology* **2014**, *59*, 1174–1197. [CrossRef]
5. Nagral, A.; Bangar, M.; Menezes, S.; Bhatia, S.; Butt, N.; Ghosh, J.; Manchanayake, J.H.; Mahtab, M.A.; Singh, S.P. Gender differences in nonalcoholic fatty liver disease. *Euroasian J. Hepatogastroenterol.* **2022**, *12*, S19–S25. [CrossRef]
6. Caddeo, A.; Spagnuolo, R.; Maurotti, S. *MBOAT7* in liver and extrahepatic diseases. *Liver Int.* **2023**, *43*, 2351–2364. [CrossRef]
7. Mancina, R.M.; Dongiovanni, P.; Petta, S.; Pingitore, P.; Meroni, M.; Rametta, R.; Borén, J.; Montalcini, T.; Pujia, A.; Wiklund, O.; et al. The *MBOAT7*-TMC4 variant rs641738 increases risk of nonalcoholic fatty liver disease in individuals of European descent. *Gastroenterology* **2016**, *150*, 1219–1230.e1216. [CrossRef]
8. Helsley, R.N.; Varadharajan, V.; Brown, A.L.; Gromovsky, A.D.; Schugar, R.C.; Ramachandiran, I.; Fung, K.; Kabbany, M.N.; Banerjee, R.; Neumann, C.K.; et al. Obesity-linked suppression of membrane-bound O-acyltransferase 7 (*MBOAT7*) drives non-alcoholic fatty liver disease. *eLife* **2019**, *8*, e49882. [CrossRef]
9. Tavaglione, F.; Kono, N.; Romeo, S. Understanding the underlying molecular pathways by which *MBOAT7*/Lpiat1 depletion induces hepatic steatosis. *J. Lipid Res.* **2021**, *62*, 100047. [CrossRef]
10. Caddeo, A.; Jamialahmadi, O.; Solinas, G.; Pujia, A.; Mancina, R.M.; Pingitore, P.; Romeo, S. *MBOAT7* is anchored to endomembranes by six transmembrane domains. *J. Struct. Biol.* **2019**, *206*, 349–360. [CrossRef]
11. Lee, H.-C.; Inoue, T.; Sasaki, J.; Kubo, T.; Matsuda, S.; Nakasaki, Y.; Hattori, M.; Tanaka, F.; Udagawa, O.; Kono, N.; et al. LPIAT1 regulates arachidonic acid content in phosphatidylinositol and is required for cortical lamination in mice. *Mol. Biol. Cell* **2012**, *23*, 4689–4700. [CrossRef]
12. Wang, K.; Lee, C.-W.; Sui, X.; Kim, S.; Wang, S.; Higgs, A.B.; Baublis, A.J.; Voth, G.A.; Liao, M.; Walther, T.C.; et al. The structure of phosphatidylinositol remodeling *MBOAT7* reveals its catalytic mechanism and enables inhibitor identification. *Nat. Commun.* **2023**, *14*, 3533. [CrossRef]
13. National Library of Medicine. Available online: https://www.ncbi.nlm.nih.gov/protein (accessed on 9 November 2023).
14. Clustal Omega. Available online: https://www.ebi.ac.uk/Tools/msa/clustalo/ (accessed on 9 November 2023).
15. Byrne, C.D.; Targher, G. NAFLD: A multisystem disease. *J. Hepatol.* **2015**, *62*, S47–S64. [CrossRef]
16. Byrne, C.D. Ectopic fat, insulin resistance and non-alcoholic fatty liver disease. *Proc. Nutr. Soc.* **2013**, *72*, 412–419. [CrossRef]
17. Cai, J.; Zhang, X.-J.; Ji, Y.-X.; Zhang, P.; She, Z.-G.; Li, H. Nonalcoholic fatty liver disease pandemic fuels the upsurge in cardiovascular diseases. *Circ. Res.* **2020**, *126*, 679–704. [CrossRef]
18. Pais, R.; Redheuil, A.; Cluzel, P.; Ratziu, V.; Giral, P. Relationship among fatty liver, specific and multiple-site atherosclerosis, and 10-year Framingham Score. *Hepatology* **2019**, *69*, 1453–1463. [CrossRef]
19. Cheung, A.; Ahmed, A. Nonalcoholic fatty liver disease and chronic kidney disease: A review of links and risks. *Clin. Exp. Gastroenterol.* **2021**, *14*, 457–465. [CrossRef]
20. Buzzetti, E.; Pinzani, M.; Tsochatzis, E.A. The multiple-hit pathogenesis of non-alcoholic fatty liver disease (NAFLD). *Metabolism* **2016**, *65*, 1038–1048. [CrossRef]
21. Massey, W.J.; Varadharajan, V.; Banerjee, R.; Brown, A.L.; Horak, A.J.; Hohe, R.C.; Jung, B.M.; Qiu, Y.; Chan, E.R.; Pan, C.; et al. *MBOAT7*-driven lysophosphatidylinositol acylation in adipocytes contributes to systemic glucose homeostasis. *J. Lipid Res.* **2023**, *64*, 100349. [CrossRef]
22. Xia, M.; Chandrasekaran, P.; Rong, S.; Fu, X.; Mitsche, M.A. Hepatic deletion of *MBOAT7* (LPIAT1) causes activation of SREBP-1c and fatty liver. *J. Lipid Res.* **2021**, *62*, 100031. [CrossRef]
23. Ipsen, D.H.; Lykkesfeldt, J.; Tveden-Nyborg, P. Molecular mechanisms of hepatic lipid accumulation in non-alcoholic fatty liver disease. *Cell. Mol. Life Sci.* **2018**, *75*, 3313–3327. [CrossRef]
24. Alharthi, J.; Bayoumi, A.; Thabet, K.; Pan, Z.; Gloss, B.S.; Latchoumanin, O.; Lundberg, M.; Twine, N.A.; McLeod, D.; Alenizi, S.; et al. A metabolic associated fatty liver disease risk variant in *MBOAT7* regulates toll like receptor induced outcomes. *Nat. Commun.* **2022**, *13*, 7430. [CrossRef]
25. Zahr, T.; Sun, K.; Qiang, L. The polarizable and reprogrammable identity of Kupffer cells in nonalcoholic steatohepatitis. *Med. Rev.* **2022**, *2*, 324–327. [CrossRef]

26. Duan, Y.; Pan, X.; Luo, J.; Xiao, X.; Li, J.; Bestman, P.L.; Luo, M. Association of inflammatory cytokines with non-alcoholic fatty liver disease. *Front. Immunol.* **2022**, *13*, 880298. [CrossRef]
27. Zhu, B.; Chan, S.L.; Li, J.; Li, K.; Wu, H.; Cui, K.; Chen, H. Non-alcoholic steatohepatitis pathogenesis, diagnosis, and treatment. *Front. Cardiovasc. Med.* **2021**, *8*, 742382. [CrossRef]
28. Mehal, W.Z. The Gordian Knot of dysbiosis, obesity and NAFLD. *Nat. Rev. Gastroenterol. Hepatol.* **2013**, *10*, 637–644. [CrossRef]
29. Galatou, E.; Mourelatou, E.; Hatziantoniou, S.; Vizirianakis, I.S. Nonalcoholic steatohepatitis (NASH) and atherosclerosis: Explaining their pathophysiology, association and the role of incretin-based drugs. *Antioxidants* **2022**, *11*, 1060. [CrossRef]
30. Godoy-Matos, A.F.; Silva Júnior, W.S.; Valerio, C.M. NAFLD as a continuum: From obesity to metabolic syndrome and diabetes. *Diabetol. Metab. Syndr.* **2020**, *12*, 60. [CrossRef]
31. Varadharajan, V.; Massey, W.J.; Brown, J.M. Membrane-bound O-acyltransferase 7 (*MBOAT7*)-driven phosphatidylinositol remodeling in advanced liver disease. *J. Lipid Res.* **2022**, *63*, 100234. [CrossRef]
32. Yuki, T.; Yuta, S.; Andrea, C.; Takuya, K.; Yanli, M.; Tetsuya, K.; Naoto, K.; Toshimasa, Y.; Rosellina Margherita, M.; Guido, B.; et al. LPIAT1/*MBOAT7* depletion increases triglyceride synthesis fueled by high phosphatidylinositol turnover. *Gut* **2021**, *70*, 180. [CrossRef]
33. Lee, H.-C.; Inoue, T.; Imae, R.; Kono, N.; Shirae, S.; Matsuda, S.; Gengyo-Ando, K.; Mitani, S.; Arai, H. *Caenorhabditis elegans* mboa-7, a member of the MBOAT family, is required for selective incorporation of polyunsaturated fatty acids into phosphatidylinositol. *Mol. Biol. Cell* **2007**, *19*, 1174–1184. [CrossRef]
34. Meroni, M.; Longo, M.; Fracanzani, A.L.; Dongiovanni, P. *MBOAT7* down-regulation by genetic and environmental factors predisposes to MAFLD. *eBioMedicine* **2020**, *57*, 102866. [CrossRef]
35. Sharpe, M.C.; Pyles, K.D.; Hallcox, T.; Kamm, D.R.; Piechowski, M.; Fisk, B.; Albert, C.J.; Carpenter, D.H.; Ulmasov, B.; Ford, D.A.; et al. Enhancing hepatic *MBOAT7* expression in mice with nonalcoholic steatohepatitis. *Gastro Hep Adv.* **2023**, *2*, 558–572. [CrossRef]
36. Longo, M.; Meroni, M.; Paolini, E.; Erconi, V.; Carli, F.; Fortunato, F.; Ronchi, D.; Piciotti, R.; Sabatini, S.; Macchi, C.; et al. TM6SF2/PNPLA3/*MBOAT7* Loss-of-function genetic variants impact on NAFLD development and progression both in patients and in in vitro models. *Cell. Mol. Gastroenterol. Hepatol.* **2022**, *13*, 759–788. [CrossRef]
37. Krawczyk, M.; Rau, M.; Schattenberg, J.M.; Bantel, H.; Pathil, A.; Demir, M.; Kluwe, J.; Boettler, T.; Lammert, F.; Geier, A. Combined effects of the PNPLA3 rs738409, TM6SF2 rs58542926, and *MBOAT7* rs641738 variants on NAFLD severity: A multicenter biopsy-based study. *J. Lipid Res.* **2017**, *58*, 247–255. [CrossRef]
38. Raja, A.M.; Ciociola, E.; Ahmad, I.N.; Dar, F.S.; Naqvi, S.M.S.; Moaeen-Ud-Din, M.; Kaukab Raja, G.; Romeo, S.; Mancina, R.M. Genetic susceptibility to chronic liver disease in individuals from Pakistan. *Int. J. Mol. Sci.* **2020**, *21*, 3558. [CrossRef]
39. Sookoian, S.; Flichman, D.; Garaycoechea, M.E.; Gazzi, C.; Martino, J.S.; Castaño, G.O.; Pirola, C.J. Lack of evidence supporting a role of TMC4-rs641738 missense variant—*MBOAT7*- intergenic downstream variant—In the susceptibility to nonalcoholic fatty liver disease. *Sci. Rep.* **2018**, *8*, 5097. [CrossRef]
40. Teo, K.; Abeysekera, K.W.M.; Adams, L.; Aigner, E.; Anstee, Q.M.; Banales, J.M.; Banerjee, R.; Basu, P.; Berg, T.; Bhatnagar, P.; et al. rs641738C>T near *MBOAT7* is associated with liver fat, ALT and fibrosis in NAFLD: A meta-analysis. *J. Hepatol.* **2021**, *74*, 20–30. [CrossRef]
41. Sivell, C. Nonalcoholic fatty liver disease: A silent epidemic. *Gastroenterol. Nurs.* **2019**, *42*, 428–434. [CrossRef]
42. Meroni, M.; Longo, M.; Rustichelli, A.; Dongiovanni, P. Nutrition and genetics in NAFLD: The perfect binomium. *Int. J. Mol. Sci.* **2020**, *21*, 2986. [CrossRef]
43. Arab, J.P.; Díaz, L.A.; Dirchwolf, M.; Mark, H.E.; Lazarus, J.V.; Vaughan, E.; Méndez-Sánchez, N.; Oliveira, C.P.; Gadano, A.; Arrese, M. NAFLD: Challenges and opportunities to address the public health problem in Latin America. *Ann. Hepatol.* **2021**, *24*, 100359. [CrossRef]
44. Donati, B.; Dongiovanni, P.; Romeo, S.; Meroni, M.; McCain, M.; Miele, L.; Petta, S.; Maier, S.; Rosso, C.; De Luca, L.; et al. *MBOAT7* rs641738 variant and hepatocellular carcinoma in non-cirrhotic individuals. *Sci. Rep.* **2017**, *7*, 4492. [CrossRef]
45. Thangapandi, V.R.; Knittelfelder, O.; Brosch, M.; Patsenker, E.; Vvedenskaya, O.; Buch, S.; Hinz, S.; Hendricks, A.; Nati, M.; Herrmann, A.; et al. Loss of hepatic *MBOAT7* leads to liver fibrosis. *Gut* **2021**, *70*, 940–950. [CrossRef]
46. Bril, F.; Biernacki, D.M.; Kalavalapalli, S.; Lomonaco, R.; Subbarayan, S.K.; Lai, J.; Tio, F.; Suman, A.; Orsak, B.K.; Hecht, J.; et al. Role of vitamin E for nonalcoholic steatohepatitis in patients with type 2 diabetes: A randomized controlled trial. *Diabetes Care* **2019**, *42*, 1481–1488. [CrossRef]
47. Iacono, A.; Raso, G.M.; Canani, R.B.; Calignano, A.; Meli, R. Probiotics as an emerging therapeutic strategy to treat NAFLD: Focus on molecular and biochemical mechanisms. *J. Nutr. Biochem.* **2011**, *22*, 699–711. [CrossRef]
48. Fiorucci, S.; Biagioli, M.; Sepe, V.; Zampella, A.; Distrutti, E. Bile acid modulators for the treatment of nonalcoholic steatohepatitis (NASH). *Expert Opin. Investig. Drugs* **2020**, *29*, 623–632. [CrossRef]
49. Jmol: An Open-Source Java Viewer for Chemical Structures in 3D with Features for Chemicals, Crystals, Materials and Biomolecules. Available online: https://jmol.sourceforge.net/ (accessed on 9 November 2023).
50. PubChem. National Library of Medicine. Available online: https://pubchem.ncbi.nlm.nih.gov/ (accessed on 9 November 2023).
51. Lange, N.F.; Graf, V.; Caussy, C.; Dufour, J.F. PPAR-targeted therapies in the treatment of non-alcoholic fatty liver disease in diabetic patients. *Int. J. Mol. Sci.* **2022**, *23*, 4305. [CrossRef]

52. Neuschwander-Tetri, B.A.; Loomba, R.; Sanyal, A.J.; Lavine, J.E.; Van Natta, M.L.; Abdelmalek, M.F.; Chalasani, N.; Dasarathy, S.; Diehl, A.M.; Hameed, B.; et al. Farnesoid X nuclear receptor ligand obeticholic acid for non-cirrhotic, non-alcoholic steatohepatitis (FLINT): A multicentre, randomised, placebo-controlled trial. *Lancet* **2015**, *385*, 956–965. [CrossRef]
53. Carr, R.M.; Reid, A.E. FXR agonists as therapeutic agents for non-alcoholic fatty liver disease. *Curr. Atheroscler. Rep.* **2015**, *17*, 500. [CrossRef]
54. Lefebvre, E.; Moyle, G.; Reshef, R.; Richman, L.P.; Thompson, M.; Hong, F.; Chou, H.L.; Hashiguchi, T.; Plato, C.; Poulin, D.; et al. Antifibrotic effects of the dual CCR2/CCR5 antagonist Cenicriviroc in animal models of liver and kidney fibrosis. *PLoS ONE* **2016**, *11*, e0158156. [CrossRef]
55. Harrison, S.A.; Wong, V.W.; Okanoue, T.; Bzowej, N.; Vuppalanchi, R.; Younes, Z.; Kohli, A.; Sarin, S.; Caldwell, S.H.; Alkhouri, N.; et al. Selonsertib for patients with bridging fibrosis or compensated cirrhosis due to NASH: Results from randomized phase III STELLAR trials. *J. Hepatol.* **2020**, *73*, 26–39. [CrossRef] [PubMed]
56. Meroni, M.; Dongiovanni, P.; Longo, M.; Carli, F.; Baselli, G.; Rametta, R.; Pelusi, S.; Badiali, S.; Maggioni, M.; Gaggini, M.; et al. *MBOAT7* down-regulation by hyper-insulinemia induces fat accumulation in hepatocytes. *eBioMedicine* **2020**, *52*, 102658. [CrossRef] [PubMed]
57. Sayed, N.; Allawadhi, P.; Khurana, A.; Singh, V.; Navik, U.; Pasumarthi, S.K.; Khurana, I.; Banothu, A.K.; Weiskirchen, R.; Bharani, K.K. Gene therapy: Comprehensive overview and therapeutic applications. *Life Sci.* **2022**, *294*, 120375. [CrossRef] [PubMed]
58. Kairuz, D.; Singh, P.; Smith, T.; Arbuthnot, P.; Ely, A.; Bloom, K. Synthetic mRNA gene therapies and hepatotropic non-viral vectors for the treatment of chronic HBV infections. In *Messenger RNA Therapeutics, RNA Technologies*; Jurga, S., Barciszewski, J., Eds.; Springer: Cham, Switzerland, 2022; Volume 13. [CrossRef]
59. Khurana, A.; Sayed, N.; Singh, V.; Khurana, I.; Allawadhi, P.; Rawat, P.S.; Navik, U.; Pasumarthi, S.K.; Bharani, K.K.; Weiskirchen, R. A comprehensive overview of CRISPR/Cas 9 technology and application thereof in drug discovery. *J. Cell. Biochem.* **2022**, *123*, 1674–1698. [CrossRef]
60. Burra, P.; Becchetti, C.; Germani, G. NAFLD and liver transplantation: Disease burden, current management and future challenges. *JHEP Rep.* **2020**, *2*, 100192. [CrossRef]

MDPI AG
Grosspeteranlage 5
4052 Basel
Switzerland
Tel.: +41 61 683 77 34

Livers Editorial Office
E-mail: livers@mdpi.com
www.mdpi.com/journal/livers

www.ingramcontent.com/pod-product-compliance
Lightning Source LLC
Chambersburg PA
CBHW040750250926
51850CB00007BB/1455